# Student Study Guide for use with

# Administrative Medical Assisting

## A Workforce Readiness Approach

**Helen J. Houser, RN, MSHA, RMA (AMT)**
*Phoenix College*
*Phoenix, AZ*

**Terri D. Wyman, CPC, CMRS**
*Financial Applications Analyst*
*Wing Memorial Hospital*
*Palmer, MA*

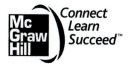

*Connect*
*Learn*
*Succeed™*

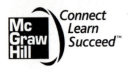

Student Study Guide for use with
ADMINISTRATIVE MEDICAL ASSISTING, FIRST EDITION
Helen Houser and Terri D. Wyman

Published by McGraw-Hill, a business unit of The McGraw-Hill Companies, Inc., 1221 Avenue of the
Americas, New York, NY 10020. Copyright © 2012 by The McGraw-Hill Companies, Inc. All rights
reserved.

1 2 3 4 5 6 7 8 9 0 QDB/QDB 1 0 9 8 7 6 5 4 3 2 1

ISBN      978-0-07-742044-4
MHID     0-07-742044-6

Cover credit: (clockwise starting with Administrative Medical Assistant): © Jack Hollingsworth/
Getty Images; © Tom Grill/Corbis; © Jose Luis Pelaez Inc/Getty Images; © TRBfoto/Getty Images

WARNING NOTICE: The clinical procedures, medicines, dosages, and other matters described in
this publication are based upon research of current literature and consultation with knowledgeable
persons in the field. The procedures and matters described in this text reflect currently accepted
clinical practice. However, this information cannot and should not be relied upon as necessarily
applicable to a given individual's case. Accordingly, each person must be separately diagnosed to
discern the patient's unique circumstances. Likewise, the manufacturer's package insert for current
drug product information should be consulted before administering any drug. Publisher disclaims
all liability for any inaccuracies, omissions, misuse, or misunderstanding of the information
contained in this publication. Publisher cautions that this publication is not intended as a substitute
for the professional judgment of trained medical personnel.

The Internet addresses listed in the text were accurate at the time of publication. The inclusion of
a Web site does not indicate an endorsement by the authors or McGraw-Hill, and McGraw-Hill does
not guarantee the accuracy of the information presented at these sites.

# Table of Contents

# Demonstrate Your Knowledge

## Procedure Check

# Procedure/Documentation Forms

# Practice Application Forms

# Preface

This *Student Study Guide* provides you with an opportunity to review and master the concepts and skills introduced in your textbook, *Administrative Medical Assisting: A Workforce Readiness Approach*. Chapter by chapter, the workbook provides the following sections.

## Test Your Knowledge

- **Vocabulary Review,** which tests your knowledge of key terms introduced in the chapter.
- **Multiple-Choice Certification Questions,** which tests your knowledge of key concepts introduced in the chapter and assists in national certification exam preparation.
- **True or False,** which tests your comprehension of the key concepts introduced in the chapter.
- **Sentence Completion,** which tests your retention of the material presented in the chapter.

## Apply Your Knowledge

- **Short Answer,** which tests not only your comprehension of the material presented in the chapter but your written communication skills and the ability to clearly express your thoughts.
- **Problem-Solving Activities,** which provide an opportunity to transition situations from the classroom to the workforce.
- **Thinking Critically,** which are case studies that provide opportunities to apply the concepts introduced in the chapter to lifelike situations you will encounter as an administrative medical assistant.

## Demonstrate Your Knowledge

- **Procedure Competency Checklists,** which enable you to monitor your mastery of the steps in the procedure(s) introduced in a chapter, such as coding from the CPT and ICD manuals and scheduling appointments, are available at the end of each chapter of the study guide. Each procedure is correlated with the CAAHEP and ABHES competencies you will need to know to become an administrative medical assistant.

At the back of the study guide are forms for practicing and testing your skills. Make extra copies since you may wish to use them more than once. This section helps tie together the learning between the textbook and Student Study Guide.

- Procedure Forms
- Application Activity Forms

Together, your textbook and the Student Study Guide form a complete learning package. *Administrative Medical Assisting: A Workforce Readiness Approach* will prepare you to enter the administrative medical assisting field with the knowledge and skills necessary to become a useful resource to patients and a valued asset to employers and to the administrative medical assisting profession.

# Medical Assisting as a Career

## Test Your Knowledge

### Vocabulary Review

Match the key terms in the right column with the definitions in the left column by placing the letter of each correct answer in the space provided.

_____ **1.** one who practices a profession

_____ **2.** an organization that offers a variety of certifications including Medical Transcriptionist (CMT) and EKG/ECG Technician (CET)

_____ **3.** a computer-generated document that summarizes your employment and educational history

_____ **4.** the process by which programs are officially authorized

_____ **5.** learning new skills and working various aspects of a facility

_____ **6.** large health-care providers who can make health care more cost-effective

_____ **7.** a national association created in 1956 that certifies medical assistants as CMA, Certified Medical Assistant

_____ **8.** an independent agency that certifies medical assistants as NCMA, National Certified Medical Assistant

_____ **9.** a regulatory agency that oversees health and safety in the workplace

_____ **10.** a certification agency and professional membership association that certifies medical assistants as RMA, Registered Medical Assistant

**a.** accreditation [LO1.5]

**b.** Occupational Safety and Health Administration (OSHA) [LO1.5]

**c.** Certified Medical Assistant (CMA) [LO1.3]

**d.** professional development [LO1.7]

**e.** Registered Medical Assistant (RMA) [LO1.3]

**f.** practitioner [LO1.5]

**g.** Health Insurance Portability and Accountability Act [LO1.5]

**h.** cross-training [LO1.5]

**i.** American Association of Medical Assistants (AAMA) [LO1.6]

**j.** National Healthcareer Association (NHA) [LO1.3]

**k.** American Medical Technologists (AMT) [LO1.3]

**l.** Clinical Laboratory Improvement Amendments of 1988 (CLIA '88) [LO1.5]

**m.** managed care organization (MCO) [LO1.3]

_____ **11.** organization that offers multiple credentials for health-care professionals including the nationally registered title of Certified Administrative Health Assistant (NRCAHA)

_____ **12.** federal legislation that regulates the protection of personal health information

_____ **13.** federal legislation that sets the standards of practice and personnel qualifications in the medical laboratory

_____ **14.** skills and knowledge attained for both personal development and career advancement

_____ **15.** the credential awarded to medical assistants who pass the certification examination of the American Medical Technologists organization

_____ **16.** the credential awarded by the Certifying Board of the AAMA to medical assistants who pass their certification exam

_____ **17.** education and training that occurs after you have entered a profession that promotes professional development and meets requirements of your certification or registration

_____ **18.** a health-care business that, through mergers and buyouts, can deliver health care more cost-effectively

**n.** National Association for Health Professionals (NAHP) **[LO1.3]**

**o.** résumé **[LO1.5]**

**p.** National Center for Competency Testing (NCCT) **[LO1.3]**

**q.** continuing education

**r.** externship

## Multiple-Choice Certification Questions

There may be more than one answer; circle the letter of the choice that best completes each statement or answers each question.

**1.** **[LO1.5]** An accredited medical assisting program is one that
a. is at least 1,000 clock hours in length.
b. is competency based.
c. is reaccredited every 10 years.
d. has an optional externship course.
e. requires completion of 1,500 clock hours.

**2.** **[LO1.3]** Which of the following is *not* a characteristic of the AAMA organization?
a. It provides a code of ethics for the medical assisting profession.
b. It has developed a medical assistant creed.
c. It oversees the functions of the American Medical Association.
d. It exists to raise the standards of the medical assisting profession.
e. It passes state laws regulating the practice of medical assisting.

**3.** [LO1.3] A main function of professional medical assistant associations is to
   a. accredit medical programs.
   b. set high standards for quality and performance for medical assistants.
   c. provide textbooks for medical assisting schools.
   d. guarantee employment for medical assistants.
   e. provide professional résumés for students.

**4.** [LO1.5] A person that is *not* a likely candidate to become a mentor for a medical assistant externship student is
   a. a recent medical assistant graduate.
   b. a nurse manager.
   c. an experienced medical assistant.
   d. a nurse practitioner.
   e. a physician.

**5.** [LO1.5] A document that provides historical information about your employment and education is a/an
   a. affiliation agreement.
   b. scope of practice.
   c. résumé.
   d. medical assistant occupation analysis.
   e. employment advertisement.

**6.** [LO1.5] The best example of a cross-trained medical assistant is one who has the ability to
   a. work efficiently in one department of the medical clinic.
   b. be an expert when rooming patients for the physician.
   c. use appropriate communication skills with patients.
   d. utilize many skills in various departments of a facility.
   e. complete tasks in a timely manner.

**7.** [LO1.3] One requirement to qualify for the certification as an RMA through the AMT is the applicant
   a. must be of good moral character.
   b. should have financial stability.
   c. has completed a program of no more than 500 clock hours.
   d. must show proof of 10 years' experience in the field.
   e. must have someone recommend them to the AMT.

**8.** [LO1.7] Which of the following would *not* be classified as professional development?
   a. Volunteering for a local community health organization
   b. Applying for a medical assisting position in a local clinic
   c. Attending a continuing education seminar
   d. Subscribing to *CMAJ*
   e. Completing a college course in health education

**9.** [LO1.5] A period of practical work experience performed by a medical assisting student in a physician's office, hospital, or other health-care facility is known as
   a. an externship.
   b. employment.
   c. accreditation.
   d. a training program.
   e. documentation.

**10.** [LO1.5] Which of the following is *not* considered an entry-level laboratory duty?
   a. Performing waived lab tests
   b. Performing high-complexity lab tests
   c. Performing a urine pregnancy test
   d. Collecting and transmitting specimens to the lab
   e. Completing a microscopic urine analysis

11. **[LO1.5]** Entry-level clinical duties of the medical assistant include
    a. handling correspondence.
    b. arranging hospital admissions.
    c. scheduling appointments.
    d. assisting the doctor during examinations.
    e. All of the above.

12. **[LO1.7]** A cross-trained team member who is able to handle many different duties is called a/an
    a. multi-skilled health-care professional.
    b. administrative assistant.
    c. practitioner.
    d. clinical assistant.
    e. specialist.

13. **[LO1.7]** A significant benefit of volunteering is that it
    a. might take time away from your family and friends.
    b. will get you a better paying job.
    c. will be a rewarding experience.
    d. should not be included on your résumé.
    e. will not count as professional development.

14. **[LO1.3]** Agencies that provide accreditation for medical assistant programs are the
    a. NHA and NCCT.
    b. ABHES and CAAHEP.
    c. AMT and AAMA.
    d. NAHP and MCO.
    e. AMT and ABHES.

15. **[LO1.7]** A Certified Medical Assistant (CMA) must recertify the credential
    a. when promoted to a new position in the medical assisting field.
    b. when continuing education is completed.
    c. annually.
    d. every 5 years.
    e. every 10 years.

16. **[LO1.2]** Under the provisions of CLIA '88, a medical assistant may perform moderately complex laboratory tests
    a. when the supervisor requests they be completed by the medical assistant.
    b. if no one else is available and the physician needs the results right away.
    c. only if the medical assistant is trained with the necessary skills to perform the tests.
    d. after the medical assistant becomes certified as an NCMA.
    e. after 5 years working in the laboratory.

17. **[LO1.5]** An activity that would be described as networking is
    a. applying for a medical assisting position.
    b. attending a professional seminar.
    c. completing an online education course.
    d. receiving a promotion at work.
    e. becoming proficient at operating a computer.

18. **[LO1.3]** The purpose of the Medical Assistant Occupational Analysis is it
    a. describes the field of medical assisting.
    b. identifies entry-level competencies.
    c. aids in developing continuing education programs.

d. sets the salary structure for medical assistants.
e. encompasses all of the above.

**19.** [LO1.5] Which of the following is *not* true of the externship expectation?
a. Completion of an externship is optional in most medical assisting programs.
b. The medical assistant student may work under the supervision of a licensed practitioner.
c. The medical facility used for externship signs an affiliation agreement with the school.
d. The medical assistant will gain experience utilizing the skills learned while in the medical assistant program courses.
e. The externship student must submit time cards to validate hours completed.

**20.** [LO1.2] Advanced administrative duties include
a. greeting patients.
b. participating in practice analysis.
c. scheduling patient appointments.
d. arranging hospital admissions.
e. All the above.

**21.** [LO1.5] A major purpose for managed care organizations is to
a. dissolve mergers of large medical companies.
b. require medical clinics to hire only credentialed medical assistants.
c. make delivery of health care more cost-effective.
d. support single-physician practices in all communities.
e. set up hospitals.

**22.** [LO1.6] Which of the following is *not* a benefit to membership in a professional association?
a. The medical assistant can attend association-sponsored seminars.
b. Professional publications are available from most associations.
c. Association members have access to legal information pertinent to the field of medical assisting.
d. Associations are not involved in promoting networking.
e. The medical assistant can obtain professional development through membership.

**23.** [LO1.2] Shredding documents that contain personal medical information is an example of maintaining compliance with
a. OSHA regulations.
b. HIPAA standards.
c. NAHP eligibility requirements.
d. NCCT certification.
e. CAAHEP standards.

**24.** [LO1.2] The best way to understand the medical assistant's scope of practice is to
a. complete the mandated externship requirements.
b. talk with another medical assistant who is employed in a medical clinic.
c. contact the AAMA organization for information on this topic.
d. discuss the scope of practice with the career services department of your school.
e. review the OSHA guidelines.

**25.** [LO1.2] Which of the following individuals may function as a HIPAA compliance officer?
a. Advanced administrative medical assistant
b. Entry-level administrative medical assistant
c. Mid-level administrative medical assistant
d. Clinical medical assistant
e. General medical assistant

# True or False

Decide whether each statement is true or false. In the space at the left, write "T" for true or "F" for false. On the lines provided, rewrite the false statements to make them true.

_____ **1.** [LO1.3] A Certified Medical Assistant, CMA (AAMA), credential is automatically renewed.

_____

_____ **2.** [LO1.5] Externships are voluntary in most accredited medical assistant programs.

_____

_____ **3.** [LO1.5] A practitioner is someone who practices a profession.

_____

_____ **4.** [LO1.5] OSHA sets up standards for medical facilities to follow when destroying confidential documents.

_____

_____ **5.** [LO1.4] To qualify as a Registered Medical Assistant (RMA), you need to pass a certification examination.

_____

_____ **6.** [LO1.5] The Medical Assistant Occupational Analysis identifies entry-level competencies for medical assistants.

_____

_____ **7.** [LO1.5] The scope of practice for all medical assistants includes starting IVs.

_____

_____ **8.** [LO1.3] Accredited medical assistant programs must be at least 2 years in length.

_____

_____ **9.** [LO1.2] Medical assistants are described as multi-skilled health-care professionals.

_____

_____ **10.** [LO1.2] Performing duties as an OSHA compliance officer is the responsibility of the entry-level medical assistant.

_____

## Sentence Completion

In the space provided, write the word or phrase that best completes each sentence.

1. **[LO1.2]** There is no single national definition for the medical assistant's scope of _____

2. **[LO1.1]** _____ habits will help you with concentration and retention of materials in school.

3. **[LO1.5]** A statement in the AAMA Creed says I will be _____ to my employer.

4. **[LO1.7]** The medical assistant profession today requires a commitment to self-directed, _____ learning.

5. **[LO1.4]** CLIA '88 is making mandatory credentialing for medical assistants a _____ step in the hiring process.

6. **[LO1.3]** A medical assistant program may be accredited by either the _____ or _____.

7. **[LO1.7]** If certified after 2006, an RMA (AMT) must accumulate _____ contact hours for continuing education units (CEU) every _____ years.

8. **[LO1.6]** The professional publication of the AAMA is the _____.

9. **[LO1.7]** When you build alliances socially and professionally, you are _____.

10. **[LO1.5]** The knowledge base of the modern medical assistant includes compliance to _____ and _____ guidelines.

1. _____
   _____
2. _____
   _____
3. _____
   _____
4. _____
   _____
5. _____
   _____
6. _____
   _____
7. _____
   _____
8. _____
   _____
9. _____
   _____
10. _____
    _____

# Apply Your Knowledge
## Short Answer

Write the answer to each question on the lines provided.

1. **[LO1.1]** List four examples of organizational skills that would help the medical assistant student.

   _____

   _____

   _____

**2.** [LO1.2] What is a managed care organization?

_____

_____

_____

**3.** [LO1.2] To ensure HIPAA compliance, what is the best way to dispose of paper in the medical office?

_____

_____

_____

**4.** [LO1.5] List three areas of competence from the CAAHEP and/or ABHES list/s of competencies.

_____

_____

_____

**5.** [LO1.2] List two clinical and two laboratory duties performed by the entry-level medical assistant.

_____

_____

_____

## Problem-Solving Activities

Follow the directions for each activity.

**1.** [LO1.1] Goal Setting
   a. Set up a table following the sample given in Chapter 1, Table 1–1.

| GOAL(S) | STUDY STRATEGIES | WHO? (PERSONS INVOLVED IN CARRYING OUT YOUR STRATEGIES) | SPECIFIC CONCERNS? | COMPLETION DATE? |
|---------|------------------|-------------------------------------------------------|--------------------|------------------|
|         |                  |                                                       |                    |                  |
|         |                  |                                                       |                    |                  |

   b. State two specific personal education goals you have.
   c. Determine at least one strategy you will need to use to achieve this goal.
   d. Establish a completion date for each goal.

**2.** [LO1.2] In a group discussion, review the belief statements of the AAMA Creed and determine at least two ways the medical assistant can uphold each of these beliefs. On your own, think of other ways you can fulfill the expectations of this creed.

## Thinking Critically

Write your response to each case study question on the lines provided.

### Case 1 [LO1.1]

A medical assistant student has started the first week of externship at a medical clinic where the assigned mentor is a 2-year experienced medical assistant who is now the clinic's administrative assistant. The back-office clinical assistant is out ill today so the mentor says to the student, "You are on your own" and asks the student to start rooming patients, taking and charting vital signs, and determining the patient's chief complaint. The mentor leaves the student alone to do these tasks while she resumes her position at the reception desk, greeting patients and answering telephone calls. As the student is rooming the patients, the mentor says, "You are not keeping up with the patient flow and need to speed up your pace."

**1.** How should the medical assistant extern student approach the mentor about this problem?

_____

_____

_____

**2.** What organizational skills will assist the extern student to improve performance?

_____

_____

_____

### Case 2 [LO1.2]

Bill is a 22-year-old medical assistant employed at an orthopedic clinic. He overhears Sue, a fellow medical assistant, tell an elderly female patient that if the doctor's treatment does not help her, she can contact Sue for the name of her mother's physician, who really helped cure her back problems.

**1.** What approach should Bill take with Sue concerning the interaction she had with the patient?

_____

_____

_____

**2.** What responsibility does Bill have to report this to the physician and to his employer?

_____

_____

_____

**Case 3** [LO1.2]

Karen is a 25-year-old administrative medical assistant. Today at the medical clinic where she is employed she is assigned to cover the front office reception desk, answering phone calls, pulling patient files, and filing documents into patient files. She is highly organized and professional in her work. Other clinic employees recognize that she is a very good and loyal employee and knowledgeable in her job. When her coworkers ask about her work ethics, she discusses her professional development activities that help her stay abreast of the changes and expectations in the medical field.

1. What are Karen's attributes that contribute to her success as an administrative medical assistant?

_____

_____

_____

2. What organizational skills do you believe Karen uses to assist in the performance of her job?

_____

_____

_____

# Demonstrate Your Knowledge

**Student Name:** _____

## Procedure 1–1: Obtaining Certification Information through the Internet

**GOAL:** To obtain information from the Internet regarding professional credentialing

**MATERIALS:** Computer with Internet access and printer

**METHOD:** To pass this procedure the minimum required score is _____% or all elements must meet "satisfactory" ability on the final demonstration. The first box may be used as a practice or final demonstration, with the evaluator placing **S for Satisfactory** or **U for Unsatisfactory** if that is the grading criteria. The second box may be used as a final demonstration with a **grade point** written in the box.

| STEPS | POSSIBLE POINTS | S/U | POINTS EARNED |
|---|---|---|---|
| 1. Open your Internet browser and locate a search engine. Search for the credential you would like to pursue. For example, Certified Medical Assistant, Registered Medical Assistant, or Certified Medical Assistant Specialist. If you are unsure of the credential you would like to pursue, you may just want to search for "Medical Assisting Credentials." | 8 | | |
| 2. Select the site for the credential you are pursuing. Avoid sponsored links. These links are paid for and will not typically bring you to the site of a credentialing organization. | 8 | | |
| 3. Navigate to the home page. For the CMA (AAMA) credential, enter the site www. aama-ntl.org. For the RMA (AMT) or CMAS (AMT) credential, enter the site www.amt1.com. | 8 | | |
| 4. Determine the steps you must take to obtain the selected credential.<br><br>a. For CMA (AAMA) go to the drop-down menu "CMA (AAMA) Exam" and select the link "How to Become a CMA (AAMA)."<br><br>b. For RMA (AMT) go to the drop-down menu on the left, click "Certification," and then select "Medical Assistant" for RMA (AMT) or "Medical Administrative Specialist" for CMAS (AMT). | 9 | | |
| 5. Print or write down the qualifications you must obtain. | 5 | | |

*(Continued)*

| STEPS | POSSIBLE POINTS | S/U | POINTS EARNED |
|---|---|---|---|
| 6. Once you have met the qualifications you will need to apply for the examination or certification. Download the application and the application instructions for the RMA (AMT) or the CMAS (AMT) or the candidate application and handbook for the CMA (AAMA). | 10 | | |
| 7. To view or print these instructions you may need to download Adobe Reader. You can click on a link to download Adobe Reader after you click on the "Apply for Certification" link for AMT or the "Apply for the CMA (AAMA) Exam" for AAMA. | 9 | | |
| 8. Before or after you apply for the examination, you will need to prepare for the examination. Select the link "Prepare for the CMA (AAMA) Exam" on the AAMA site or the "Prepare for Exam" link under the "Medical Assistant" or "Medical Assistant Specialist" drop-down menus on the AMT site. | 10 | | |
| 9. Prepare for the exam by reviewing the content outline, obtaining additional study resources, or taking a practice exam online. | 9 | | |
| 10. Print or save downloaded information in a file folder on your desktop labeled "credentials" or something that you can recognize. To print, click the printer icon found at the bottom of the Web page or just simply click the printer icon in your browser. | 8 | | |
| 11. Return to the appropriate site if you have additional questions. For the CMA (AAMA) site you may want to check the "FAQs on CMA (AAMA) Certification" link. On the AMT site for RMA or CMAS, click the "Take the Exam" link and download the FAQs regarding the testing process. | 8 | | |
| 12. Any questions you have that are not addressed on the sites can be e-mailed to the organizations. For CMAS send an e-mail to the link cmas@amt1.com. For RMA send an e-mail to the link rma@amt1.com. On the AAMA site for the CMA credential, click the "Contact" link on the top right-hand side of the screen. | 8 | | |
| **Total Points (if applicable)** | 100 | | |

**Comments:** _____

_____

_____

**Final Evaluator's Signature:** _____

**Date:** _____

## CAAHEP Competencies Achieved

IX. C (5) Discuss licensure and certification as it applies to health-care providers

## ABHES Competencies Achieved

1. c. Understand medical assistant credentialing requirements and the process to obtain the credential; comprehend the importance of credentialing

8. ll. Apply electronic technology

# Professional Behaviors

## Test Your Knowledge

### Vocabulary Review

Match the key terms in the right column with the definitions in the left column by placing the letter of each correct answer in the space provided.

_____ **1.** a set of values of hard work held by employees

_____ **2.** specific technical and operational proficiencies

_____ **3.** adhering to the appropriate code of law and ethics; trustworthy and honest

_____ **4.** time-off given back for working extra without pay

_____ **5.** a manner of carrying oneself

_____ **6.** a computerized system of the patient's medical record allowing tracking and transmission of documentation of histories, care, orders, results, reports, and administrative functions

_____ **7.** credits given by a professional organization for participating in approved educational offerings to maintain certification

_____ **8.** working with others in the best interest of completing the job

_____ **9.** integration of activities

_____ **10.** striving for excellence in doing the job; pride in one's performance

_____ **11.** showing up on appointed days and at appointed times

**a.** attitude [LO2.2]

**b.** communication [LO2.2]

**c.** compensation time [LO2.2]

**d.** comprehension [LO2.2]

**e.** continuing education units (CEU) [LO2.1]

**f.** constructive criticism [LO2.2]

**g.** cooperation [LO2.2]

**h.** coordination [LO2.2]

**i.** critical thinking [LO2.2]

**j.** cultural diversity [LO2.2]

**k.** electronic health record (EHR) [LO2.2]

**l.** empathy [LO2.2]

**m.** hard skills [LO2.2]

**n.** integrity [LO2.2]

**o.** judgment [LO2.2]

_____ **12.** the variety of human social structures, belief systems, and strategies for adapting to situations in different parts of the world

_____ **13.** feeling and understanding another's experience without having the experience oneself

_____ **14.** a member of a vocation requiring specialized educational training

_____ **15.** exhibiting the traits or features that correspond with some model of that profession

_____ **16.** personal attributes that enhance an individual's interactions, job performance, and career prospects

_____ **17.** learning, retaining, and processing information

_____ **18.** continuing in spite of difficulty; determined; overcoming obstacles

_____ **19.** counseling or advice that is intended to be useful with the goal of improving something

_____ **20.** believing in oneself; assured

_____ **21.** coming to an appropriate conclusion and acting accordingly; critical thinking

_____ **22.** purposeful; judgment resulting from analysis and evaluation

_____ **23.** understanding gained through study and experience; associating theory with practice

_____ **24.** planning and coordinating information and tasks in an orderly manner to efficiently complete the job in a given time

_____ **25.** utilizing time in an effective manner to accomplish the desired results

_____ **26.** sorting and dealing with matters in the order of urgency and importance

_____ **27.** giving and receiving accurate information

**p.** knowledge [LO2.2]

**q.** organization [LO2.2]

**r.** persistence [LO2.2]

**s.** professional [LO2.1]

**t.** professionalism [LO2.1]

**u.** prioritizing [LO2.2]

**v.** punctuality [LO2.2]

**w.** self-confidence [LO2.2]

**x.** soft skills [LO2.2]

**y.** time management [LO2.2]

**z.** work ethic [LO2.2]

**aa.** work quality [LO2.2]

# Multiple-Choice Certification Questions

There may be more than one answer; circle the letter of the choice that best completes each statement or answers each question.

1. **[LO2.2]** In your medical assisting classes, when you are learning, retaining, and processing information, you are
   a. persisting.
   b. comprehending.
   c. cooperating.
   d. organizing.
   e. relating.

2. **[LO2.2]** When you are observing a patient, evaluating the situation, and taking action, you are demonstrating
   a. good time management.
   b. honesty and integrity.
   c. verbal communication.
   d. critical thinking skills.
   e. cooperation and teamwork.

3. **[LO2.2]** To avoid becoming excessively friendly with a patient, the medical assistant must maintain
   a. professional boundaries.
   b. self-confidence.
   c. an empathic attitude.
   d. persistence.
   e. continuing education.

4. **[LO2.3]** A frequent reason for termination from an externship or a job is when the medical assistant is
   a. maintaining appropriate personal hygiene.
   b. showing respect and integrity.
   c. not punctual on a daily basis.
   d. demonstrating professionalism.
   e. setting professional boundaries.

5. **[LO2.2]** Which of the following is an example of a hard skill?
   a. Professionalism
   b. Integrity
   c. Cooperation
   d. Appointment scheduling
   e. All of the above

6. **[LO2.1]** What could happen if a medical assistant does not give a patient proper instructions prior to a test?
   a. The test may have to be cancelled.
   b. The test may need to be repeated.
   c. There is a potential for litigation against the medical practice.
   d. There may be inaccurate test results.
   e. All of the above.

7. **[LO2.3]** A major reason a medical assistant may not successfully complete his education is
   a. having poor or weak soft skills.
   b. possessing strong hard skills.
   c. understanding cultural diversity.
   d. demonstrating integrity.
   e. All of the above.

8. **[LO2.2]** Which of the following is *not* an attribute of a medical assistant who possesses good work ethics?
   a. The medical assistant uses good organizational skills.
   b. The medical assistant was absent and forgot to contact the medical office.
   c. The medical assistant is able to accept constructive criticism.
   d. The medical assistant is self-confident.
   e. All of the above.

9. **[LO2.2]** A medical assistant who is adhering to laws in the state where she is employed is demonstrating
   a. persistence.
   b. self-confidence.
   c. integrity.
   d. comprehension.
   e. cooperation.

10. **[LO2.1]** When a patient and the physician are feeling more comfortable that you know what you are doing, you are demonstrating
   a. self-confidence.
   b. tenacity and persistence.
   c. nonverbal communication.
   d. organizational skills.
   e. honesty and integrity.

11. **[LO2.2]** Which of the following is required in order to properly prioritize tasks?
   a. An understanding of cultural diversity
   b. Effective communication skills
   c. A belief in oneself
   d. Good organizational skills
   e. Acceptance of constructive criticism

12. **[LO2.2]** When you willingly receive feedback and suggestions about improving your performance of a skill, you are demonstrating how to
   a. be persistent.
   b. accept constructive criticism.
   c. practice time management.
   d. be punctual.
   e. All of the above.

13. **[LO2.2]** Which of the following is an example of compensation time?
   a. Working from 9 A.M. to 6 P.M. with a 1-hour lunch break
   b. Applying for a 2-week paid vacation from work
   c. Working every other Saturday during office hours
   d. Taking a paid holiday off work
   e. Receiving 4 hours off work in exchange for working 4 hours of extra time at the medical office

14. **[LO2.2]** Which of the following is an example of cooperation in a work setting?
   a. Earning continuing education credits
   b. Working together as a team
   c. Showing confidence
   d. Demonstrating integrity
   e. None of the above

15. **[LO2.2]** To properly work with electronic health records, a medical assistant must have specific attributes including
   a. cooperation and coordination.
   b. punctuality and good attendance.
   c. appropriate professional appearance.
   d. acceptance of criticism.
   e. All of the above.

**16.** [LO2.2] When you are doing things for another person that that person should be doing for himself, you are
   a. showing empathy toward the other person.
   b. cooperating with the other person.
   c. coordinating activities for the other person.
   d. enabling the other person.
   e. trusting the other person.

**17.** [LO2.2] Which of the following is a good example of accepting criticism?
   a. Blaming other co-workers for your mistake
   b. Thanking a co-worker for showing you how to do a procedure
   c. Becoming defensive with your instructor
   d. Believing that other co-workers do not like you
   e. Telling co-workers that they cannot perform a procedure as well as you can

**18.** [LO2.2] Performing insurance coding and medical records management are examples of
   a. soft skills.
   b. time management.
   c. coordination.
   d. teamwork.
   e. hard skills.

**19.** [LO2.2] Employers are seeking employees that have good work ethics including
   a. persistence.
   b. self-confidence.
   c. integrity.
   d. punctuality.
   e. All of the above.

**20.** [LO2.2] Judgment is also known as
   a. tenacity.
   b. critical thinking.
   c. integrity.
   d. ethics.
   e. prioritizing.

**21.** [LO2.2] The most important key to good communication is to
   a. ensure the information communicated is accurate.
   b. be persistent when delivering a message.
   c. practice good time management.
   d. employ hard skills you have learned.
   e. accept constructive criticism.

**22.** [LO2.1] Falsifying a time card while an extern is an example of
   a. lacking good time management.
   b. applying good work ethics.
   c. failing to cooperate with your extern supervisor.
   d. not adhering to the principles of integrity.
   e. not being punctual.

**23.** [LO2.1] An example of earning continuing education units is
   a. attending seminars.
   b. reading articles.
   c. taking courses online.
   d. writing an article for publication.
   e. All of the above.

**24.** [LO2.2] One way to set professional boundaries is
   a. to offer others advice on personal matters.
   b. to use only tasteful, appropriate humor with patients.
   c. to obtain continuing education units.
   d. to meet with patients outside of the workplace.
   e. None of the above.

**25.** [LO2.2] Which of the following is an example of applying the principles of cultural diversity?
   a. Requiring all patients to look at you when you are questioning them
   b. Showing respect to all individuals regardless of their culture
   c. Allowing patients with a higher socioeconomic status to be scheduled first
   d. Asking everyone to agree with your belief system
   e. Having good relationships only with those patients that speak English

## True or False

Decide whether each statement is true or false. In the space at the left, write "T" for true or "F" for false. On the lines provided, rewrite the false statements to make them true.

_____ **1.** [LO2.1] Coming to work every day that you are scheduled is optional.

_____

_____ **2.** [LO2.1] A professional is a member of a vocation requiring specialized educational training.

_____

_____ **3.** [LO2.3] Weakness in the soft skills is one of the major reasons that students do not successfully complete their medical assisting education.

_____

_____ **4.** [LO2.2] The attribute of tenacity allows you to better overcome obstacles.

_____

_____ **5.** [LO2.2] Comprehension is the ability to get along with people.

_____

_____ **6.** [LO2.2] Self-confidence is a trait that puts people at ease.

_____

_____ **7.** [LO2.2] Effective communication is always a one-way process.

_____

_____ **8.** [LO2.2] Knowledge is the only requirement to be an effective organizer.

_____

_____ **9.** [LO2.3] If a medical assistant student is caught taking cash or supplies from an externship site, immediate removal from the site is possible and the student may be terminated from his or her program of study.

_____

_____**10.** [LO2.2] Cooperation is working with others in the best interest of completing the job.

_____

## Sentence Completion

In the space provided, write the word or phrase that best completes each sentence.

**1.** [LO2.1] In the medical practice, the overall goal should be providing _____ patient care.

**2.** [LO2.2] Appointment scheduling, insurance coding, and medical records management are examples of _____.

**3.** [LO2.2] The majority of soft skills are about working with _____.

**4.** [LO2.2] A medical assistant must give _____ information in order to properly communicate with patients.

**5.** [LO2.2] The attribute of organization has many aspects including _____ and _____.

**6.** [LO2.2] Growth is an ongoing effort to learn and _____.

**7.** [LO2.2] Relations with others involves treating everyone with _____ and _____ even when it is difficult.

**8.** [LO2.1] Maintaining professional boundaries requires that you avoid becoming _____ friendly.

**9.** [LO2.2] Relations with others includes respect for the individual and the individual's _____.

**10.** [LO2.3] Medical assisting education and the medical practice are an examples of a _____ partnership.

**1.** _____
_____

**2.** _____
_____

**3.** _____
_____

**4.** _____
_____

**5.** _____
_____

**6.** _____
_____

**7.** _____
_____

**8.** _____
_____

**9.** _____
_____

**10.** _____
_____

# Apply Your Knowledge

## Short Answer

Write the answer to each question on the lines provided.

1. [LO2.1] List four habits or items that contribute to a professional appearance.

_____

_____

_____

2. [LO2.2] What are the requirements for good communication?

_____

_____

_____

3. [LO2.2] Explain how you can acquire self-confidence.

_____

_____

_____

4. [LO2.3] Visit the AAMA or AMT Web site and discover at least two ways to earn continuing education credit with the organization to maintain certification.

_____

_____

_____

5. [LO2.2] Describe a situation in which the medical assistant needs to demonstrate empathy toward a patient.

_____

_____

_____

## Problem-Solving Activities

Follow the directions for each activity.

1. [LO2.2] Professional Behaviors
   a. Refer to Chapter 2, Table 2–1.

**TABLE 2-1 Professional Behaviors**

| BEHAVIOR | DEFINITION |
|---|---|
| Comprehension | Learning, retaining, and processing information |
| Persistence (tenacity) | Continuing in spite of difficulty; determined; overcoming obstacles |
| Self-confidence | Believing in oneself; assured |
| Judgment | Evaluating a situation and coming to an appropriate conclusion, then acting accordingly; critical thinking |
| Knowledge | Understanding gained through study and experience; putting theory into practice |
| Organization | Planning and coordinating information and tasks in an orderly manner to efficiently complete the job in the given time |
| Communication | Giving and receiving accurate information |
| Integrity (honesty) | Adhering to the appropriate code of law and ethics; trustworthy |
| Growth | Ongoing efforts to learn and improve |
| Cooperation | Working with others in the best interest of completing the job |
| Acceptance of criticism | Willingness to consider feedback and suggestions to improve; taking responsibility for one's actions |
| Relations with others | Getting along with people |
| Work quality | Striving for excellence in doing the job; pride in one's performance |
| Punctuality and attendance | Showing up on appointed days and at appointed times |
| Professional appearance | Adhering to the standards and codes of dress, including rules on body art and the practicing of good personal hygiene |

  b.  Select five of the professional behaviors listed.
  c.  For each behavior selected, give an example of how you will further develop this behavior as a practicing medical assistant.

2.  [LO2.3] In a group, discuss the reasons a medical assisting student would not successfully complete his or her medical assistant education. List the reasons and give an example of the behavior that would lead to the problem.

## Thinking Critically

Write your response to each case study question on the lines provided.

### Case 1 [LO2.3]

Mary and Joanne are administrative medical assistant students in the same classroom and sit by each other during the administration of a written examination. Mary observes that Joanne is looking at her friend's answer sheet and copying down answers. When the instructor returns the graded exams for the students to review, Joanne discovers that she has failed the examination.

1.  How should Mary, who witnessed the event, deal with or interact with Joanne, who cheated?

_____

_____

_____

**2.** Should Mary report this activity to the instructor? Why or why not?

_____

_____

_____

## Case 2 [LO2.2]

Bill and Nancy are administrative medical assistants working at the same medical clinic. Nancy, who is not very organized, is assigned to perform the supply inventory. Every time she carries out this function, she forgets something that is needed for the office to run smoothly. Bill sees that Nancy needs some help with her organizational skills and offers advice to Nancy. Nancy tells Bill that he is not her supervisor and to mind his own business. She says that she just has her own way of doing things.

**1.** What can Bill do to convince Nancy that her job would be easier and more efficient if she improved her organizational skills?

_____

_____

_____

**2.** What can Nancy do to improve her acceptance of constructive criticism?

_____

_____

_____

## Case 3 [LO2.2]

Susan is an administrative medical assistant who works in a multipractice medical clinic. The clinic has many patients of different cultures that have relocated from other countries. Susan feels awkward and uncomfortable talking and working with these patients.

**1.** What are some things that Susan can do to become more comfortable with these patients?

_____

_____

_____

**2.** What avenues can Susan seek to find out more about different cultures?

_____

_____

_____

# Demonstrate Your Knowledge

**Student Name:** _____

## Procedure 2–1: Professional Behavior Self-Assessment

**GOAL:** To conduct a self-assessment of professional behaviors as a baseline for personal and professional growth and development

**MATERIALS:** Professional behavior rubric (Figure 2–8, which is also available at the end of this study guide), pen or pencil

**METHOD:** To pass this procedure the minimum required score is _____% or all elements must meet "satisfactory" ability on the final demonstration. The first box may be used as a practice, or final demonstration with the evaluator placing **S for Satisfactory** or **U for Unsatisfactory** if that is the grading criteria. The second box may be used as a final demonstration with a **grade point** written in the box.

| STEPS | POSSIBLE POINTS | S/U | POINTS EARNED |
|---|:---:|:---:|:---:|
| 1. Rate yourself according to the four possible choices on the professional behavior rubric (Figure 2–8) | 30 | | |
| 2. Create a self-improvement plan for any of your behaviors that are unacceptable or questionable (ask your instructor or the program director for assistance if needed). | 30 | | |
| 3. Tell an instructor, classmate, family member, or friend the areas you are focused on improving. Research demonstrates that telling someone, especially in public, increases the chances of success. | 10 | | |
| 4. Review your original self-assessment at specific intervals selected by you to monitor your improvement (mark your calendar now for the interval you chose; suggestions are weekly, monthly, or by class). | 10 | | |
| 5. (Optional) Ask a colleague or instructor to rate you using the rubric after one month into your medical assisting program. Print or write down the qualification you must obtain. | 10 | | |
| 6. File the rubric in a safe place for further use prior to your externship. | 10 | | |
| **Total Points (if applicable)** | 100 | | |

**Comments:** _____

_____

_____

_____

**Final Evaluator's Signature:** _____

**Date:** _____

## CAAHEP Compentencies Achieved

IV. A (6) Demonstrate awareness of how an individual's personal appearance affects anticipated responses

IV. C (13) Identify the role of self boundaries in the health care environment

X. C (5) Identify the effect personal ethics may have on professional performance

X. A (1) Apply ethical behaviors, including honesty/integrity in performance of medical assisting practice

## ABHES Compentencies Achieved

11. b. Demonstrate professionalism by:

    (1) Exhibiting dependability, punctuality, and positive work ethic

    (2) Exhibiting a positive attitude and a sense of responsibility

    (3) Maintaining confidentiality at all times

    (5) Exhibiting initiative

    (6) Adapting to change

    (7) Expressing a positive attitude

    (8) Being courteous and diplomatic

# The Health-Care Team

## Test Your Knowledge

### Vocabulary Review

Match the key terms in the right column with the definitions in the left column by placing the letter of each correct answer in the space provided.

_____ **1.** a specialist who diagnoses and treats diseases of the heart and blood vessels

_____ **2.** an individual trained to use pressure, kneading, and stroking to promote muscle and full-body relaxation

_____ **3.** a specialist who identifies tumors and treats patients who have cancer

_____ **4.** a specialist who diagnoses and treats diseases of the ear, nose, and throat

_____ **5.** a doctor who focuses special attention on the musculoskeletal system and uses hands and eyes to identify and adjust structural problems, supporting the body's natural tendency toward health and self-healing

_____ **6.** a specialist who studies, diagnoses, and manages diseases of the kidney

_____ **7.** a specialist who diagnoses and treats physical reactions to substances including mold, dust, fur, pollen, foods, drugs, and chemicals

_____ **8.** a specialist who diagnoses and treats childhood diseases and teaches parents skills for keeping their children healthy

_____ **9.** a system of hands-on techniques that help relieve pain, restore motion, support the body's natural functions, and influence the body's structure

**a.** acupuncturist [LO3.1]

**b.** allergist [LO3.1]

**c.** American Board of Medical Specialties (ABMS) [LO3.1]

**d.** anesthetist [LO3.1]

**e.** autopsy [LO3.1]

**f.** biopsy [LO3.1]

**g.** cardiologist [LO3.1]

**h.** chiropractor [LO3.1]

**i.** dermatologist [LO3.1]

**j.** doctor of osteopathy [LO3.1]

**k.** endocrinologist [LO3.1]

**l.** family practitioner [LO3.1]

**m.** gastroenterologist [LO3.1]

**n.** gerontologist [LO3.1]

**o.** gynecologist [LO3.1]

_____ 10. a specialist who reconstructs, corrects, or improves body structures

_____ 11. a specialist who diagnoses and treats disorders of the endocrine system, which regulates many body functions by circulating hormones that are secreted by glands throughout the body

_____ 12. a specialist who diagnoses and treats diseases and disorders of the muscles and bones

_____ 13. a specialist who studies the aging process

_____ 14. a practitioner who treats people with pain or discomfort by inserting thin, hollow needles under the skin

_____ 15. a physician who provides routine medical care and referrals to specialists

_____ 16. a medical doctor who studies the changes a disease produces in the cells, fluids, and processes of the entire body

_____ 17. a specialist who uses medications to cause patients to lose sensation or feeling during surgery

_____ 18. a physician who diagnoses and treats disorders of the anus, rectum, and intestines

_____ 19. a physical medicine specialist, who diagnoses and treats diseases and disorders with physical therapy

_____ 20. a physician who does not specialize in a branch of medicine but treats all types and ages of patients; also called a general practitioner

_____ 21. a physician who specializes in taking and reading x-rays

_____ 22. a specialist who performs routine physical care and examinations of the female reproductive system

_____ 23. a specialist who diagnoses and treats diseases of the kidney, bladder, and urinary system

_____ 24. the removal and examination of a sample of tissue from a living body for diagnostic purposes

**p.** internist **[LO3.1]**

**q.** massage therapist **[LO3.1]**

**r.** nephrologist **[LO3.1]**

**s.** neurologist **[LO3.1]**

**t.** oncologist **[LO3.1]**

**u.** orthopedist **[LO3.1]**

**v.** osteopathic manipulative medicine (OMM) **[LO3.1]**

**w.** otorhinolaryngologist **[LO3.1]**

**x.** pathologist **[LO3.1]**

**y.** pediatrician **[LO3.1]**

**z.** physiatrist **[LO3.1]**

**aa.** plastic surgeon **[LO3.1]**

**bb.** podiatrist **[LO3.1]**

**cc.** primary care physician **[LO3.1]**

**dd.** proctologist **[LO3.1]**

**ee.** radiologist **[LO3.1]**

**ff.** surgeon **[LO3.1]**

**gg.** triage **[LO3.1]**

**hh.** urologist **[LO3.1]**

_____ **25.** a physician who uses hands and medical instruments to diagnose and correct deformities and treat external and internal injuries or disease

_____ **26.** a physician who uses a system of therapy, including manipulation of the spine, to treat illness or pain

_____ **27.** a doctor who specializes in diagnosing and treating problems related to the internal organs

_____ **28.** an organization whose purpose is to maintain and improve the quality of medical care and certify doctors in various specialties

_____ **29.** to assess the urgency and types of conditions patients present as well as their immediate medical needs

_____ **30.** a specialist who diagnoses and treats diseases of the skin, hair, and nails

_____ **31.** a physician who specializes in the study and treatment of the foot and ankle

_____ **32.** the examination of a cadaver to determine or confirm the cause of death

_____ **33.** a specialist who diagnoses and treats disorders and diseases of the nervous system, including the brain, spinal cord, and nerves

_____ **34.** a specialist who diagnoses and treats disorders of the entire gastrointestinal tract including the stomach, intestines, and associated digestive organs

## Multiple-Choice Certification Questions

There may be more than one answer; circle the letter of the choice that best completes each statement or answers each question.

**1.** [LO3.1] The first year of residency for a physician in medical school is called
   a. an internship.
   b. an externship.
   c. a freshman assignment.
   d. a first-year student rotation.
   e. None of the above.

**2.** [LO3.1] A family practitioner is also called a
   a. gerontologist.
   b. gynecologist.
   c. general practitioner.
   d. physician assistant.
   e. physiatrist.

**3.** [LO3.2] The physician who specializes in reading electrocardiograms is a/an
   a. internist.
   b. primary care physician.
   c. osteopath.
   d. endocrinologist.
   e. cardiologist.

**4.** [LO3.2] A patient with stomach or intestinal problems would be referred to
   a. a bariatric specialist.
   b. a proctologist.
   c. an endocrinologist.
   d. a gastroenterologist.
   e. None of the above.

**5.** [LO3.2] A patient who is suspected of having a stroke would be seen by a/an
   a. oncologist.
   b. neurologist.
   c. nephrologist.
   d. physiatrist.
   e. pathologist.

**6.** [LO3.1] The physician who specifically deals with pregnancy, labor, and delivery is a/an
   a. primary care physician.
   b. internist.
   c. pediatrician.
   d. gynecologist.
   e. obstetrician.

**7.** [LO3.1] Nuclear medicine is a specialty that is related to the field of
   a. radiology.
   b. oncology.
   c. pathology.
   d. nephrology.
   e. physical medicine.

**8.** [LO3.1] An optometric doctor is trained to
   a. perform cataract surgery.
   b. treat eye infections.
   c. fit eye glasses.
   d. repair detached retina.
   e. All of the above.

**9.** [LO3.2] Skin grafting is a procedure performed by a/an
   a. allergist.
   b. physiatrist.
   c. osteopath.
   d. plastic surgeon.
   e. endocrinologist.

**10.** [LO3.2] A physician who specializes in treating benign and malignant growths is an
   a. orthopedist.
   b. oncologist.
   c. osteopath.
   d. ophthalmologist.
   e. otorhinolaryngologist.

**11.** [LO3.2] When an athlete fractures a bone in the ankle, the specialist who should be consulted is a/an
   a. primary care physician.
   b. physiatrist.

    c. chiropractor.
    d. podiatrist.
    e. internist.

**12.** [LO3.2] A female patient who discovers a lump in her breast would be referred to see a/an
    a. gynecologist.
    b. obstetrician.
    c. oncologist.
    d. plastic surgeon.
    e. primary care physician.

**13.** [LO3.2] Which of the following specialty areas uses radiation to diagnose and treat disease?
    a. Nuclear medicine
    b. Internal medicine
    c. Physical medicine
    d. Electroencephalographic medicine
    e. Sports medicine

**14.** [LO3.3] Which of the following would be a career opportunity for a medical assistant who wants to work with patients that have physical injuries or illnesses, to help the patients attain their maximum physical and mental health?
    a. Mental health technician
    b. Acupuncturist
    c. Electroencephalographic technologist
    d. Optician
    e. Occupational therapist

**15.** [LO3.3] A technologist who has the letters RHIA after her name would work with
    a. laboratory specimens.
    b. radioactive substances.
    c. medical records.
    d. pregnant patients.
    e. None of the above.

**16.** [LO3.2] Frequently, a physician who is an obstetrician is also a/an
    a. oncologist.
    b. gynecologist.
    c. nephrologist.
    d. internist.
    e. pathologist.

**17.** [LO3.2] A physician who would repair a cleft lip and cleft palate is a/an
    a. dermatologist.
    b. internist.
    c. pathologist.
    d. plastic surgeon.
    e. oncologist.

**18.** [LO3.2] The subspecialty of medicine that deals with the treatment and preventative care of amateur and professional athletes is
    a. internal medicine.
    b. physical medicine.
    c. sports medicine.
    d. adolescent medicine.
    e. podiatric medicine.

**19.** [LO3.2] The physician specialist that is also referred to as an ENT is a/an
    a. otorhinolaryngologist.
    b. pediatrician.
    c. primary care physician.

        d. gastroenterologist.
        e. gerontologist.

**20.** [LO3.2] What type of surgery is required for a patient who needs gastric bypass?
   a. Orthopedic surgery
   b. Plastic surgery
   c. Vascular surgery
   d. Bariatric surgery
   e. Proctologic surgery

**21.** [LO3.2] A pathologist's duties include
   a. studying changes a disease produces in the body's cells.
   b. performing autopsies.
   c. reading biopsies.
   d. examining cadavers.
   e. All of the above.

**22.** [LO3.2] A specialist who treats people without drugs or surgery is a/an
   a. chiropractor.
   b. family practitioner.
   c. cardiologist.
   d. endocrinologist.
   e. dermatologist.

**23.** [LO3.2] The specialist who treats scars and performs hair transplants is
   a. a gerontologist.
   b. a dermatologist.
   c. an endocrinologist.
   d. a physiatrist.
   e. None of the above.

**24.** [LO3.2] A radiographer may be employed in
   a. a hospital.
   b. a clinic.
   c. a physician's office.
   d. a mobile medical facility.
   e. All of the above.

**25.** [LO3.2] A health-care specialist who supplies emergency oxygen equipment and services to home-care patients is
   a. a radiologic technologist.
   b. a physical therapist.
   c. a medical laboratory technologist.
   d. a respiratory therapist.
   e. None of the above.

## True or False

Decide whether each statement is true or false. In the space at the left, write "T" for true or "F" for false. On the lines provided, rewrite the false statements to make them true.

_____ **1.** [LO3.3] A dietician is sometimes confused with a nutritionist.

_____

_____ **2.** [LO3.2] A physiatrist specializes in taking and reading x-rays.

_____

_____ **3.** [LO3.2] A pediatrician diagnoses and treats childhood diseases.

_____

_____ **4.** [LO3.2] An otorhinolaryngologist diagnoses and treats illnesses of the ear, nose, and throat.

_____

_____ **5.** [LO3.2] A nephrologist uses medications to cause patients to lose sensation during surgery.

_____

_____ **6.** [LO3.2] A gynecologist specializes in the treatment of problems and diseases of older adults.

_____

_____ **7.** [LO3.2] An otorhinolaryngologist diagnoses and treats illnesses dealing with hormonal imbalance.

_____

_____ **8.** [LO3.2] A doctor of osteopathy holds the title DO and focuses attention on the musculoskeletal system as it relates to the body as a whole.

_____

_____ **9.** [LO3.2] An allergist diagnoses and treats physical reactions to substances such as dust and pollen.

_____

_____ **10.** [LO3.2] Obstetrics involves the study of pregnancy, labor delivery, and the period following labor called postpartum.

_____

## Sentence Completion

In the space provided, write the word or phrase that best completes each sentence.

**1.** [LO3.3] Membership in a(n) _____, such as the American Medical Technologists, enables one to get involved in relevant issues and activities.

**2.** [LO3.3] _____ are allied health professionals trained to draw blood for diagnostic laboratory testing.

**3.** [LO3.2] A family practitioner is also called a(n) _____ by insurance companies.

**4.** [LO3.2] An example of a disorder treated by a(n) _____ is thyroidism.

**5.** [LO3.2] _____, who hold the title of DO, practice a "whole-person" approach to health care.

**1.** _____
_____

**2.** _____
_____

**3.** _____
_____

**4.** _____
_____

**5.** _____
_____

6. **[LO3.2]** The theory of _____ relates to Chinese beliefs about how the body works.

7. **[LO3.2]** _____ is used to diagnose diseases and irregularities of the brain.

8. **[LO3.3]** Professional medical _____ and _____ review patient insurance coverage.

9. **[LO3.3]** Two types of allied health professionals who work in medical technology are the _____ and the medical technologist.

10. **[LO3.3]** _____ is one of the oldest methods of promoting healing and is used to treat strains, bruises, muscle soreness or tightness, lower back pain, and dislocations.

6. _____
   _____

7. _____
   _____

8. _____
   _____

9. _____
   _____

10. _____
    _____

# Apply Your Knowledge

## Short Answer

Write the answer to each question on the lines provided.

1. **[LO3.2]** What are the benefits of learning about the medical specialties and subspecialties?

   _____

   _____

   _____

2. **[LO3.2]** What are the differences between medical assistants and physician assistants?

   _____

   _____

   _____

3. **[LO3.2]** Why are patients referred to specialty physicians?

   _____

   _____

   _____

4. **[LO3.2]** Compare DOs and chiropractors. How are their practices different? How are they similar or the same?

   _____

   _____

   _____

**5.** [LO3.2] Discuss how a medical assistant may interact with other health-care professionals or specialists.

_____

_____

_____

## Problem-Solving Activities

Follow the directions for each activity.

**1.** [LO3.2] Medical Specialties
   a. Research the Internet for specialties in which a medical assistant may be employed.
   b. Research the credentials needed and the experience required for the job.
   c. Find a position within the specialty and research what duties are performed by the position and how you may gain those skills.

**2.** [LO3.3] Using the Internet, research the AMT, the AAMA, and the National Healthcareer Association (NHA). Select two certifications that you would like to complete upon graduation. Research the eligibility requirements and process for making applications to the certifications.

## Thinking Critically

Write your response to each case study question on the lines provided.

### Case 1 [LO3.2]

You are currently working for an internist who treats a variety of skin conditions, such as acne, eczema, and hives. A patient presents with a small lesion that has not healed in several months. The physician requests that you submit a referral to a dermatologist. Why would this patient seek medical care from a dermatologist instead of being treated by the internist?

_____

_____

_____

_____

_____

_____

## Case 2 [LO3.2]

You are working in a family practice office. A longtime patient makes an appointment for a diabetes follow-up. She weighs more than 500 pounds and is having difficulty controlling her diabetes as well as problems with general mobility. She asks you what options she has to lose the extra weight. What specialist will she be referred to? What surgical options might be available to her? Do you believe her insurance would pay for weight-control surgery?

_____

_____

_____

_____

_____

_____

## Case 3 [LO3.2]

You are employed by a primary care physician but you are interested in pursuing other avenues of specialty in your medical assisting career. What are some of the ways you can proceed to find out what other areas of practice are of interest to you?

_____

_____

_____

_____

_____

_____

# Professional Communication

## Test Your Knowledge

### Vocabulary Review

Match the key terms in the right column with the definitions in the left column by placing the letter of each correct answer in the space provided.

_____ **1.** the end result of prolonged periods of stress without relief

_____ **2.** verbal and nonverbal evidence that a message was received and understood

_____ **3.** volunteers who work with terminally ill patients and their families

_____ **4.** a harmonious, positive relationship

_____ **5.** a certain area that surrounds an individual and within which another person's physical presence is felt as an intrusion

_____ **6.** nonverbal communication, including facial expressions, eye contact, posture, touch, and attention to personal space

_____ **7.** a term that pertains to Abraham Maslow's hierarchy of needs stating that human beings are motivated by unsatisfied needs that must be satisfied before higher needs are met

_____ **8.** attitudes, qualities, and abilities that influence the level of success and satisfaction achieved in interacting with other people

_____ **9.** a position that conveys the feeling of not being totally receptive to what is being said; arms are often rigid or folded across the chest

**a.** active listening [LO4.1]

**b.** aggressive [LO4.1]

**c.** assertive [LO4.1]

**d.** body language [LO4.1]

**e.** boundaries [LO4.1]

**f.** burnout [LO4.1]

**g.** closed posture [LO4.1]

**h.** conflict [LO4.1]

**i.** feedback [LO4.1]

**j.** hierarchy [LO4.1]

**k.** homeostasis [LO4.1]

**l.** hospice [LO4.1]

**m.** interpersonal skills [LO4.1]

**n.** open posture [LO4.1]

**o.** passive listening [LO4.1]

_____ **10.** part of two-way communication, such as offering feedback or asking questions

**p.** personal space **[LO4.1]**

_____ **11.** an opposition of opinions or ideas

**q.** rapport **[LO4.1]**

_____ **12.** hearing what a person has to say without responding in any way

_____ **13.** being firm and standing up for oneself while showing respect for others

_____ **14.** a position that conveys a feeling of receptiveness and friendliness; facing another person with arms comfortably at the sides or in the lap

_____ **15.** a balanced, stable state within the body

_____ **16.** a physical or psychological space that indicates the limit of appropriate versus inappropriate behavior

_____ **17.** imposing one's position on others or trying to manipulate them

## Multiple-Choice Certification Questions

There may be more than one answer; circle the letter of the choice that best completes each statement or answers each question.

**1.** **[LO4.1]** Which of the following is an example of negative communication?
   a. Maintaining eye contact
   b. Displaying open posture
   c. Listening carefully
   d. Asking questions
   e. Mumbling

**2.** **[LO4.1]** The communication circle involves
   a. a message, noise, and good customer service.
   b. a message, a response, and an answer.
   c. feedback, noise, and an answer.
   d. a message, a source, and a receiver.
   e. None of the above.

**3.** **[LO4.2]** According to Maslow's hierarchy, the basic needs include
   a. physiological needs.
   b. the need for safety.
   c. a sense of belonging.
   d. love.
   e. All of the above.

**4.** **[LO4.3]** An example of positive verbal communication is to
   a. look directly at a patient when you speak to them.
   b. discourage patients to ask questions since they will not understand.
   c. be sure to use technical medical terms when speaking to patients.

d. speak very quickly in order to get your message across clearly.

e. avoid eye contact when talking with patients since some cultures may not like you staring at them.

**5.** [LO4.4] To improve your listening skills, you should
   a. avoid eye contact with the person you are speaking with.
   b. prepare yourself to listen to the message.
   c. ignore personal space while the other person is talking.
   d. pretend to listen to what is being said especially if you have heard the message before.
   e. interrupt the speaker and respond to the message before you think about what you will say.

**6.** [LO4.1] Compensation is a defense mechanism that occurs when there is
   a. an unconscious attempt to reject unacceptable feelings, needs, thoughts, wishes, or external reality factors.
   b. an unconscious transfer of unacceptable thoughts, feelings, or desires from the self to a more acceptable external substitute.
   c. overemphasis placed on a trait to make up for a perceived or actual failing.
   d. a disconnect of emotional significance from specific ideas or events.
   e. an unconscious replacing of an unreachable or unacceptable goal with another, more acceptable one.

**7.** [LO4.5] When you are standing by your principles while still showing respect for others, you are demonstrating
   a. repression.
   b. assertiveness.
   c. aggression.
   d. substitution.
   e. dissociation.

**8.** [LO4.6] When working with a patient who is anxious, he may exhibit signs of anxiety including
   a. a tense appearance.
   b. sweaty palms.
   c. increased breathing.
   d. increased blood pressure.
   e. All of the above.

**9.** [LO4.6] When a person makes a negative statement about the specific traits of a group that is applied unfairly to an entire population, the person is
   a. stereotyping.
   b. reflecting.
   c. generalizing.
   d. rationalizing.
   e. customizing.

**10.** [LO4.6] Which of the following is *not* an accurate statement regarding elderly patients?
   a. Elderly patients should be treated with respect.
   b. Elderly patients may be confused if they have some impairment in memory, judgment, or other mental abilities.
   c. Elderly people may become dependent, passive, or anxious.
   d. Elderly people have multiple health issues and like to complain frequently.
   e. Elderly patients may have difficulty understanding instructions.

**11.** [LO4.6] Which of the following actions are among the stages of dying or grief?
   a. Denial and identification
   b. Denial and anger
   c. Bargaining and substitution
   d. Acceptance and projection
   e. Substitution and anger

**12.** [LO4.7] Which of the following is *not* an action that is used to develop good rapport with co-workers?
   a. Have respect.
   b. Use active listening skills.
   c. Employ good communication techniques.
   d. Be open and friendly.
   e. None of the above.

**13.** [LO4.7] Which of the following would be an acceptable way to communicate with your manager or supervisor?
   a. When the office copy machine breaks down, don't tell the manager but just call the repair company and hope it is repaired before the manager finds out.
   b. If you are uncertain about performing a certain task, go ahead and perform the task the way you think it should be done without admitting to your manager that you don't know how to do the task.
   c. Do not recommend more efficient ways to do tasks in the office because your manager will think you are just trying to show off.
   d. When you have a question, avoid interrupting your supervisor if the question can wait until a more appropriate time when your supervisor is not as busy.
   e. You should go ahead with a new project without consulting your manager first; then when you are finished you can brag about how well you did completing the project.

**14.** [LO4.7] When dealing with conflict in the workplace you should
   a. not feed into other people's negative attitudes.
   b. agree with a co-worker who is criticizing a physician in the practice.
   c. not volunteer to assist a co-worker if she is having a bad day.
   d. not show respect for a co-worker if he is being judgmental.
   e. jump to conclusions quickly to end the conflict between two co-workers.

**15.** [LO4.7] Which of the following is a professional behavior that a medical assistant should demonstrate at the workplace?
   a. Be judgmental at all times.
   b. Show aggression, not assertiveness.
   c. Treat patients impersonally so you are not getting too friendly.
   d. Set physical and psychological boundaries.
   e. Make patients feel like they are taking up too much of your time.

**16.** [LO4.6] Which of the following would *not* be appropriate customer service in a physician's office?
   a. Using proper telephone techniques
   b. Asking patients to read health information brochures instead of explaining procedures to them
   c. Ensuring that patients are comfortable in your office
   d. Responding to telephone messages promptly
   e. Creating a warm and reassuring environment

**17.** [LO4.2] The expected development of an adolescent includes
   a. ego identity.
   b. thinking about marriage, family, and career.
   c. having an active imagination and curiosity about everything.
   d. beginning to trust the world around them.
   e. starting to explore the environment at home and everywhere else.

**18.** [LO4.2] Maslow's hierarchy level of self-actualization includes
   a. morality.
   b. creativity.
   c. spontaneity.
   d. problem solving.
   e. All of the above.

**19.** [LO4.3] Which of the following is *not* an example of negative communication?
   a. Speaking sharply
   b. Avoiding eye contact
   c. Encouraging patients to ask questions
   d. Showing boredom
   e. Rushing through explanations or instructions

**20.** [LO4.3] Which statement is accurate when describing the difference between open and closed posture?
   a. Closed posture conveys a feeling of friendliness.
   b. When a person has her hands in her lap she is displaying closed posture.
   c. Open posture creates a feeling of receptiveness.
   d. A person with his arms folded across his chest is demonstrating open posture.
   e. Open posture is a form of negative communication.

**21.** [LO4.6] When you are being empathetic with a patient you are
   a. showing a lack of respect toward the patient.
   b. just going through the motions of being kind.
   c. being silent and allowing the patient to talk.
   d. sensitive to the other person's feelings.
   e. providing feedback to the patient.

**22.** [LO4.3] Ineffective therapeutic communication results from roadblocks that can interfere with communication, including
   a. reassuring patients that there is no need to worry.
   b. giving approval for the patient's behavior that may lead to the patient striving for praise rather than progress.
   c. overtly disapproving of a patient's behavior implying that you have the right to pass judgment on the patient's thoughts and actions.
   d. not adhering to the principles of integrity.
   e. All of the above.

**23.** [LO4.3] Defense mechanisms are also referred to as
   a. stereotyping.
   b. coping strategies.
   c. psychological needs.
   d. interpersonal skills.
   e. body language.

**24.** [LO4.2] The physiological needs of Maslow's hierarchy include
   a. breathing.
   b. food.
   c. sleep.
   d. excretion.
   e. All of the above.

**25.** [LO4.5] Characteristics of assertive behavior includes feelings of
   a. anger.
   b. righteousness.
   c. resentment.
   d. confidence.
   e. guilt.

# True or False

Decide whether each statement is true or false. In the space at the left, write "T" for true or "F" for false. On the lines provided, rewrite the false statements to make them true.

_____ **1.** [LO4.4] Passive listening is hearing without the need for a reply.

_____

_____ **2.** [LO4.4] Active listening involves two-way communication.

_____

_____ **3.** [LO4.2] Maslow's hierarchy level of esteem includes security of body and employment.

_____

_____ **4.** [LO4.3] A good way to avoid negative communication is to close your eyes and ears to others.

_____

_____ **5.** [LO4.6] Empathy is a process of feeling sorry for someone.

_____

_____ **6.** [LO4.1] Feedback is a verbal or nonverbal response from a patient that she understands what has been communicated.

_____

_____ **7.** [LO4.4] Patients will see a medical assistant as standoffish and reserved when he portrays an open posture.

_____

_____ **8.** [LO4.5] When a person demonstrates aggressive behavior, others will feel angry and resentful toward that person.

_____

_____ **9.** [LO4.6] Stereotyping is a positive statement about the specific traits of a group of people.

_____

_____ **10.** [LO4.6] When interacting with a patient who is visually impaired you should speak louder so they can hear you clearly.

_____

## Sentence Completion

In the space provided, write the word or phrase that best completes each sentence.

1. [LO4.6] _____ workers often go to the home of the terminally ill.

2. [LO4.7] It is important to build a good _____ with co-workers in order to have a harmonious and positive relationship.

3. [LO4.7] Conflict, or _____, in the workplace can result from opposition of opinions.

4. [LO4.8] Stress can be a barrier to _____.

5. [LO4.8] Burnout is a/an _____ condition that will affect your health and career.

6. [LO4.3] Good communication supports a _____-centered approach in a medical office.

7. [LO4.4] One way to improve active listening skills is to maintain _____ contact.

8. [LO4.1] Touch is a powerful form of _____ communication.

9. [LO4.6] Being _____ in your interactions with patients mean that you refrain from "putting on an act" or just going through the motions.

10. [LO4.6] Patients may develop defense mechanisms, which are _____, to protect themselves from anxiety, guilt, and shame.

1. _____
   _____

2. _____
   _____

3. _____
   _____

4. _____
   _____

5. _____
   _____

6. _____
   _____

7. _____
   _____

8. _____
   _____

9. _____
   _____

10. _____
    _____

# Apply Your Knowledge

## Short Answer

Write the answer to each question on the lines provided.

1. **[LO4.3]** List four examples of customer service in a physician's office.

   _____

   _____

   _____

2. **[LO4.2]** Explain why learning developmental life span models can help you communicate with patients.

   _____

   _____

   _____

3. **[LO4.7]** What are three rules for establishing positive communication with co-workers?

   _____

   _____

   _____

4. **[LO4.6]** Describe three things you might do when dealing with very young patients.

   _____

   _____

   _____

5. **[LO4.6]** What are three things you can do to improve communication with a hearing-impaired patient?

   _____

   _____

   _____

# Problem-Solving Activities

Follow the directions for each activity.

1. **[LO4.8]** Reducing Stress
   a. Refer to Chapter 4, Table 4–3: Tips for Reducing Stress

| |
|---|
| • Maintain a healthy balance in your life among work, family, and leisure activities. |
| • Exercise regularly. |
| • Eat balanced, nutritious meals and healthful snacks. |
| • Avoid foods high in caffeine, salt, sugar, and fat. |
| • Get enough sleep. |
| • Allow time for yourself, and plan time to relax. |
| • Rely on the support that family, friends, and co-workers have to offer. Don't be afraid to share your feelings. |
| • Try to be realistic about what you can and cannot do. Do not be afraid to admit that you cannot take on another responsibility. |
| • Try to set realistic goals for yourself. Remember that there are always choices, even when there appear to be none. |
| • Be organized. Good planning can help you manage your workload. |
| • Redirect excess energy constructively—clean your closet, work in the garden, do volunteer work, have friends over for dinner, exercise. |
| • Change some of the things you have control over. Keep yourself focused. Finish one project before starting another. |
| • Identify sources of conflict, and try to resolve them. |
| • Learn and use relaxation techniques, such as deep breathing, meditation, or imagining yourself in a quiet, peaceful place. Choose what works for you. |
| • Maintain a healthy sense of humor. Laughter can help relieve stress. |
| • Try not to overreact. Ask yourself if a situation is really worth getting upset or worried about. |
| • The only person you can change is yourself. Take full responsibility and do not blame others for your dissatisfaction and stress. |
| • Seek help from social or professional support groups, if necessary. |

   b. Review the tips listed and select at least five that you know you could improve or change in your life that would help you to better manage stress.
   c. For each item selected, write down activities or habits that you can develop or change that will address each of these areas.

2. **[LO4.3]** Work with a fellow student to develop a role-play scenario that will be presented to the rest of the class. The scenario should represent one of the communication topics presented in Chapter 4 and should be a realistic event that could be experienced in the medical office workplace. You and your partner will present the scenario through role-play and have the class critique your presentation. They will need to determine if your presentation represented positive or negative communication.

# Thinking Critically

Write your response to each case study question on the lines provided.

## Case 1 [LO4.6]

A young child is about to receive an injection. He is scared and tearful. You know the injection will hurt slightly, but you decide to put the child's mind at ease by telling him that it won't hurt a bit. Is this the best way to handle the situation? Explain.

_____

_____

_____

## Case 2 [LO4.7]

You are having a problem with a co-worker. Both of you have the same job title and often work together to interview and prepare patients. This co-worker cuts you off when you speak and contradicts you in front of patients. Her actions are affecting the way patients see you as a professional. How should you handle the situation?

_____

_____

_____

## Case 3 [LO4.6]

A male patient is waiting in the exam room to see the physician. He is seeing the physician for sexual dysfunction. You and several medical assistants are outside his room at the workstation and burst into laughter about a comment unrelated to the patient. A few minutes later, the patient leaves without being seen by the physician. What could have happened to cause the patient to leave? How could this have been avoided?

_____

_____

_____

# Demonstrate Your Knowledge

**Student Name:** _____

## Procedure 4–1: Communicating with the Anxious Patient

**GOAL:** To use communication and interpersonal skills to calm an anxious patient

**MATERIALS:** None

**METHOD:** To pass this procedure the minimum required score is _____% or all elements must meet "satisfactory" ability on the final demonstration. The first box may be used as a practice or final demonstration, with the evaluator placing **S for Satisfactory** or **U for Unsatisfactory** if that is the grading criteria. The second box may be used as a final demonstration with a **grade point** written in the box.

| STEPS | POSSIBLE POINTS | S/U | POINTS EARNED |
|---|---|---|---|
| 1. Identify signs of anxiety in the patient. | 5 | | |
| 2. Acknowledge the patient's anxiety. (Ignoring a patient's anxiety often makes it worse.) | 5 | | |
| 3. Identify possible sources of anxiety, such as fear of a procedure or test result, along with supportive resources available to the patient, such as family members and friends. Understanding the source of anxiety in a patient and identifying the supportive resources available can help you communicate with the patient more effectively. | 10 | | |
| 4. Do what you can to alleviate the patient's physical discomfort. For example, find a calm, quiet place for the patient to wait, a comfortable chair, or access to the bathroom (Figure 4–4). | 10 | | |
| 5. Allow ample personal space for conversation. *Note:* You would normally allow a 1½- to 4-foot distance between yourself and the patient. Adjust this space as necessary. | 5 | | |
| 6. Create a climate of warmth, acceptance, and trust. | | | |
|    a. Recognize and control your own anxiety. Your air of calm can decrease the patient's anxiety. | 2 | | |
|    b. Provide reassurance by demonstrating genuine care, respect, and empathy. | 7 | | |
|    c. Act confidently and dependably, maintaining truthfulness and confidentiality at all times. | 10 | | |
| 7. Using the appropriate communication skills, have the patient describe the experience that is causing anxiety, her thoughts about it, and her feelings. Proceeding in this order allows the patient to describe what is causing the anxiety and to clarify her thoughts and feelings about it. | | | |
|    a. Maintain an open posture. | 1 | | |
|    b. Maintain eye contact, if culturally appropriate. | 2 | | |

*(Continued)*

| STEPS | POSSIBLE POINTS | S/U | POINTS EARNED |
|---|---|---|---|
| c. Use active listening skills. | 5 | | |
| d. Listen without interrupting. | 5 | | |
| 8. Do not belittle the patient's thoughts and feelings. This can cause a breakdown in communication, increase anxiety, and make the patient feel isolated. | 9 | | |
| 9. Be empathic to the patient's concerns. | 10 | | |
| 10. Help the patient recognize and cope with the anxiety. | | | |
| a. Provide information to the patient. Patients are often fearful of the unknown. Helping them understand their disease or the procedure they are about to undergo will help decrease their anxiety. | 2 | | |
| b. Suggest coping behaviors, such as deep breathing or other relaxation exercises. | 2 | | |
| 11. Notify the doctor of the patient's concerns. The physician must be aware of all aspects of the patient's health, including anxiety, to allow for optimal patient care. Part of your job as a medical assistant is to act as a liaison between the patient and the physician. | 10 | | |
| **Total Points (if applicable)** | **100** | | |

**Comments:** _____

_____

_____

**Final Evaluator's Signature:** _____

**Date:** _____

## CAAHEP Competencies Achieved

IV. C (2) Identify nonverbal communication

IV. C (3) Recognize communication barriers

IV. C (7) Identify resources and adaptations that are required based on an individual's needs, i.e., culture and environment, developmental life stage, and physical threats to communication

IV. A (2) Apply active listening

IV. A (3) Use appropriate body language and other nonverbal skills in communicating with patients, family and staff

IV. A (4) Demonstrate awareness of territorial boundaries of the person with whom you are communicating

IV. A (6) Demonstrate recognition of the patient's level of understanding in communications

IV. A (9) Recognize and protect personal boundaries in communicating with others

IV. A (11) Respond to nonverbal communication

IV. P (2) Report relevant information to others succinctly and accurately

## ABHES Competencies Achieved

5. b. Identify and respond appropriately when working/caring for patients with special needs

5. g. Analyze the effect of hereditary, cultural and environmental influences

**Student Name:** _____

## Procedure 4–2: Obtaining Information from the Patient with a Hearing Aid

**GOAL:** To learn techniques to enhance communication with the patient with a hearing aid

**MATERIALS:** Dependent on materials required for the task such as specific forms, pen, or computer; include a writing tablet, which may be necessary for communication

**METHOD:** To pass this procedure the minimum required score is _____% or all elements must meet "satisfactory" ability on the final demonstration. The first box may be used as a practice or final demonstration, with the evaluator placing **S for Satisfactory** or **U for Unsatisfactory** if that is the grading criteria. The second box may be used as a final demonstration with a **grade point** written in the box.

| STEPS | POSSIBLE POINTS | S/U | POINTS EARNED |
|---|---|---|---|
| 1. Approach from the patient's front in order to be seen and confirm the name. | 9 | | |
| 2. Introduce yourself to the patient and give your title. | 9 | | |
| 3. Escort the patient to a quiet area with little or no background noise. | 9 | | |
| 4. Face the patient; speak in a normal, clear tone and ask if he or she is able to hear you. | 9 | | |
| 5. If the patient is having difficulty hearing you, speak slower and louder, avoiding using a high pitch since this sometimes increases the problem. | 9 | | |
| 6. Determine if the patient uses other tools for communication such as a computer or writing tablet or other devices and access one if appropriate. | 9 | | |
| 7. Explain to the patient verbally or in writing what you will be doing and why. Inform the patient to ask questions if he or she cannot hear or does not understand. It is important for you to get accurate information. | 9 | | |
| 8. Show any forms that you will be using and have the patient verify what you write. | 10 | | |
| 9. Use other visual aids that may be appropriate. | 9 | | |
| 10. When the task is completed, inquire if there are questions. If not, thank the patient for his or her time and ask if there is anything further you can do. | 9 | | |

*(Continued)*

| STEPS | POSSIBLE POINTS | S/U | POINTS EARNED |
|---|---|---|---|
| 11. Document in the patient's medical record in the appropriate area, such as the billing information, that the patient was wearing a hearing aid, answered appropriately, reviewed the material, and acknowledged understanding. | 9 | | |
| **Total Points (if applicable)** | **100** | | |

**Comments:** _____

_____

_____

**Final Evaluator's Signature:** _____

**Date:** _____

## CAAHEP Competencies Achieved

IV. C (2) Identify nonverbal communication

IV. C (3) Recognize communication barriers

IV. C (4) Identify techniques for overcoming communication barriers

IV. C (7) Identify resources and adaptations that are required based on an individual's needs, i.e., culture and environment, developmental life stage, and physical threats to communication

IV. A (3) Use appropriate body language and other nonverbal skills in communicating with patients, family, and staff

## ABHES Competencies Achieved

5. b. Identify and respond appropriately when working/caring for patients with special needs

**Student Name:** _____

## Procedure 4–3: Obtaining Information from a Geriatric Patient

**GOAL:** To obtain accurate information while demonstrating respect and caring

**MATERIALS:** Dependent on materials required for the task such as specific forms, pen, or computer; include a writing tablet, which may be necessary for communication

**METHOD:** To pass this procedure the minimum required score is _____% or all elements must meet "satisfactory" ability on the final demonstration. The first box may be used as a practice or final demonstration, with the evaluator placing **S for Satisfactory** or **U for Unsatisfactory** if that is the grading criteria. The second box may be used as a final demonstration with a **grade point** written in the box.

| STEPS | POSSIBLE POINTS | S/U | POINTS EARNED |
|---|---|---|---|
| 1. Introduce yourself to the patient and give your title. | 10 | | |
| 2. Identify the patient with "Mr.," "Mrs.," "Ms.," or "Miss," unless the patient asks to be called by his or her first name. Do not use terms such as "honey" or "sweetie." | 10 | | |
| 3. When interviewing the patient to obtain a medical history, before you begin, explain the type of questions you will ask, and how the information will be used. | 10 | | |
| 4. Follow the form you are using related to the needed information; determine if you need to speak slower or louder. | 10 | | |
| 5. Pay attention to the patient's verbal and nonverbal cues. Do not interrupt the patient. After the patient finishes giving each answer, repeat it for accuracy. | 15 | | |
| 6. If you need to use medical terminology, try also to express the same information in lay terms. For example, you might ask "Do you have any other insurance besides Medicare?" instead of using the terms "medigap" or "Medicare supplement." | 10 | | |
| 7. If copying insurance or other information, assure the patient that you will return them quickly. | 10 | | |
| 8. Explain documents and ask if there are questions. | 10 | | |

*(Continued)*

| STEPS | POSSIBLE POINTS | S/U | POINTS EARNED |
|---|---|---|---|
| 9. Provide copies of the documents in an envelope and labeled with a brief description of what they are; for example, "consent form treatment," "privacy policy." | 10 | | |
| 10. Thank the patient for his or her time and explain what will happen next. | 5 | | |
| **Total Points (if applicable)** | **100** | | |

**Comments:** _____

_____

_____

**Final Evaluator's Signature:** _____

**Date:** _____

## CAAHEP Competencies Achieved

I. A (2) Use language/verbal skills that enable patients' understanding

I. A (3) Demonstrate respect for diversity in approaching patients and families

IV. C (4) Identify techniques for overcoming communication barriers

IV. C (7) Identify resources and adaptations that are required based on an individual's needs, i.e., culture and environment, developmental life stage, and physical threats to communication

IV. A (1) Demonstrate empathy in communicating with patients, family and staff

IV. A (2) Apply active listening skills

IV. A (3) Use appropriate body language and other nonverbal skills in communicating with patients, family, and staff

IV. A (9) Recognize and protect personal boundaries in communicating with others

IV. A (10) Demonstrate respect for individual diversity, incorporating awareness of one's own biases in areas including gender, race, religion, age and economic status

IV. C (5) Recognize the elements of oral communication using a sender-receiver process

## ABHES Competencies Achieved

5. a. Define and understand abnormal behavior patterns

5. b. Identify and respond appropriately when working/caring for patients with special needs

5. g. Analyze the effect of hereditary, cultural, and environmental influences

8. cc. Communicate on the recipient's level of comprehension

8. kk. Adapt to individualized needs

9. q. Instruct patients with special needs

Student Name: _____

**GOAL:** To demonstrate techniques to effectively communicate with a non-English speaking patient through an interpreter

**MATERIALS:** Materials needed for the task such as pen, forms, or computer and appropriate pictures and other visual aids if available

**METHOD:** To pass this procedure the minimum required score is _____ % or all elements must meet "satisfactory" ability on the final demonstration. The first box may be used as a practice or final demonstration, with the evaluator placing **S for Satisfactory** or **U for Unsatisfactory** if that is the grading criteria. The second box may be used as a final demonstration with a **grade point** written in the box.

| STEPS | POSSIBLE POINTS | S/U | POINTS EARNED |
|---|---|---|---|
| 1. Identify the patient by name and ask if you pronounced it correctly. Be sure to smile, even if you are feeling slightly awkward or unsure of yourself. | 9 | | |
| 2. Introduce yourself with your title to the patient and the interpreter. | 9 | | |
| 3. Ask the interpreter to spell his or her full name and provide identification such as his agency's identification or a business card. Retain this business card to file in the patient's medical record. If he or she does not have a business card, obtain contact information, which should also be filed in the patient's medical record. | 9 | | |
| 4. Do not take it personally if the patient appears abrupt or even rude; ascertain from the interpreter if there is a problem. This behavior may be considered appropriate in the patient's culture. In some cultures, male patients may not deal with a female staff member and that should be respected if possible. | 9 | | |
| 5. Inquire of the interpreter if the patient speaks or understands any English and if there are any communication or other customs that you should know. For example, traditional Navajos consider it rude to have direct eye contact. | 10 | | |
| 6. Provide a quiet area. | 9 | | |
| 7. Speak directly to the patient and speak slowly if the patient has any understanding of English. | 9 | | |
| 8. If forms are to be completed, instruct the interpreter to translate with appropriate intervals and give the patient opportunities to ask questions and ensure understanding (for example, providing general consent for treatment, permission to send information to and receive payment directly from the insurance company, and privacy decisions). Have one area translated at a time and inquire if there are any questions and ensure understanding. | 9 | | |

*(Continued)*

| STEPS | POSSIBLE POINTS | S/U | POINTS EARNED |
|---|---|---|---|
| 9. If the patient and interpreter are discussing an issue in depth or appear to be leaving you out of the conversation, ask the translator what is being said. | 9 | | |
| 10. Provide the information and services that you would to a native English speaker with the same courtesies. If possible, give written information in the patient's native language. | 9 | | |
| 11. Document what you would ordinarily document and on all forms; note that "translation was done by" and include the name, credential, and agency of the interpreter, the date, and time. | 9 | | |
| **Total Points (if applicable)** | **100** | | |

Comments: _____

_____

_____

Final Evaluator's Signature: _____

Date: _____

## CAAHEP Competencies Achieved

IV. C (2) Identify nonverbal communication

IV. C (3) Recognize communication barriers

IV. C (7) Identify resources and adaptations that are required based on an individual's needs, i.e., culture and environment, developmental life stage, and physical threats to communication

IV. A (2) Apply active listening

IV. A (3) Use appropriate body language and other nonverbal skills in communicating with patients, family, and staff

IV. A (4) Demonstrate awareness of territorial boundaries of the person with whom you are communicating

IV. A (6) Demonstrate recognition of the patient's level of understanding in communications

IV. A (9) Recognize and protect personal boundaries in communicating with others

IV. A (11) Respond to nonverbal communication

## ABHES Competencies Achieved

5. b. Identify and respond appropriately when working/caring for patients with special needs

5. g. Analyze the effect of hereditary, cultural, and environmental influences

# 5 Patient Education

## Test Your Knowledge

### Vocabulary Review

Match the key terms in the right column with the definitions in the left column by placing the letter of each correct answer in the space provided.

_____ 1. the process of teaching the patient a new skill by having the patient observe and imitate it

_____ 2. a participatory teaching method in which the technique is first described to the patient and then demonstrated to the patient; the patient is then asked to repeat the demonstration

_____ 3. the process by which the average person learns to make informed decisions about goods and services, including health care

_____ 4. the system of values and principles an office has adopted in its everyday practice

_____ 5. a method of teaching that provides the patient with details of the information that is being taught

_____ 6. a method of teaching that provides the patient with a description of the physical sensations he or she may have as part of the learning or the procedure involved

_____ 7. a method of teaching that includes demonstrations of techniques that may be necessary to show that something has been learned

_____ 8. the performing of a diagnostic test on a person who is typically free of symptoms

**a.** consumer education [LO5.5]

**b.** factual teaching [LO5.3]

**c.** modeling [LO5.2]

**d.** participatory teaching [LO5.3]

**e.** philosophy [LO5.4]

**f.** return demonstration [LO5.2]

**g.** screening [LO5.5]

**h.** sensory teaching [LO5.3]

# Multiple-Choice Certification Questions

There may be more than one answer; circle the letter of the choice that best completes each statement or answers each question.

1. **[LO5.6]** Which of the following is *not* a printed form of patient education materials?
   a. Sheet of paper
   b. Booklet
   c. Brochure
   d. Fact sheet
   e. None of the above

2. **[LO5.4]** Types of patient education information given to patients include all of the following *except*
   a. explanation of medical procedures.
   b. information about specific diseases.
   c. information about medical conditions.
   d. postoperative exercise sheets.
   e. All of the above.

3. **[LO5.4]** The primary benefit of providing patients visual materials over other forms of education materials is that visual materials
   a. make it easier for the patient to understand complicated medical information.
   b. are easier to create.
   c. are less expensive to produce.
   d. can include more complex, higher level medical terminology.
   e. can be mailed to patients who don't want to come to the office.

4. **[LO5.1]** Which of the following is a benefit of providing patients health education?
   a. Promoting wellness
   b. Providing information on health habits
   c. Assisting patients with information to protect them from injury
   d. Discussing preventive measures
   e. All of the above

5. **[LO5.4]** A patient information packet for a medical practice would *not* include the
   a. description of the medical practice.
   b. medical office hours of operation.
   c. physician's home phone and address.
   d. payment policy of the office.
   e. insurance plans accepted by the practice.

6. **[LO5.4]** In a patient information packet there *must* be a copy of the office
   a. fee schedule.
   b. OSHA standards.
   c. welcome statement.
   d. HIPAA regulations.
   e. list of community resources.

7. **[LO5.7]** When working with elderly patients, it is important to remember that you
   a. cannot rely on elderly patients to remember basic instructions.
   b. must treat all elderly patients as if they are incapable of caring for themselves.
   c. must talk at the lowest level of understanding.
   d. should adjust procedures as needed to accommodate each patient.
   e. need to talk down to elderly patients.

8. **[LO5.6]** Which of the following terms is used to describe an office's set of values and principles?
   a. Screening technique
   b. Benefits
   c. Confidentiality
   d. Philosophy
   e. Privacy rules

9. **[LO5.4]** Which of the following topics would most likely be found in an educational newsletter?
   a. Current health-care tips
   b. A physician's list of credentials
   c. A list of the office staff's phone numbers
   d. A community resource directory
   e. Insurance company phone numbers

10. **[LO5.5]** The process of diagnostic screening
   a. doesn't allow an early diagnosis.
   b. differs according to patient age.
   c. is only advisable when symptoms are present.
   d. is free of charge.
   e. can't be performed in a private medical practice.

11. **[LO5.4]** When developing a patient education plan, the first thing to do is to
   a. discuss the plan with the patient.
   b. decide the type of printed materials to use.
   c. identify the patient's education needs.
   d. identify how intelligent the patient is.
   e. perform the instruction with the patient.

12. **[LO5.4]** A community assistance directory would include information about
   a. visiting nurse services.
   b. local day-care centers.
   c. weight-loss clinics in the area.
   d. meals-on-wheels food service programs.
   e. All of the above.

13. **[LO5.5]** Patient education includes promoting healthy habits such as the amount of rest that is considered adequate. How many hours of sleep each night are recommended?
   a. 5 to 6 hours
   b. 6 to 7 hours
   c. 7 to 8 hours
   d. 8 to 9 hours
   e. Over 9 hours

14. **[LO5.1]** When a patient is prescribed a new prescription, it is critical that the physician question the patient about
   a. herbal products and over-the-counter medication they take.
   b. the pharmacy they want to use.
   c. whether the new medication is covered by the patient's insurance.
   d. the number of refills the patient wants.
   e. None of the above.

15. **[LO5.6]** When communicating the policies about patient confidentiality, you *must*
   a. use legal jargon and terminology in the written patient materials.
   b. specify that the confidentiality policy is effective immediately.
   c. state that the office will not ever change its privacy practices.
   d. describe an individual's rights under the Privacy Rule.
   e. inform the patient that the medical office can release information without a signature.

16. **[LO5.7]** When developing patient education materials it is necessary to consider the patient's
   a. age.
   b. cultural background.
   c. learning style.
   d. educational background.
   e. All of the above.

**17.** [LO5.8] One of the primary benefits of providing preoperative education is to
   a. increase the amount of postoperative pain medication required.
   b. decrease the patient's anxiety.
   c. lengthen the recovery time.
   d. protect the physician from a lawsuit.
   e. obtain the patient's personal history and insurance information.

**18.** [LO5.8] Which of the following is *not* included on a patient surgical consent form?
   a. The patient's agreement to have his or her name and identity released
   b. The patient's permission to receive anesthesia as needed
   c. The name of the surgical procedure
   d. The patient's or legal guardian's signature
   e. The surgeon's signature

**19.** [LO5.2] To ensure that the patient has understanding of the educational information, the medical assistant should ask the patient
   a. to state that he understands the information.
   b. to sign a document stating that he understands the information.
   c. to repeat back to you his expectations from the patient education information.
   d. to send a letter back to the office stating that he read the materials.
   e. None of the above.

**20.** [LO5.5] When educating patients about good health, you can teach patients the importance of
   a. learning about the anatomy and physiology of the body.
   b. living a balanced lifestyle of work and leisure activities.
   c. understanding medical terminology.
   d. drinking alcohol without becoming intoxicated.
   e. starting an exercise program before it is too late to matter.

**21.** [LO5.5] Tips for preventing injuries in the workplace include the following *except*
   a. using protective gear as required.
   b. making sure hallways and entrance areas are well lit.
   c. practicing proper posture when sitting.
   d. keeping your knees straight when lifting heavy boxes.
   e. never attempting to move furniture on your own.

**22.** [LO5.4] A patient information packet may include the physician's qualifications, which includes the physician's
   a. age and marital status.
   b. private phone number and address.
   c. religious affiliation.
   d. membership in private clubs.
   e. education and residency.

**23.** [LO5.5] Which of the following is *not* considered part of an annual screening for health maintenance?
   a. Routine blood work
   b. Chest x-ray
   c. Upper GI studies
   d. Electrocardiogram
   e. Urinalysis

**24.** [LO5.7] Rehabilitation is a level of disease prevention that involves working with patients that
   a. have had a stroke.
   b. are recovering from a heart attack.
   c. need pain management.
   d. have arthritis.
   e. experience any of the above.

# True or False

Decide whether each statement is true or false. In the space at the left, write "T" for true or "F" for false. On the lines provided, rewrite the false statements to make them true.

_____ 1. [LO5.5] Many accidents happen because people fail to see potential risks and do not develop plans of action.

_____

_____ 2. [LO5.2] Many patients are better able to comprehend complicated medical information when it is presented in a written format.

_____

_____ 3. [LO5.5] Good nutrition includes eating an adequate amount of fruits, vegetables, and high-fat foods.

_____

_____ 4. [LO5.5] To prevent injury at home, a parent should rely on bath seats or rings as a safety device for babies and children.

_____

_____ 5. [LO5.6] A patient information packet is a good way to acquaint new office staff members with office policies.

_____

_____ 6. [LO5.4] Providing the office's telephone policies in the information packet can help reduce the number of unnecessary calls to the office.

_____

_____ 7. [LO5.3] The psychomotor domain of learning influences physical movement, coordination, and the use of motor skills to complete tasks.

_____

_____ 8. [LO5.3] When providing education, three types of teaching can occur: factual, sensory, and beneficial.

_____

_____ 9. [LO5.6] For an information packet to be effective, you must make sure that new patients sign for receipt of the packet.

_____

_____10. [LO5.7] When working with elderly patients, try to communicate with them at the highest level they can understand.

_____

## Sentence Completion

In the space provided, write the word or phrase that best completes each sentence.

1. **[LO5.1]** The ultimate goal of all medical professionals is to encourage and teach _____ habits.

2. **[LO5.1]** When patients are suffering from illness, disease, or injury, _____ can help them regain their health and independence more quickly.

3. **[LO5.1]** Any time written materials of any kind are given to a patient, it must be noted in the _____.

4. **[LO5.4]** Educational newsletters are often written by the _____ or the _____.

5. **[LO5.1]** Maintaining or improving your health is the best way to protect yourself against _____ and _____.

6. **[LO5.7]** Always ask a patient if he has told the doctor about all the medications he is already taking, including _____, _____, and _____ medications.

7. **[LO5.4]** An information packet should include the office payment policies listing the forms of payment accepted such as _____, _____, and _____.

8. **[LO5.4]** It is important to match the learning materials to the patient's needs and the level of _____.

9. **[LO5.8]** The purpose of preoperative patient education is to prepare the patient for the procedure and to aid the patient during the _____.

1. _____
   _____

2. _____
   _____

3. _____
   _____

4. _____
   _____

5. _____
   _____

6. _____
   _____

7. _____
   _____

8. _____
   _____

9. _____
   _____

# Apply Your Knowledge
## Short Answer

Write the answer to each question on the lines provided.

1. **[LO5.3]** List the three types of teaching and the corresponding domains of learning.

_____

_____

_____

**2.** [LO5.5] List five tips for preventing injury in the workplace.

_____

_____

_____

**3.** [LO5.7] What are three tips for preventing injury in the home that the medical assistant could share with a mother of young children?

_____

_____

_____

**4.** [LO5.7] List three suggestions that a medical assistant could use when working with elderly patients.

_____

_____

_____

**5.** [LO5.8] What are three things a medical assistant can do to help relieve a patient's anxiety prior to a surgical procedure?

_____

_____

_____

## Problem-Solving Activities

Follow the directions for each activity.

**1.** [LO5.6] Community Resources
   a. Using Internet resources, research three agencies or organizations in your community that would be beneficial in providing information and services to patients with small children.
   b. For each of the resources, list two services that could be used in patient education for parents of small children.

**2.** [LO5.1] Preventing Injury at Home
   a. Develop a trifold patient education brochure that will present five tips for preventing injury at home.
   b. The brochure should be written for 7- to 8-year-old children to read and understand. The tips you select should also be applicable to that age child.

# Thinking Critically

Write your response to each case study question on the lines provided.

## Case 1 [LO5.1]

A medical assistant is preparing a teenage patient for a high school sports physical examination. The patient admits that he lives "mainly on hamburgers, fries, and snacks from the school vending machine," and that he usually gets fewer than six hours of sleep a night, except on weekends. He states, "I'll worry about my health when I'm older."

   **1.** What can the medical assistant say to the patient to encourage him to start adopting healthier habits now?

_____

_____

_____

## Case 2 [LO5.7]

A physician has asked a medical assistant to have a discussion with one of their elderly patients about the steps in preparing for admission to the hospital for invasive tests. As the medical assistant starts to inform the patient about what she will need to do, the patient appears to be confused and overwhelmed, and then starts crying. How should the medical assistant handle this patient?

   **1.** What can be done to help alleviate the patient's anxiety?

_____

_____

_____

## Case 3 [LO5.8]

A patient calls the office with questions about her upcoming surgery. Her patient record reflects that the physician has already discussed the nature of the surgery with her.

   **1.** As a medical assistant, what are your responsibilities for ensuring that the patient is fully prepared for the surgery?

_____

_____

_____

# Demonstrate Your Knowledge

**Student Name:** _____

## Procedure 5–1: Creating Electronic Patient Instructions

**GOAL:** To create and administer patient instructions electronically

**MATERIALS:** An electronic health records software program that includes a patient instructions feature

**METHOD:** To pass this procedure the minimum required score is _____% or all elements must meet "satisfactory" ability on the final demonstration. The first box may be used as a practice or final demonstration, with the evaluator placing **S for Satisfactory** or **U for Unsatisfactory** if that is the grading criteria. The second box may be used as a final demonstration with a **grade point** written in the box.

| STEPS | POSSIBLE POINTS | S/U | POINTS EARNED |
|---|:---:|:---:|:---:|
| 1. Search the EHR to find the button or icon to create Patient Instructions. (Check the Help button or training manual.) | 10 | | |
| 2. Determine if you will need to write your own or select from a previously created list of patient instructions. Select the correct button to proceed. (See Figure 5–1 on page 114 of the student text for an example using Springcharts™ EHR) | 10 | | |
| 3. Create new instructions by either of the following methods: <br><br>a. Type your patient instructions directly in the open window or a word processor program. This will depend on the EHR you are using. <br><br>b. Open the Web browser and navigate to a credible Internet site for patient instruction. (Review Procedure 5–3 before selecting this option.) If available on the site, select the printer-friendly version. Highlight the information you want to use from the Web site, place your cursor at the beginning of the text, and with your left mouse button depressed, drag the cursor to the end of the instruction page. Right-click on any highlighted area and choose "Copy." Click in the patient instruction window or in the word processor program, and using the keypad, press the [Ctrl] + [V] keys. Close the Web page and return to the EHR. | 30 | | |
| 4. Import instructions by opening a previously created document saved as an RTF or other word processing file type. Import the document by selecting the "Import from file" option. | 16 | | |
| 5. Use existing instructions by selecting them from a list within EHR or a file folder on your computer. Check the specific directions for the EHR program you are using. See Figure 5–7 for an example of how to enter the existing Patient Instruction from SpringCharts™. | 14 | | |

*(Continued)*

| STEPS | POSSIBLE POINTS | S/U | POINTS EARNED |
|---|---|---|---|
| 6. Record in the EHR that patient instructions were provided. In most programs this will occur when you generate the instructions and it becomes a permanent record in the patient's chart. See Figure 5–8 for an example charting entry using SpringCharts™. | 20 | | |
| **Total Points (if applicable)** | 100 | | |

Comments: _____

_____

_____

_____

**Final Evaluator's Signature:** _____

**Date:** _____

### CAAHEP Competencies Achieved

IV. P (9) Document patient education

V. P (5) Execute data management using electronic health-care records such as the EMR

### ABHES Competencies Achieved

4. a. Document accurately

7. b. Identify and properly utilize office machines, computerized systems, and medical software such as:

    (2) Apply computer application skills using a variety of different electronic programs including both practice management software and EMR software

Student Name: _____

## Procedure 5–2: Identifying Community Resources

**GOAL:** To create a list of useful community resources for patient referrals

**MATERIALS:** Computer with Internet access, phone directory, printer

**METHOD:** To pass this procedure the minimum required score is _____% or all elements must meet "satisfactory" ability on the final demonstration. The first box may be used as a practice or final demonstration, with the evaluator placing **S for Satisfactory** or **U for Unsatisfactory** if that is the grading criteria. The second box may be used as a final demonstration with a **grade point** written in the box.

| STEPS | POSSIBLE POINTS | S/U | POINTS EARNED |
|---|---|---|---|
| 1. Determine the needs of your medical office and formulate a list of community resources. The specific needs of your patients will help you formulate your list. Being able to assist them with finding outside assistance, when necessary, is the goal. | 20 | | |
| 2. Use the Internet to research the names, addresses, Web addresses, and phone numbers of local resources such as state and federal agencies, home health-care agencies, long-term nursing facilities, mental health agencies, and local charities. Use the phone directory to assist in locating local agencies such as Meals on Wheels; Alcoholics Anonymous; shelters for abused individuals; hospice care; Easter Seals; Women, Infants, and Children (WIC); and support groups for grief, obesity, and various diseases. | 20 | | |
| 3. Contact each resource and request information such as business cards and brochures. Some agencies may send a representative to meet with you regarding their services. If patients can access information easily, they are more likely to avail themselves of the services available to them. | 25 | | |
| 4. Compile a list of community resources with the proper name, address, phone number, e-mail address, and contact name. Include any information that may be helpful to the office. | 15 | | |
| 5. Update and add to the information often because outdated information will only frustrate you and your patients, creating even more anxiety. | 15 | | |
| 6. Post the information in a location where it is readily available. | 5 | | |
| **Total Points (if applicable)** | 100 | | |

**Comments:** _____

_____

_____

**Final Evaluator's Signature:** _____

**Date:** _____

### CAAHEP Competencies Achieved

IV. P (12) Develop and maintain a current list of community resources related to patient's health-care needs

XI. P (12) Maintain a current list of community resources for emergency preparedness

### ABHES Competencies Achieved

8. dd. Serve as a liaison between physician and others

11. b. Demonstrate professionalism by:

    (5) Exhibit initiative

## Procedure 5–3: Locating Credible Patient Education Information on the Internet

**GOAL:** To determine the credibility of patient education information on the Internet

**MATERIALS:** Computer with Internet access

**METHOD:** To pass this procedure the minimum required score is _____% or all elements must meet "satisfactory" ability on the final demonstration. The first box may be used as a practice or final demonstration, with the evaluator placing **S for Satisfactory** or **U for Unsatisfactory** if that is the grading criteria. The second box may be used as a final demonstration with a **grade point** written in the box.

| STEPS | POSSIBLE POINTS | S/U | POINTS EARNED |
|---|---|---|---|
| 1. Open your Internet browser and locate a search engine. Search engines vary in the way they search so you may want to use more than one search engine for different results. | 5 | | |
| 2. Search the topic. Be specific to the topic. For example, if you want to know about the proper diet for high cholesterol, you should type, "high cholesterol diet." For different or more medical sites, try using different terms, instead of "high cholesterol" try "hyperlipidemia." | 8 | | |
| 3. Select a site from the list of results and evaluate the source. | | | |
| a. Click the "About Us" link to find out who developed the site. Sites should have an active link available to contact the Webmaster and verify the source. | 8 | | |
| b. Sites developed by professional organizations, educational institutions, or a branch of the federal government are generally better than those developed by an individual or a commercial company. | 5 | | |
| 4. Review the Web site's "About Us" page to determine the quality of the information. | | | |
| a. Review the mission statement or other detailed information about the developer. | 8 | | |
| b. Look for information about the writers or authors of the site. Make sure they are medical professionals. | 8 | | |
| 5. Check the content of the site. | | | |
| a. Avoid sites that have sensational writing or make claims that are too good to be true. | 10 | | |
| b. Make sure the language of the information is at a level that you can understand. Avoid sites with lots of technical jargon for patient instruction. | 10 | | |

*(Continued)*

| STEPS | POSSIBLE POINTS | S/U | POINTS EARNED |
|---|---|---|---|
| 6. Make sure the information is current by checking the copyright or by checking with the contact information on the site. Medical information changes frequently so check the date and avoid information over five years old. | 11 | | |
| 7. Avoid Web sites with bias. For example, if the site is written by a pharmaceutical company, the site will only present information about the medication manufactured by that company. There may be alternative medications. Sites written by individuals are interesting but will be biased as well. | 11 | | |
| 8. Protect your privacy. If the sites require you to register, review their Privacy Policy. They may be able to share your or your patient's information with other companies. | 11 | | |
| 9. Once you have evaluated the site and decide to use it, you may want to have your supervisor or licensed practitioner review the information you will be providing to the patient. | 5 | | |
| **Total Points (if applicable)** | **100** | | |

**Comments:** _____

_____

_____


**Final Evaluator's Signature:** _____


**Date:** _____

## CAAHEP Competencies Achieved

V. P (7) Use the Internet to access information related to the medical office

## ABHES Competencies Achieved

8. e. Locate resources and information for patients and employers

8. ll. Apply electronic technology

## Procedure 5–4: Developing a Patient Education Plan

**GOAL:** To create and implement a patient teaching plan

**MATERIALS:** Pen, paper, various educational aids (such as instructional pamphlets and brochures), and/or visual aids (such as posters, videotapes, or DVDs)

**METHOD:** To pass this procedure the minimum required score is _____% or all elements must meet "satisfactory" ability on the final demonstration. The first box may be used as a practice or final demonstration, with the evaluator placing **S for Satisfactory** or **U for Unsatisfactory** if that is the grading criteria. The second box may be used as a final demonstration with a **grade point** written in the box.

| STEPS | POSSIBLE POINTS | S/U | POINTS EARNED |
|---|:---:|:---:|:---:|
| 1. Identify the patient's educational needs in order to provide instruction at the patient's point of need. Consider the following: | | | |
| a. The patient's current knowledge | 4 | | |
| b. Any misconceptions the patient may have | 4 | | |
| c. Any obstacles to learning (loss of hearing or vision, limitations of mobility, language barriers, and so on) | 4 | | |
| d. The patient's willingness and readiness to learn (motivation) | 4 | | |
| e. How the patient will use the information | 4 | | |
| 2. Develop and outline a plan using the various educational aids available and that address all the patient's needs. Include the following areas in the outline: | | | |
| a. What you want to accomplish (your goal) | 4 | | |
| b. How you plan to accomplish it | 4 | | |
| c. How you will determine if the teaching was successful | 4 | | |
| 3. Write the plan. Try to make the information interesting for the patient. | 15 | | |
| 4. Before carrying out the plan, share it with the physician to get approval and suggestions for improvement. | 10 | | |
| 5. Perform the instruction. Be sure to use more than one teaching method. For instance, if written material is being given, be sure to explain or demonstrate the material instead of simply telling the patient to read the educational materials. | 15 | | |
| 6. Document the teaching in the patient's chart for continuity of care and a legal document. | 4 | | |

*(Continued)*

| STEPS | POSSIBLE POINTS | S/U | POINTS EARNED |
|---|---|---|---|
| 7. Evaluate the effectiveness of your teaching session. Ask yourself: | | | |
|   a. Did you cover all the topics in your plan? | 4 | | |
|   b. Was the information well received by the patient? | 4 | | |
|   c. Did the patient appear to learn? | 4 | | |
|   d. How would you rate your performance? | 4 | | |
| 8. Revise your plan as necessary to make it even more effective. To be an effective teacher you must evaluate the methods you use. | 8 | | |
| **Total Points (if applicable)** | 100 | | |

**Comments:** _____

_____

_____

**Final Evaluator's Signature:** _____

**Date:** _____

## CAAHEP Competencies Achieved

I. A (2) Use language/verbal skills that enable patients' understanding

IV. C (12) Organize technical information and summaries

IV. P (5) Instruct patients according to their needs to promote health maintenance and disease prevention

## ABHES Competencies Achieved

5. b. Identify and respond appropriately when working/caring for patients with special needs

5. e. Advocate on behalf of family/patients, having the ability to deal and communicate with family

5. g. Analyze the effect of hereditary, cultural, and environmental influences

8. aa. Graduates are attentive, listen, and learn

8. bb. Graduates are impartial and show empathy when dealing with patients

8. cc. Communicate on the recipient's level of comprehension

8. dd. Serve as liaison between physician and others

8. gg. Use pertinent medical terminology

8. ii. Recognize and respond to verbal and nonverbal communication

8. jj. Perform fundamental writing skills including correct grammar, spelling, and formatting techniques when writing prescriptions, documenting medical records, etc.

8. kk. Adapt to individualized needs

## Procedure 5–5: Outpatient Surgery Teaching

**GOAL:** To inform a preoperative patient of the necessary guidelines to follow prior to surgery

**MATERIALS:** Patient chart, surgical guidelines

**METHOD:** To pass this procedure the minimum required score is _____% or all elements must meet "satisfactory" ability on the final demonstration. The first box may be used as a practice or final demonstration, with the evaluator placing **S for Satisfactory** or **U for Unsatisfactory** if that is the grading criteria. The second box may be used as a final demonstration with a **grade point** written in the box.

| STEPS | POSSIBLE POINTS | S/U | POINTS EARNED |
|---|---|---|---|
| 1. Review the patient's chart to determine the type of surgery to be performed and then ask the patient what procedure is being performed. This confirms the patient's knowledge of the procedure. | 8 | | |
| 2. Tell the patient that you will be providing both verbal and written instructions that should be followed prior to surgery. | 5 | | |
| 3. Inform the patient about policies regarding makeup, jewelry, contact lenses, wigs, dentures, and so on. | 5 | | |
| 4. Tell the patient to leave money and valuables at home. | 5 | | |
| 5. If applicable, suggest appropriate clothing for the patient to wear for postoperative ease and comfort. | 5 | | |
| 6. Explain the need for someone to drive the patient home following an outpatient surgical procedure. Driving after even simple surgery can be very dangerous. Surgery can be canceled if a patient does not identify a responsible driver before surgery occurs. | 5 | | |
| 7. Tell the patient the correct time to arrive at the office surgery center or the hospital for the procedure. | 5 | | |
| 8. Inform the patient of dietary restrictions. Be sure to use specific, clear instructions about what may or may not be ingested and at what time the patient must abstain from eating or drinking. Also explain these points: | | | |
|    a. The reasons for the dietary restrictions | 3 | | |
|    b. The possible consequences of not following the dietary restrictions | 3 | | |
|    c. That surgery can be canceled if the patient has not followed dietary restrictions | 1 | | |
| 9. Ask patients who smoke to refrain from or reduce cigarette smoking during at least the 8 hours prior to the procedure. Explain to the patient that reducing smoking improves the level of oxygen in the blood during surgery. | 4 | | |

*(Continued)*

| STEPS | POSSIBLE POINTS | S/U | POINTS EARNED |
|---|---|---|---|
| 10. Suggest that the patient shower or bathe the morning of the procedure or the evening before. | 4 | | |
| 11. Instruct the patient about medications to take or avoid before surgery. Surgery can be canceled if the patient has not followed medication instructions. | 10 | | |
| 12. If necessary, clarify any information about which the patient is unclear. | 10 | | |
| 13. Provide written surgical guidelines, and suggest that the patient call the office if additional questions arise. Patients may not understand or remember verbal instructions. Written instructions can be taken home and reviewed again. | 10 | | |
| 14. Document the instruction in the patient's chart for continuity of care and as a legal record. | 10 | | |
| **Total Points (if applicable)** | 100 | | |

Comments: _____

_____

_____

**Final Evaluator's Signature:** _____

**Date:** _____

## CAAHEP Competencies Achieved

IV. P (2) Report relevant information to others succinctly and accurately

IV. P (5) Instruct patients according to their needs to promote health maintenance and disease prevention

IV. P (9) Document patient education

IV. A (7) Demonstrate recognition of the patient's level of understanding in communications

## ABHES Competencies Achieved

5. b. Identify and respond appropriately when working/caring for patients with special needs

5. e. Advocate on behalf of family/patients, having the ability to deal and communicate with family

5. g. Analyze the effect of hereditary, cultural, and environmental influences

8. aa. Graduates are attentive, listen, and learn

8. bb. Graduates are impartial and show empathy when dealing with patients

8. cc. Communicate on the recipient's level of comprehension

8. dd. Serve as liaison between physician and others

# 6 Law and Ethics in the Medical Office

## Test Your Knowledge

### Vocabulary Review

Match the key terms in the right column with the definitions in the left column by placing the letter of each correct answer in the space provided.

_____ **1.** the speaking of defamatory words intended to prejudice others against an individual in a manner that jeopardizes his or her reputation or means of livelihood

_____ **2.** the legal basis for informed consent, usually outlined in a state's medical practice act

_____ **3.** a less serious crime such as theft under a certain dollar amount or disturbing the peace

_____ **4.** principles of right and wrong in issues that arise from medical advances

_____ **5.** a situation in which a health-care professional stops caring for a patient without arranging for care by an equally qualified substitute

_____ **6.** individually identifiable health information that is transmitted or maintained by electronic or other media, such as computer storage devices

_____ **7.** a type of business group, such as a medical practice, that is established by law and managed by a board of directors

**a.** abandonment [LO6.2]

**b.** agent [LO6.10]

**c.** arbitration [LO6.2]

**d.** assault [LO6.1]

**e.** authorization [LO6.7]

**f.** battery [LO6.1]

**g.** bioethics [LO6.1]

**h.** breach of contract [LO6.2]

**i.** civil law [LO6.1]

**j.** consent [LO6.2]

**k.** contract [LO6.2]

**l.** controlled substances [LO6.9]

**m.** corporation [LO6.9]

**n.** crime [LO6.1]

**o.** criminal law [LO6.1]

_____ **8.** a form of medical practice management in which a physician practices alone, assuming all benefits and liabilities of the business

_____ **9.** a law stating that an employee is considered to be acting on the physician's behalf while performing professional duties

_____ **10.** a Latin term meaning a legal document that requires the recipient to provide testimony under penalty

_____ **11.** the technical safeguards that protect the confidentiality, integrity, and availability of health information covered by HIPAA

_____ **12.** a principle under which a physician can exercise judgment as to whether to show patients who are being treated for mental or emotional conditions their records

_____ **13.** anyone under the age of majority—18 in most states, 21 in some jurisdictions

_____ **14.** the violation of or failure to live up to a contract's terms

_____ **15.** a person who acts on a physician's behalf while performing professional tasks

_____ **16.** a common name for the HIPAA Standards for Privacy of Individually Identifiable Health Information, which provides the first comprehensive federal protection for the privacy of health information

_____ **17.** an offense against the state committed or omitted in violation of public law

_____ **18.** a written court order that is addressed to a specific person and requires that person's presence in court on a specific date at a specific time

_____ **19.** a rule of conduct established and enforced by an authority or governing body, such as the federal government

_____ **20.** a Latin term meaning a legal document that requires the recipient to bring certain written records to court to be used as evidence in a lawsuit

_____ **21.** the act or practice of controlling risk

**p.** defamation [LO6.1]

**q.** disclosure [LO6.7]

**r.** doctrine of informed consent [LO6.2]

**s.** doctrine of professional discretion [LO6.2]

**t.** durable power of attorney [LO6.4]

**u.** electronic transaction record [LO6.8]

**v.** ethics [LO6.1]

**w.** expressed contract [LO6.2]

**x.** felony [LO6.1]

**y.** fraud [LO6.1]

**z.** group practice [LO6.9]

**aa.** implied consent [LO6.2]

**bb.** implied contract [LO6.2]

**cc.** informed consent [LO6.2]

**dd.** law [LO6.1]

**ee.** law of agency [LO6.10]

**ff.** liable [LO6.2]

**gg.** libel [LO6.1]

**hh.** malpractice claim [LO6.2]

**ii.** minors [LO6.1]

**jj.** misdemeanor [LO6.1]

**kk.** moral values [LO6.1]

**ll.** negligence [LO6.1]

**mm.** Notice of Privacy Practices (NPP) [LO6.7]

**nn.** partnership [LO6.9]

**oo.** Privacy Rule [LO6.7]

**pp.** protected health information (PHI) [LO6.7]

_____ **22.** a document naming the person who will make decisions regarding medical care on behalf of another person if that person becomes unable to do so

_____ **23.** a lawsuit brought by a patient against a physician for errors in diagnosis or treatment

_____ **24.** an area of law that involves crimes against a person; a person can sue another person, business, or the government

_____ **25.** a process in which opposing sides choose a person or persons outside the court system, often someone with special knowledge in the field, to hear and decide a dispute

_____ **26.** the portion of HIPAA that allows the provider to use and share patient health-care information for treatment, payment, and operations, such as quality improvement

_____ **27.** a form of medical practice management in which two or more parties practice together under a written agreement, specifying the rights, obligations, and responsibilities of each partner

_____ **28.** an area of law that involves crimes against the state; when a state or federal law is violated, the government brings criminal charges against the alleged offender

_____ **29.** the patient's right to receive all information relative to his or her condition and then make a decision regarding treatment based upon that knowledge

_____ **30.** an act of deception that is used to take advantage of another person or entity

_____ **31.** a Latin term meaning "let the master answer," a doctrine under which an employer is legally liable for the acts of his or her employees, if such acts were performed within the scope of the employee's duties

_____ **32.** the standardized codes and formats used for the exchange of medical data

_____ **33.** a voluntary agreement in which a patient gives a medically trained person the permission to touch, examine, and perform a treatment on that patient

**qq.** _qui tam_ [LO6.5]

**rr.** _res ipsa loquitur_ [LO6.3]

**ss.** _respondeat superior_ [LO6.3]

**tt.** risk management [LO6.2]

**uu.** Security Rule [LO6.7]

**vv.** slander [LO6.1]

**ww.** sole proprietorship [LO6.9]

**xx.** subpoena [LO6.3]

**yy.** _subpoena duces tecum_ [LO6.1]

**zz.** _subpoena ad testificandum_ [LO6.1]

**aaa.** tort [LO6.1]

**bbb.** treatment, payment, and operations (TPO) [LO6.7]

**ccc.** uniform donor card [LO6.4]

**ddd.** use [LO6.2]

**eee.** void [LO6.1]

_____ **34.** the open threat of bodily harm to another

_____ **35.** a document that informs patients of their rights as outlined under HIPAA

_____ **36.** damaging a person's reputation by making public statements that are both false and malicious

_____ **37.** a contract that is created by the acceptance or conduct of the parties rather than by the written word

_____ **38.** a serious crime, such as murder or rape, that is punishable by imprisonment

_____ **39.** the sharing, employing, applying, utilizing, examining, or analyzing of individually identifiable health information by employees or other members of an organization's workforce

_____ **40.** a Latin term meaning "the thing speaks for itself," which is also known as the doctrine of common knowledge

_____ **41.** general principles of right and wrong, as opposed to requirements of law

_____ **42.** a false publication, as in writing, print, signs, or pictures, that damages a person's reputation

_____ **43.** a voluntary agreement between two parties in which specific promises are made

_____ **44.** a form that explains in detail the standards for the use and disclosure of patient information for purposes other than treatment, payment, or health-care operations

_____ **45.** a medical professional's failure to perform an essential action or performance of an improper action that directly results in the harm of a patient

_____ **46.** the release of, the transfer of, the provision of access to, or the divulgence in any manner of patient information

_____ **47.** a form of consent that is not expressly granted by a person, but rather inferred from a person's actions and the facts and circumstances of a particular situation

_____ **48.** a legal document that states a person's wish to make a gift upon death of one or more organs for medical research, organ transplants, or placement in a tissue bank

_____ **49.** a term used to describe something that is not legally enforceable

_____ **50.** in civil law, a breach of some obligation that causes harm or injury to someone

_____ **51.** a contract clearly stated in written or spoken words

_____ **52.** legally responsible

_____ **53.** a Latin term meaning "to bring action for the king and for one's self."

_____ **54.** a drug or drug product that is categorized as potentially dangerous and addictive

_____ **55.** an action that causes bodily harm to another

_____ **56.** values or types of behavior that serve as a basis for ethical conduct and are formed through the influence of the family, culture, or society

_____ **57.** a medical management system in which a group of three or more licensed physicians share their collective income, expenses, facilities, equipment, records, and personnel.

## Multiple-Choice Certification Questions

There may be more than one answer; circle the letter of the choice that best completes each statement or answers each question.

**1.** [LO6.3] The term _res ipsa loquitur_ refers to cases in which
a. the patient has a previously existing condition.
b. the physician abandons the patient.
c. the patient has already filed a lawsuit.
d. the doctor's error was caused by faulty record keeping.
e. the doctor's mistake is clear to everyone.

**2.** [LO6.3] If the physician decides to terminate his care of a patient, the physician must
a. tell the patient face to face.
b. leave a message for the patient on the patient's answering machine.
c. obtain the patient's consent.
d. inform the patient's family.
e. send the patient a certified letter.

**3.** [LO6.1] Which of the following is not a legal procedure for administrative medical assistants to perform?
   a. Maintain certification and continuing education
   b. Recruit qualified medical assistants for the medical office
   c. Determine needs for documentation and reporting
   d. Change a diagnosis while coding the medical record
   e. File a grievance with the employer

**4.** [LO6.7] A physician's receptionist asks a patient to sign in and list the reason for his visit. This receptionist is violating the patient's rights to
   a. confidentiality.
   b. a second opinion.
   c. sue for malpractice.
   d. be seen by the physician in a timely manner.
   e. follow the physician's recommendation for treatment.

**5.** [LO6.2] While practicing within the context of an implied contract with a patient, the physician is obligated to do all the following *except*
   a. use due care.
   b. provide complete information and instructions to the patient about diagnoses, options, and methods of treatment.
   c. promise the patient that he or she will recover completely.
   d. stay current regarding technology and treatments available.
   e. treat the patient within the scope of the physician's practice.

**6.** [LO6.1] Crimes such as attempted burglary and disturbing the peace are examples of
   a. felonies.
   b. misdemeanors.
   c. civil law.
   d. intentional crimes.
   e. social crimes.

**7.** [LO6.1] If a provider gives a patient an injection after the patient refused the procedure, it could result in a charge of
   a. assault.
   b. battery.
   c. false imprisonment.
   d. libel.
   e. slander.

**8.** [LO6.2] Preventing a patient from leaving the medical facility after administration of an allergy injection could be seen as
   a. an invasion of privacy.
   b. false imprisonment.
   c. an acceptable practice as long as it was documented in the chart.
   d. malpractice.
   e. negligence.

**9.** [LO6.3] If a patient can prove that she felt "reasonable apprehension of bodily harm," it can result in what kind of charge?
   a. Defamation of character
   b. Battery
   c. Assault
   d. Negligence
   e. Slander

**10.** [LO6.2] Parties who enter into an agreement must be capable of fully understanding all its terms and conditions. This is referred to as a/an
   a. consideration.
   b. implied contract.

c. contractual capacity.

d. intentional contract.

e. breach of contract.

**11.** [LO6.2] While practicing within the context of an implied contract with the patient, the physician is bound to

a. make a correct diagnosis in every case.

b. restore a patient to his or her original state of health.

c. promise a cure to all patients.

d. not release patient information without permission.

e. guarantee the successful result of any treatment or operation.

**12.** [LO6.1] Child abuse, elder abuse, and domestic violence are examples of

a. a tort.

b. a felony.

c. an intentional tort.

d. a misdemeanor.

e. misfeasance.

**13.** [LO6.10] To safeguard employees, medical facilities are required to have an exposure plan that includes all the following *except*

a. training and updates every other year regarding hazardous materials and infectious substances.

b. immunizations against hepatitis B virus.

c. labeling for biohazard wastes.

d. personal protective equipment.

e. information on how to dispose of sharp equipment.

**14.** [LO6.8] Following the principles for preventing improper release of information from the medical office, which of the following is appropriate practice?

a. When in doubt, it is better not to release information.

b. It is the patient's right to keep patient information confidential.

c. All patients should be treated with the same degree of confidentiality.

d. Get written approval from the patient before releasing information.

e. All of the above.

**15.** [LO6.2] Which of the following is *false* regarding an agreement?

a. It must be made in good faith.

b. It must contain high-level medical jargon and terminology.

c. It must be communicated.

d. It must be clear enough to be understood by both parties.

e. It must define what each party will do if accepted.

**16.** [LO6.10] Which of the following practice models is now the least popular?

a. Sole proprietorship

b. Partnership

c. Group practice

d. Professional corporation

e. Clinic

**17.** [LO6.7] If HIPAA privacy and security regulations are violated, it could result in

a. criminal penalties of $100 with annual caps of $25,000.

b. civil penalties resulting in 10 years in prison.

c. civil penalties of up to $25,000 per year for repeated violations of the same requirement.

d. civil penalties if the offense is to sell the information for profit or do malicious harm.

e. criminal penalties only if the information was released by accident, not intentionally.

**18.** [LO6.7] Which of the following is *not* appropriate when trying to maintain security in the reception area of a medical office?

a. Log off or lock your computer or terminal when leaving the area.

b. Have a sign-in sheet at the reception desk that is left out on the counter for all patients to access with ease.

c. Place patient charts on the counter face down so the patient's name does not show.

d. When discussing a patient, step away from the reception area and move the conversation into a private office area.

e. Place the computer in an area where patients cannot see the screen.

**19.** [LO6.3] Professional liability coverage is specialty coverage that protects the physician and staff against

a. having a lawsuit brought against the practice.

b. performing procedures not covered by insurance.

c. financial losses from lawsuits.

d. being served with a subpoena.

e. None of the above.

**20.** [LO6.1] Defamation of character can take the form of

a. slander and libel.

b. fraud.

c. battery.

d. assault.

e. a felony.

**21.** [LO6.2] If a physician enters into a contract with a patient to pay for the services of a physician but the physician is not licensed to practice medicine, it would result in a/an

a. voided contract.

b. implied contract.

c. expressed contract.

d. unintentional contract.

e. legal contract.

**22.** [LO6.9] What is the purpose of obtaining and maintaining CEUs for medical professionals such as physicians, nurses, and certified medical assistants?

a. Keeping the ability to keep "initials after your name"

b. Maintaining a minimum standard of knowledge

c. Keeping abreast of the latest medical advances

d. Increasing patient confidence in the ability of medical professionals

e. Providing a means of termination for incompetent employees

**23.** [LO6.2] The doctrine of informed consent implies that the patient understands

a. the proposed treatment.

b. the reasons why the treatment is necessary.

c. the risks involved if treatment is refused.

d. available alternative modes of treatment.

e. All of the above.

**24.** [LO6.3] A postoperative patient experiences internal bleeding in the recovery room, and it is discovered that the physician did not properly complete the closure of all the blood vessels during the surgery. This could possibly lead to a case of

a. negligence.

b. fraud.

c. slander.

d. defamation.

e. None of the above.

**25.** [LO6.3] Which of the following would *not* be a reason a physician would terminate medical care of a patient?

a. The patient refuses to follow the physician's instructions.

b. The patient's family members complain incessantly to or about the physician.

c. The patient pays the remainder of all the bills once the insurance company has paid its share.

d. The patient fails to keep appointments.

e. The patient has a personality conflict with the physician that cannot be reasonably resolved.

# True or False

Decide whether each statement is true or false. In the space at the left, write "T" for true or "F" for false. On the lines provided, rewrite the false statements to make them true.

_____ 1. [LO6.2] If you communicate with patients in a professional manner, the patient will not sue the physician.

_____

_____ 2. [LO6.1] Battery may be charged for any unauthorized touching of a patient.

_____

_____ 3. [LO6.5] The Federal False Claims Act requires financial records be kept for 10 years.

_____

_____ 4. [LO6.3] Improper documentation in a patient chart can contribute to or cause a case to be lost in court.

_____

_____ 5. [LO6.4] A patient's medical records are considered the property of the patient and his or her family.

_____

_____ 6. [LO6.2] An advance medical directive instructs health-care providers to only resuscitate a patient if the family wants it done.

_____

_____ 7. [LO6.2] A uniform donor card is a legal document that states one's wish to be an organ donor.

_____

_____ 8. [LO6.5] It is legal to bill for medical services that were not performed.

_____

_____ 9. [LO6.4] A durable power of attorney is put in place when a person wants to hire a different lawyer.

_____

_____ 10. [LO6.5] The Health Care Quality Improvement Act of 1986 established a peer review of physicians.

_____

## Sentence Completion

In the space provided, write the word or phrase that best completes each sentence.

1. **[LO6.1]** Misfeasance refers to a lawful act that is done _____.

2. **[LO6.3]** The four Ds of negligence are duty, derelict, _____, and damages.

3. **[LO6.2]** The relationship between a doctor and a patient is called an implied _____.

4. **[LO6.1]** Damaging a person's reputation by making public statements that are both false and malicious is considered _____.

5. **[LO6.2]** Health-care practitioners who promise patients miracle cures or accept fees from patients while using mystical or spiritual powers to heal is considered _____.

6. **[LO6.2]** A contract that is stated in written or spoken words is considered a/an_____.

7. **[LO6.1]** Torts that are committed without the intention to cause harm but are committed unreasonably or with a disregard for the consequences are _____.

8. **[LO6.2]** A patient who rolls up her sleeve and offers her arm for an injection is entering into a/an _____contract.

9. **[LO6.7]** A document that communicates patient rights under HIPAA is called _____.

10. **[LO6.10]** According to the law of agency, an employee is considered to be acting as the doctor's _____.

1. _____
   _____

2. _____
   _____

3. _____
   _____

4. _____
   _____

5. _____
   _____

6. _____
   _____

7. _____
   _____

8. _____
   _____

9. _____
   _____

10. _____
    _____

# Apply Your Knowledge

## Short Answer

Write the answer to each question on the lines provided.

1. **[LO6.1]** Explain the difference between malfeasance and misfeasance.

_____

_____

_____

2. **[LO6.7]** List eight types of personal information that is considered individually identifiable health information under HIPAA.

_____

_____

_____

3. **[LO6.3]** Explain how effective communication helps prevent lawsuits.

_____

_____

_____

4. **[LO6.2]** List and briefly define the four essential elements of a contract.

_____

_____

_____

5. **[LO6.2]** List three reasons why a patient might not be able to give informed consent and how you could obtain consent from patients in these circumstances.

_____

_____

_____

# Problem-Solving Activities

Follow the directions for each activity.

1. **[LO6.2]** Writing a Letter of Withdrawal
   a. Refer to the sample Letter of Withdrawal from Care in Chapter 6, Figure 6–3.

## LETTER OF WITHDRAWAL FROM CARE

December 12, 2012

Jack Smallwood
PO Box 3457C
Funton, XY 12345-6789

Dear Mr. Smallwood:

This is to inform you of our intent to discontinue providing medical care to you due to the habitual and continued noncompliance in your treatment plan. Our records indicate that you have missed several appointments and have not complied with ordered testing. This discontinuance will go into effect 30 days from the date of this letter in order to allow you sufficient time to locate another physician. We will be happy to forward your medical records to the physician of your choice. There is 24-hour medical care available to you at the hospital.

If you need assistance in locating a new physician, please contact your insurance carrier or the Tennessee Medical Society at 1-800-666-9898.

Sincerely,

*Matthew Rodriguez, MD*

Matthew Rodriguez, MD

   b. Choose one of the reasons for termination of a patient and compose a letter that could be sent to a patient.
   c. Ensure that the content is appropriate, grammar is correct, and there are no spelling errors.
   d. Place the letter in an envelope and put it in a box provided by your instructor.
   e. Each student will complete this assignment and then will randomly select one of the letters to read aloud to the class.
   f. As a group, discuss how the recipient of the letter might feel about receiving this letter.

2. **[LO6.9]** The bioethics section on page 157 of your student textbook uses the following scenarios of bioethical issues. For each issue, write a paragraph or two discussing your personal feelings about each issue. Include how your feelings may affect your professional development and employment decisions.
   a. A treatment for Parkinson's disease was developed that uses fetal tissue. Some women, upon learning about this treatment, might get pregnant just to have an abortion and sell the fetal tissue. Is this ethical?
   b. If a couple cannot have a baby because of a medical condition of the mother, using a surrogate mother is an option some couples choose. The surrogate mother is artificially inseminated with the sperm of the husband and carries the baby to term. The couple then raises the child. Ethically speaking, who is the real mother, the woman who bears the child or the woman who raises the child? If the surrogate mother wants to keep the baby after it is born, does she have a right to do so?

c. When a liver transplant is needed by both a famous patient who has had a history of alcohol abuse and a woman who is a recipient of public assistance, what criteria are considered when determining who receives the organ? Who makes the decision?

## Thinking Critically

Write your response to each case study question on the lines provided.

### Case 1 [LO6.7]

A patient has a sexually transmitted disease but does not want you or the doctor to contact any former sex partners. The doctor has asked the medical assistant to handle this case to try to contact the former partners.

**1.** What are the appropriate methods to try to contact the sex partners?

_____

_____

_____

**2.** What information is the medical assistant able to disclose when contacting these people?

_____

_____

_____

### Case 2 [LO6.7]

You work as a medical assistant in a medical practice with three other medical assistants. During lunch, in the employee break room, one of the other assistants discusses the patients that were seen that morning. You realize that one of the patients is your neighbor.

**1.** What, if anything, has the medical assistant done wrong by discussing these patients?

_____

_____

_____

**2.** What, if anything, should you do about this situation?

_____

_____

_____

**Case 3** [LO6.10]

Mary is a medical assistant in your office. She is assigned to perform all the phlebotomy procedures today. As she prepares to obtain blood on a patient, you observe that she does not have gloves on. She completes the blood draw and then discards the needle and used supplies in the trash can. After the patient leaves the office, you approach Mary and question her about the techniques she used. She states that "I was taught to do it that way, and gloves just get in my way. I cannot feel the veins with them on."

**1.** What was wrong with the techniques that Mary used to perform phlebotomy?

_____

_____

_____

**2.** What should you do about this situation?

_____

_____

_____

# Demonstrate Your Knowledge

**Student Name:** _____

## Procedure 6–1: Obtaining Signature for Receipt of Privacy Practices

**GOAL:** To follow HIPAA guidelines and obtain the patient's signature that they have received and understand the office privacy policies

**MATERIALS:** Preprinted Receipt of Privacy Practices Information (such as Figure 6–5, which is also available at the end of this study guide), pens, copy machine

**METHOD:** To pass this procedure the minimum required score is _____% or all elements must meet "satisfactory" ability on the final demonstration. The first box may be used as a practice or final demonstration, with the evaluator placing **S for Satisfactory** or **U for Unsatisfactory** if that is the grading criteria. The second box may be used as a final demonstration with a **grade point** written in the box.

| STEPS | POSSIBLE POINTS | S/U | POINTS EARNED |
|---|---|---|---|
| 1. Explain to the patient the office privacy policy regarding protected health information. | 25 | | |
| 2. Ask the patient to read the policy carefully and feel free to ask any questions he may have regarding the policy. Answer any questions that may arise. | 25 | | |
| 3. When the patient's questions have been answered, witness the patient (or guardian) signature and printed name. Note any restrictions that may be placed on the document. | 20 | | |
| 4. Print your name and sign the document as witness, including your title. | 10 | | |
| 5. Date the document when all signatures have been completed. | 10 | | |
| 6. Make a copy of the document to file in the patient medical record and give the original to the patient. | 10 | | |
| **Total Points (if applicable)** | 100 | | |

**Comments:** _____

_____

_____

_____

**Final Evaluator's Signature:** _____

**Date:** _____

## CAAHEP Competencies Achieved

IV. P (4) Explain general office policies

IV. P (9) Document patient education

IX. C (2) Explore issue of confidentiality as it applies to the medical assistant

IX. C (3) Describe the implications of HIPAA for the medical assistant in various medical settings

IX. P (1) Respond to issues of confidentiality

IX. P (3) Apply HIPAA rules in regard to privacy/release of information

IX. P (5) Incorporate the Patient's Bill of Rights into personal practice and medical office policies and procedures

IX. P (8) Apply local, state, and federal health-care legislation and regulation appropriate to the medical assistant practice setting

IX. A (1) Demonstrate sensitivity to patient rights

IX. A (3) Recognize the importance of local, state, and federal legislation and regulations in the practice setting

## ABHES Competencies Achieved

4. a. Document accurately

4. b. Institute federal and state guidelines when releasing medical records or information

4. f. Comply with federal, state, and local health laws and regulations

8. d. Apply concepts for office procedures

## Procedure 6–2: Completing a Privacy Violation Complaint Form

**GOAL:** To assist the patient to complete a Privacy Violation Complaint Form if she feels her protected health information (PHI) has been compromised

**MATERIALS:** Privacy Violation Complaint Form (such as Figure 6–6, which is also available at the end of this study guide), pens, private room to complete form, copy machine

**METHOD:** To pass this procedure the minimum required score is _____% or all elements must meet "satisfactory" ability on the final demonstration. The first box may be used as a practice or final demonstration, with the evaluator placing **S for Satisfactory** or **U for Unsatisfactory** if that is the grading criteria. The second box may be used as a final demonstration with a **grade point** written in the box.

| STEPS | POSSIBLE POINTS | S/U | POINTS EARNED |
|---|---|---|---|
| 1. Explain to the patient that all formal complaints must be made in writing. | 20 | | |
| 2. Ask the patient if she feels assistance will be needed completing the form. If not, patient may complete the form on her own. Answer any questions she may have regarding completion of the form. | 15 | | |
| 3. When the patient completes the form, read it carefully, making sure it is complete and legible and that the information regarding the breach of privacy is clear. | 15 | | |
| 4. If the patient requires any copies be made for documentation backing the claim, make the copies, returning any originals to the patient. | 10 | | |
| 5. Make sure the patient signs and dates the complaint. | 10 | | |
| 6. As the person receiving the complaint, sign the document as indicated and date it. | 10 | | |
| 7. Explain to the patient that the office will respond to the complaint within 30 days of today's receipt. | 10 | | |
| 8. Make a copy of the document for the patient and keep the original for the office files. | 10 | | |
| **Total Points (if applicable)** | 100 | | |

**Comments:** _____

_____

_____

**Final Evaluator's Signature:** _____

**Date:** _____

## CAAHEP Competencies Achieved

IV. P (4) Explain general office policies

IV. P (9) Document patient education

IX. C (2) Explore issue of confidentiality as it applies to the medical assistant

IX. C (3) Describe the implications of HIPAA for the medical assistant in various medical settings

IX. P (1) Respond to issues of confidentiality

IX. P (3) Apply HIPAA rules in regard to privacy/release of information

IX. P (5) Incorporate the Patient's Bill of Rights into personal practice and medical office policies and procedures

IX. P (8) Apply local, state, and federal health-care legislation and regulation appropriate to the medical assistant practice setting

IX. A (1) Demonstrate sensitivity to patient rights

IX. A (3) Recognize the importance of local, state, and federal legislation and regulations in the practice setting

## ABHES Competencies Achieved

4. a. Document accurately

4. b. Institute federal and state guidelines when releasing medical records or information

4. f. Comply with federal, state, and local health laws and regulations

8. d. Apply concepts for office procedures

## Procedure 6–3: Obtaining Authorization to Release Health Information

**GOAL:** To follow HIPAA guidelines when obtaining a patient's protected health information (PHI) without violating confidentiality regulations

**MATERIALS:** Preprinted Authorization to Release Health Information (such as Figure 6–7, which is available at the end of this study guide), pens, copy machine

**METHOD:** To pass this procedure the minimum required score is _____% or all elements must meet "satisfactory" ability on the final demonstration. The first box may be used as a practice or final demonstration, with the evaluator placing **S for Satisfactory** or **U for Unsatisfactory** if that is the grading criteria. The second box may be used as a final demonstration with a **grade point** written in the box.

| STEPS | POSSIBLE POINTS | S/U | POINTS EARNED |
|---|---|---|---|
| 1. Explain to the patient the need for the requested medical information. | 15 | | |
| 2. Obtain the name and address of the practice to which the authorization is to be mailed. | 0 | | |
| 3. Fill in the patient's name, address, and DOB as required. | 10 | | |
| 4. Enter the physician's or practitioner's name from your practice who is requesting the PHI. | 0 | | |
| 5. Enter the information that is being requested. | 5 | | |
| 6. Complete the "reason for request" area explaining why the patient is requesting the information be sent to your office. | 10 | | |
| 7. Enter an expiration date for the authorization, giving a reasonable amount of time for the request to be fulfilled. | 5 | | |
| 8. Prior to signing the release, go over the information contained within the release with the patient, answering any questions that may arise. Be sure the patient understands the request may be withdrawn (in writing) at any time. | 20 | | |
| 9. Witness the patient (or guardian) signature and dating; if necessary be sure the guardian relationship area is completed. | 5 | | |
| 10. Sign the document as witness, including your title. | 10 | | |
| 11. Make a copy of the document to file in the patient medical record and, if requested, give a copy to the patient as well. | 10 | | |
| 12. Make a notation in the medical record of the document signing and note the date the authorization is mailed. | 10 | | |
| **Total Points (if applicable)** | 100 | | |

**Comments:** _____

_____

_____

**Final Evaluator's Signature:** _____

**Date:** _____

## CAAHEP Competencies Achieved

IV. P (4) Explain general office policies

IV. P (9) Document patient education

IX. C (2) Explore issue of confidentiality as it applies to the medical assistant

IX. C (3) Describe the implications of HIPAA for the medical assistant in various medical settings

IX. P (1) Respond to issues of confidentiality

IX. P (3) Apply HIPAA rules in regard to privacy/release of information

IX. P (5) Incorporate the Patient's Bill of Rights into personal practice and medical office policies and procedures

IX. P (8) Apply local, state, and federal health-care legislation and regulation appropriate to the medical assistant practice setting

IX. A (1) Demonstrate sensitivity to patient rights

IX. A (3) Recognize the importance of local, state, and federal legislation and regulations in the practice setting

## ABHES Competencies Achieved

4. a. Document accurately

4. b. Institute federal and state guidelines when releasing medical records or information

4. f. Comply with federal, state, and local health laws and regulations

8. d. Apply concepts for office procedures

# From Appointment to Payment

## Test Your Knowledge

### Vocabulary Review

Match the key terms in the right column with the definitions in the left column by placing the letter of each correct answer in the space provided.

_____ **1.** a health plan that agrees to carry the risk of paying for patient services

_____ **2.** a form that combines the charges for services rendered, an invoice for payment or insurance copayment, and all the information for submitting an insurance claim

_____ **3.** a daily journal that accounts for the total charges and payments of the day

_____ **4.** the area where patients enter the office

_____ **5.** the process for an arriving patient to list his or her name and other information on a form in the registration area

**a.** daily log [LO7.3]

**b.** encounter form, superbill [LO7.3]

**c.** reception [LO7.1]

**d.** sign in [LO7.1]

**e.** third-party payers [LO7.4]

### Multiple-Choice Certification Questions

There may be more than one answer; circle the letter of the choice that best completes each statement or answers each question.

**1.** [LO7.2] An allied health professional who works in the laboratory preparing specimens and operating centrifuges and analyzers is
a. the MLT.
b. the CMAS.
c. the HER.
d. the CLIA.
e. None of the above.

**2.** [LO7.2] The common role of the administrative medical assistant is to
   a. draw blood.
   b. operate centrifuges and analyzers.
   c. perform electrocardiograms.
   d. complete diagnostic testing.
   e. None of the above.

**3.** [LO7.1] When a patient first arrives at the medical office, what is one of the first tasks that is performed by the administrative medical assistant?
   a. Obtain the charges from the encounter form.
   b. Perform an electrocardiogram.
   c. Enter information from the encounter form to the daily log.
   d. Obtain a copy of the patient's insurance card.
   e. Set up a follow-up appointment for the patient.

**4.** [LO7.1] When a patient signs a release of information form, it allows
   a. the patient's information to be released to his or her family.
   b. the patient's information to be released to the insurance company.
   c. the physician to review the patient's former medical record.
   d. the medical assistant to perform procedures on the patient.
   e. the insurance company to bill the patient.

**5.** [LO7.3] The patient's encounter form information includes the patient's
   a. insurance coverage.
   b. laboratory results.
   c. procedures and charges.
   d. personal health history.
   e. family history.

**6.** [LO7.4] A third-party payer is
   a. a family member.
   b. the insurance company.
   c. the patient.
   d. the medical staff.
   e. the patient's spouse.

**7.** [LO7.4] The daily journal is used to
   a. account for the charges and payments for the day.
   b. provide the patient with a receipt for services that day.
   c. submit insurance claims to the insurance company.
   d. make daily deposits to the bank account.
   e. Do none of the above.

**8.** [LO7.2] The main responsibility of the medical laboratory technician (MLT) in the medical office is to
   a. obtain vital signs on the patient.
   b. diagnose the patient.
   c. prescribe medication for the patient.
   d. bill the insurance company for lab charges.
   e. perform laboratory tests.

**9.** [LO7.1, 7.2, 7.3, 7.4] Patient-related responsibilities include
   a. arranging referrals.
   b. following up with patients.
   c. calling in prescriptions.
   d. screening telephone calls.
   e. All of the above.

**10.** [LO7.1] HIPAA primarily is concerned with
   a. the physician's fee schedule.
   b. equal employment opportunities.
   c. patient confidentiality.
   d. pre-authorization for referrals.
   e. disability insurance.

# True or False

Decide whether each statement is true or false. In the space at the left, write "T" for true or "F" for false. On the lines provided, rewrite the false statements to make them true.

_____ **1.** [LO7.1] A patient is registered when he is signed in.

_____

_____ **2.** [LO7.3] The encounter form may be electronically initiated by the physician.

_____

_____ **3.** [LO7.2] A common role of the administrative medical assistant is to obtain blood from the patient for the laboratory tests ordered by the physician.

_____

_____ **4.** [LO7.2] CLIA is an agency that regulates laboratory testing performed in the medical office.

_____

_____ **5.** [LO7.1, 7.2] Medical offices have the option of adopting the HIPAA regulations.

_____

_____ **6.** [LO7.1] Under HIPAA regulations, the patient is subject to heavy fines for releasing personal information.

_____

_____ **7.** [LO7.4] Once claims are submitted to the insurance company, the company's representatives will code the procedures and tests performed on the patient.

_____

_____ **8.** [LO7.4] The electronic health record is available to all authorized staff simultaneously.

_____

_____ **9.** [LO7.3] Administrative responsibilities include assuring diagnostic testing is completed and results obtained.

_____

_____ **10.** [LO7.4] Since a medical office is not a business, there is no need to have specific requirements for personnel management.

_____

## Sentence Completion

In the space provided, write the word or phrase that best completes each sentence.

1. **[LO7.4]** Offices differ depending on size, specialty, and _____ services.

2. **[LO7.1]** Medical offices may mail the _____ materials or encourage the patient to access them through the practice's Web site.

3. **[LO7.1]** When a patient arrives at the medical office, she is usually required to _____ to become registered for the appointment.

4. **[LO7.2]** When a patient is in the screening area of the medical office, he will have his vital signs taken as well as his _____ and _____ determined.

5. **[LO7.2]** The MLT is also referred to as the _____ laboratory technician.

6. **[LO7.2]** Most MLTs work in hospitals and diagnostic laboratories called _____ laboratories.

7. **[LO7.3]** Laboratory test results may be reported to the physician's office via computer, _____, or _____.

8. **[LO7.2]** Good communication between the administrative medical assistant and the medical laboratory technician is an asset to good _____ _____.

9. **[LO7.4]** To avoid HIPAA violations in a medical office, simple actions include to _____ all documents before discarding.

10. **[LO7.1, 7.3]** Two mnemonics that may help you remember and become more conscious of patient privacy are _____ the Lip and _____ the Phone.

1. _____

_____

2. _____

_____

3. _____

_____

4. _____

_____

5. _____

_____

6. _____

_____

7. _____

_____

8. _____

_____

9. _____

_____

10. _____

_____

# Apply Your Knowledge

## Short Answer

Write the answer to each question on the lines provided.

1. [LO7.2] List four specific duties of the medical laboratory technician.

_____

_____

_____

2. [LO7.4] Why is it necessary to apply the HIPAA regulations to the medical practice?

_____

_____

_____

3. [LO7.4] List three advantages to utilizing the electronic health records method in a medical practice.

_____

_____

_____

4. [LO7.4] List three duties or responsibilities of the administrative medical assistant. Also, list three duties the administrative medical assistant will *not* perform in the medical office and explain why the assistant will not perform these functions.

_____

_____

_____

5. [LO7.1] Write an appropriate dialogue for the administrative medical assistant to use with a patient as the patient enters the medical practice reception area for her first appointment.

_____

_____

_____

## Problem-Solving Activities

Follow the directions for each activity.

1. [LO7.2] CLIA '88 Regulations
   a. Access the Web site for Centers for Medicare and Medicaid Services at www.cms.gov.
   b. At the CMS Web site, search for information regarding CLIA.
   c. Once you have located the CLIA information, search for the approved waived laboratory listing.
   d. List at least five waived laboratory tests that are included under the CLIA '88 standards.

2. [LO7.1, 7.2, 7.3] Partner with a classmate to develop a role-play scenario involving a new patient and an administrative or clinical medical assistant. The scenario can be staged in the front office, screening area, or clinical area of a mock medical office. You should role play the event using both appropriate and inappropriate techniques and communication. The scenario will be presented in front of the class for the other students to critique and give feedback about what was inappropriate and appropriate behavior and what corrective action would be indicated.

## Thinking Critically

Write your response to each case study question on the lines provided.

### Case 1 [LO7.4]

Susan and Desiree are administrative medical assistants working in the same medical practice. In the employee break room, Susan overhears Desiree talking on her cell phone about a patient that was seen in the office that morning. Susan knows that the patient is Desiree's neighbor.

1. What is the main issue with this scenario and what are the consequences of this type of action?

   _____

   _____

   _____

2. Should Susan become involved with this situation? If so, why?

   _____

   _____

   _____

### Case 2 [LO7.1]

Debbie is an administrative medical assistant who is checking in a new patient, Mr. Jamison. The reception desk is located in the area where there are several other patients. Mr. Jamison has questions about information required on the Patient Registration Form. At the reception desk, he asks Debbie whom he should put down in the space where it asks for the Subscriber's Name and Relative Emergency Contact. Debbie says, "Mr. Jamison, you can put your name in the Subscriber's Name space and your wife's name, Martha Jamison, where it asks for a Relative Emergency Contact."

**1.** Is there a problem with Debbie's communication with Mr. Jamison? If so, why?

_____

_____

_____

**2.** Explain what Debbie could have done differently to address Mr. Jamison's questions.

_____

_____

_____

## Case 3 [LO7.2]

Bill Miller is a medical laboratory technician and is obtaining blood and urine specimens from a patient who has multiple laboratory tests ordered. The patient appears to be quite anxious about the tests and tells Bill, "I am very worried about these tests. Can you tell me anything about them?" Bill tells the patient, "Don't worry, everything will be fine, and we will have the results in a day or two. If you don't hear from us, that means everything is normal."

**1.** Explain why Bill's responses were inappropriate.

_____

_____

_____

**2.** What is an appropriate response to the patient's concerns about the laboratory tests?

_____

_____

_____

# Demonstrate Your Knowledge

**Student Name:** _____

## Procedure 7–1: Registering a New Patient

**GOAL:** To accurately register the patient by obtaining all the necessary information for treatment

**MATERIALS:** Registration form (you may use Figure 7–2), Authorization for Release of Information, Assignment of Benefits and Financial Responsibility Information form (you may use Figure 7–3), pen or computer, copy machine or scanner (*Note:* The forms are available at the end of this study guide.)

**METHOD:** To pass this procedure the minimum required score is _____ % or all elements must meet "satisfactory" ability on the final demonstration. The first box may be used as a practice or final demonstration, with the evaluator placing **S for Satisfactory** or **U for Unsatisfactory** if that is the grading criteria. The second box may be used as a final demonstration with a **grade point** written in the box.

| STEPS | POSSIBLE POINTS | S/U | POINTS EARNED |
|---|---|---|---|
| 1. Greet the patient and instruct him to sign in; this may be done manually or digitally, depending on the office technology. | 10 | | |
| 2. Provide the patient with a registration form to complete or interview the patient and input the information directly into the computer. | 15 | | |
| 3. Ensure all areas are addressed. | 15 | | |
| 4. Obtain the patient's or legal representative's signature on the Authorization for Release of Information, Assignment of Benefits and Financial Responsibility Information form. (*Note:* Procedures related to privacy practices are in Chapter 6: Law and Ethics.) | 15 | | |
| 5. Provide the patient with a copy. | 10 | | |
| 6. Answer any questions and obtain the patient's or legal representative's signature. | 15 | | |
| 7. Copy or scan the patient's or insured party's insurance card and a photo identification such as a driver's license. | 15 | | |
| 8. Thank the patient and instruct him to have a seat until the clinical medical assistant calls the patient's name. | 5 | | |
| **Total Points (if applicable)** | 100 | | |

**Comments:** _____

_____

_____

**Final Evaluator's Signature:** _____

**Date:** _____

## CAAHEP Competencies Achieved

IV. C (9) Discuss applications of electronic technology in effective communication

IV. P (2) Report relevant information to others succinctly and accurately

V. P (6) Use office hardware and software to maintain office systems

VII. P (2) Apply third-party guidelines

IX. C (2) Explore issue of confidentiality as it applies to the medical assistant

## ABHES Competencies Achieved

1. d. Have knowledge of the general responsibilities of the medical assistant

4. a. Document accurately

4. c. Follow established policies when initiating or terminating medical treatment

7. a. Perform basic keyboarding skills

8. a. Perform basic clerical functions

8. ll. Apply electronic technology

# 8 The Medical Office Environment

## Test Your Knowledge

### Vocabulary Review

Match the key terms in the right column with the definitions in the left column by placing the letter of each correct answer in the space provided.

_____ **1.** a piece of equipment that is used repeatedly such as a telephone, computer, or examination table

_____ **2.** a bill for materials or services received by or services performed by the practice

_____ **3.** cash kept on hand in the office for small purchases

_____ **4.** an item that is used and must then be restocked; also known collectively as supplies

_____ **5.** a U.S. civil rights act forbidding discrimination against people because of a physical or mental handicap

_____ **6.** a person who works in the reception area at the front desk

_____ **7.** patient registration; also referred to as patient check-in

_____ **8.** a paper listing all the items ordered from a vendor that is packed in the shipment of supplies; used to ensure all supplies ordered have been received

_____ **9.** an authorization for an insurance carrier to pay a physician or practice directly

**a.** Americans with Disabilities Act (ADA) **[LO8.2]**

**b.** assignment of benefits **[LO8.3]**

**c.** copayment **[LO8.3]**

**d.** durable item **[LO8.4]**

**e.** expendable item **[LO8.4]**

**f.** inventory **[LO8.4]**

**g.** invoice **[LO8.4]**

**h.** packing slip **[LO8.4]**

**i.** petty cash **[LO8.3]**

**j.** reception **[LO8.3]**

**k.** receptionist **[LO8.3]**

**l.** requisition **[LO8.4]**

**m.** sign in **[LO8.3]**

**n.** medical identify theft **[LO8.4]**

**o.** Red Flag Rule **[LO8.4]**

_____ **10.** a formal request from a staff member or doctor for the purchase of equipment or supplies

_____ **11.** a list of supplies used regularly and the quantities in stock

_____ **12.** the point of entry to an office; an administrative area referred to as the front desk

_____ **13.** a small fee paid by the insured at the time of a medical service rather than by the insurance company

_____ **14.** when a person seeks health care using another person's name or insurance

_____ **15.** an August 1, 2009, law requiring certain businesses including most medical offices and other health-care facilities to develop written programs to detect the warning signs of identity theft

## Multiple-Choice Certification Questions

There may be more than one answer; circle the letter of the choice that best completes each statement or answers each question.

**1.** [LO8.4] Broad categories of supplies include
   a. administrative and basic.
   b. general and clinical.
   c. clinical and everyday.
   d. general and basic.
   e. administrative and office.

**2.** [LO8.4] Which group of items is considered general supplies?
   a. Lancets, tongue depressors, and sutures
   b. Lubricating jelly, alcohol swabs, and needles
   c. Paper cups, toilet paper, and liquid soap
   d. Copy paper, stamps, and pens
   e. File folders, insurance manuals, and forms

**3.** [LO8.3] Which of the following actions is *not* appropriate to maintain confidentiality?
   a. When a patient signs in on a roster at the reception desk, cross out the name with a heavy black marker once the name is acknowledged by the administrative medical assistant.
   b. Cover the name of the patient on the roster with a piece of opaque tape.
   c. Provide a clipboard with a sign-in sheet that all patients use to sign in when registering.
   d. Provide an electronic sign-in method that automatically registers that patient but others are not able to see.
   e. Provide an individual sign-in sheet that others will not see.

**4.** [LO8.3] A new patient packet should include
   a. insurance coverage information.
   b. the patient's consent for treatment.
   c. HIPAA forms.
   d. release of information form.
   e. All of the above.

**5.** [LO8.3] Certain patients should not be seated in the main reception area with other patients. These include patients that
   a. need an allergy shot.
   b. are scheduled for a complete physical.
   c. need laboratory tests and an electrocardiogram.
   d. are having difficulty breathing.
   e. are seeing the physician for a follow-up appointment.

**6.** [LO8.4] Which of the following are examples of a durable item?
   a. A computer
   b. Needles and syringes
   c. Sample medications
   d. Paper for the copy machine
   e. None of the above.

**7.** [LO8.1] When making a decision to lease or purchase equipment it is important to consider
   a. how long the equipment will last.
   b. if there is any equipment that can be traded in.
   c. whether the equipment will become outdated with advancing technology.
   d. how often the equipment will be used.
   e. All of the above.

**8.** [LO8.4] General supplies include those that are
   a. used only by the physician.
   b. purchased from an office supply store.
   c. used during patient procedures.
   d. consumed over a 1-year period of time.
   e. None of the above.

**9.** [LO8.4] Over-ordering of supplies is advised when
   a. the office receives a significant discount for ordering large quantities.
   b. there is additional storage space to accommodate large quantities.
   c. the products are due to expire in a month.
   d. the sales representative is ensured a larger commission on the order.
   e. the current inventory level is running low.

**10.** [LO8.3] When managing the petty cash for the office, it is important to
   a. keep the petty cash in the same location as the patient cash payments.
   b. use petty cash to pay for major supply orders that arrive at the office.
   c. complete a voucher for the person requesting the cash.
   d. count the petty cash fund every Friday prior to closing the office.
   e. deplete the petty cash fund each month.

**11.** [LO8.1] When determining how to set up a reception area for a medical practice that sees pediatric patients, it is important to
   a. have low, dim lighting to reduce the glare.
   b. provide a refreshment area with coffee or tea for the parents.
   c. purchase only disposable toys that can be discarded after use.
   d. provide soft, soothing music.
   e. provide many games that have small parts that the children can share.

**12.** [LO8.2] Which of the following would *not* be required to maintain compliance with the Americans with Disabilities Act?
   a. Wheelchair ramps
   b. A separate reception area
   c. Large-print patient forms
   d. Handrails in halls and bathrooms
   e. Braille elevator floor indicators

**13.** [LO8.4] The appropriate time period to consider when managing a supply level is
   a. 1 month.
   b. 1 week.
   c. 1 year.
   d. 2 weeks.
   e. 6 months.

**14.** [LO8.4] A requisition form is used to
   a. ensure all supplies are included in the shipping box.
   b. pay the bill.
   c. manage the supply inventory list.
   d. balance the petty cash for the office.
   e. order the supplies needed for the medical practice.

**15.** [LO8.5] Which of the following is *not* considered a function of the administrative medical assistant when opening the office for the day?
   a. Ensure that all equipment is working properly
   b. Check the appointment book or log for the day
   c. Disarm the security system
   d. Turn on the answering service
   e. Pull patient charts for the day

**16.** [LO8.5] Which of the following is *not* considered a function of the administrative medical assistant when closing the office for the day?
   a. Organize and straighten the reception area
   b. Ensure that the security system is disarmed
   c. Restock the administrative supplies
   d. Log off all computers
   e. Lock the doors

**17.** [LO8.3] _____ in the administrative areas of the medical office.
   a. Patients are received
   b. Appointments are made
   c. Petty cash is maintained
   d. Nonclinical activities are performed
   e. All of the above.

**18.** [LO8.4] Most durable items
   a. have a short shelf life.
   b. must be restocked often.
   c. include equipment that is used indefinitely.
   d. are disposable items that are ordered frequently.
   e. are only used in administrative areas.

**19.** [LO8.1] Which of the following is *not* considered when setting up a new office for a medical practice?
   a. The amount of expendable supplies that will be needed
   b. The number of patients that will be seen on a typical day
   c. The physician's schedule or work hours in the office
   d. The type of patients that will be seen by the physician
   e. The durable equipment that will need to be ordered

**20.** [LO8.4] Administrative supplies include
   a. paper towels.
   b. alcohol swabs.
   c. copy machine toner.
   d. tongue depressors.
   e. toilet paper.

**21.** [LO8.3] The patient's copayment is collected by the administrative medical assistant
a. when the patient returns for an annual physical examination.
b. prior to the patient seeing the physician.
c. after the insurance claim has been submitted.
d. when the patient receives his next paycheck.
e. when the collections department requests it.

**22.** [LO8.1] When furnishing a medical office, it is best to
a. purchase chairs that have stain-resistant fabrics.
b. use artificial plants to avoid problems with allergies.
c. use artwork that is appropriate for the type of practice.
d. avoid refreshment centers in practices where patients arrive for fasting lab tests.
e. All of the above.

**23.** [LO8.2] The Americans with Disabilities Act prohibits discrimination based on
a. employment qualifications.
b. age or sex of the individual.
c. level of education obtained.
d. physical or mental handicaps.
e. race and religion.

## True or False

Decide whether each statement is true or false. In the space at the left, write "T" for true or "F" for false. On the lines provided, rewrite the false statements to make them true.

_____ **1.** [LO8.3] A patient record may be electronic or a combination of electronic and hard copy.

_____

_____ **2.** [LO8.3] When there is a significant wait time to see the physician, patients should be told to wait since it is difficult to reschedule many patients.

_____

_____ **3.** [LO8.4] Supplies include durable items and dependable, disposable items.

_____

_____ **4.** [LO8.2] Service animals may include cats and monkeys.

_____

_____ **5.** [LO8.3] When the administrative medical assistant is in charge of opening the office for the day, it is appropriate to arrive at least 30 minutes ahead of the scheduled time the office will open.

_____

_____ **6.** [LO8.1] Overcrowding of a reception area is undesirable for patient comfort and for the potential of disease transmission.

_____

_____ **7.** [LO8.1] Space utilization is not dependent on the type of medical practice.

_____

_____ **8.** [LO8.3] Petty cash should be counted daily at the end of the business day.

_____

_____ **9.** [LO8.1] The color selection is critical to the overall effect of the office so the colors red and dark brown are frequently used because of their soothing effects on people.

_____

_____ **10.** [LO8.4] Over-ordering is a prudent way to manage office supplies because you do not have to order as frequently.

_____

## Sentence Completion

In the space provided, write the word or phrase that best completes each sentence.

**1.** [LO8.3] When registering a patient, HIPAA requires that information remain confidential including time of _____, time of _____, and name of _____.

**2.** [LO8.4] When supplies are received they should be checked for _____.

**3.** [LO8.3] Petty cash is used for _____ expenses.

**4.** [LO8.3] The clinical area of the medical office is where _____ patient care takes place.

**5.** [LO8.1] A pediatric office may have separate reception areas for _____ children and _____ children.

**6.** [LO8.2] When locating a vendor for office supplies, you should consider the _____ of the vendor and _____ offered.

**7.** [LO8.4] Prescription pads are _____ items.

**8.** [LO8.2] The Americans with Disabilities Act is also referred to as the _____ rights act for the _____.

**9.** [LO8.3] Third-party checks are _____ accepted by offices so the patient should write a check for the _____ amount of the bill.

**10.** [LO8.1] The _____ and _____ of the practice are among the first considerations when designing a reception area.

1. _____
   _____

2. _____
   _____

3. _____
   _____

4. _____
   _____

5. _____
   _____

6. _____
   _____

7. _____
   _____

8. _____
   _____

9. _____
   _____

10. _____
    _____

# Apply Your Knowledge

## Short Answer

Write the answer to each question on the lines provided.

1. **[LO8.1]** List four items to be considered when setting up a new medical practice and explain why each is important.

_____

_____

_____

2. **[LO8.4]** What are two consequences of running out of expendable supplies in a medical office?

_____

_____

_____

3. **[LO8.2]** How can a medical practice ensure that it is in compliance with mandated ADA requirements?

_____

_____

_____

4. **[LO8.1]** Give two examples of utilization of space and explain why it is so important in a medical office.

_____

_____

_____

5. **[LO8.1]** Color plays a significant role in the medical environment. For the following five types of practice, decide which color would be the best choice for the reception area and explain why: Family Practice, Obstetrics and Gynecology, Gerontology, Ophthalmology, and Pediatrics.

_____

_____

_____

## Problem-Solving Activities

Follow the directions for each activity.

1. **[LO8.2]** ADA Regulations
   a. Using the Internet, access the Web site www.ada.gov.
   b. Locate the section regarding the employer's responsibility to employees with disabilities.
   c. List at least three items that employers need to do to accommodate employees with declared disabilities.

2. **[LO8.4]** Comparative Shopping
   a. Locate two vendors in the local community that sell administrative supplies.
   b. Select five administrative supply items available from both vendors and obtain a price for each item.
   c. Set up a table listing each item in the left column and the vendors in each of two vertical columns.

**Sample Table**

|  | VENDOR #1 COST | VENDOR #2 COST |
|---|---|---|
| Item #1: | | |
| Item #2: | | |
| Item #3: | | |
| Item #4: | | |
| Item #5: | | |
| **Total of Supply Costs** | | |

   d. After listing all five items, using the same quantity for each item, do a total of supply costs for each vendor to determine which one has the best overall pricing.

## Thinking Critically

Write your response to each case study question on the lines provided.

### Case 1 [LO8.4]

As the administrative medical assistant in a general medical practice, you are responsible for maintaining the administrative supplies for the office. You discover that the supply cabinet is frequently depleted of supplies such as reams of paper for the copy machine, pens, and legal tablets. You suspect that someone in the office is taking supplies out of the office for personal use.

1. How will you attempt to better manage the supplies so that the office has an adequate quantity on hand?

_____

_____

_____

**2.** If you discover that one of the employees is taking supplies for home use, what should you do?

_____

_____

_____

## Case 2 [LO8.2]

The office where you are employed is located on the fourth floor of a medical complex. The landlord of the building has notified all the businesses that the elevators will be worked on for 1 hour tomorrow morning from 9 A.M.–10 A.M. After you review the patient appointment log for tomorrow morning, you discover that there are three patients scheduled to arrive during that time. All three patients require access to the elevator to get to the office. Two of the patients are willing to reschedule; however, the third patient has made special transportation arrangements to get to the appointment. This patient is extremely upset about the situation and is unwilling to reschedule. He also demands that there is a way for him to get to the fourth floor office. He further states that he knows his rights as a disabled person.

**1.** How should you handle this patient? What should you tell him?

_____

_____

_____

**2.** What, if anything, should be documented in the patient's medical record?

_____

_____

_____

## Case 3 [LO8.3]

The office manager of a general practice has resigned, and you are given the responsibility of ordering supplies. You discover that the main vendor that has been used for years is a relative of the office manager. You do some investigating and find out that the vendor's pricing is far above all other vendors in the area. For example, a case of copy paper is $50.00 per case at the popular vendor in the area, and the vendor you currently use charges $65.00 per case. Other items are also priced similarly.

**1.** What are the initial steps that you should do now that you are in charge of the ordering of administrative supplies?

_____

_____

_____

**2.** If you decide to not use the current vendor anymore, how will you handle the communication with this vendor?

_____

_____

_____

# Demonstrate Your Knowledge

**Student Name:** _____

## Procedure 8–1: Establishing and Conducting a Supply Inventory

**GOAL:** To ensure the correct supplies are on hand and to determine which supplies require reordering

**MATERIALS:** Vendor catalogs, pen and pencil or computer with Internet access

**METHOD:** To pass this procedure the minimum required score is _____% or all elements must meet "satisfactory" ability on the final demonstration. The first box may be used as a practice or final demonstration, with the evaluator placing **S for Satisfactory** or **U for Unsatisfactory** if that is the grading criteria. The second box may be used as a final demonstration with a **grade point** written in the box.

| STEPS | POSSIBLE POINTS | S/U | POINTS EARNED |
|---|---|---|---|
| 1. Create an inventory form with supply levels using Table 8–1; you may choose to create an electronic spreadsheet version or a paper version. Note that this table is available at the end of this study guide. | 20 | | |
| 2. Research appropriate vendors for each item and include a vendor for each item on your inventory form (it may be the same vendor). | 20 | | |
| 3. Use the vendor catalogs to determine costs and how quantities are supplied. | 20 | | |
| 4. Count the number of items on hand and record on the inventory form. | 20 | | |
| 5. Compare the number of each item on hand to the established supply level and determine if reorder is needed. | 20 | | |
| **Total Points (if applicable)** | 100 | | |

**Comments:** _____

_____

_____

**Final Evaluator's Signature:** _____

**Date:** _____

## CAAHEP Competencies Achieved

IV. P (2) Report relevant information to others succinctly and accurately

IV. P (4) Explain general office policies

V. P (10) Perform an office inventory

IX. A (3) Recognize the importance of local, state and federal legislation and regulations in the practice setting

## ABHES Competencies Achieved

1. d. Have knowledge of the general responsibilities of the medical assistant

4. a. Document accurately

4. f. Comply with federal, state, and local health laws and regulation

8. a. Perform basic clerical functions

8. d. Apply concepts for office procedures

8. z. Maintain inventory equipment and supplies

## Procedure 8–2: Receiving Supplies

**GOAL:** To follow an organized process when receiving supplies to ensure the order is complete and the charges correspond with those quoted during the requisition process

**MATERIALS:** Requisition or order form, packing slip, invoice (you may use Figures 8–7, 8–8, 8–9), pen, real or virtual supplies
*Note:* The figures are available at the end of this study guide.

**METHOD:** To pass this procedure the minimum required score is _____% or all elements must meet "satisfactory" ability on the final demonstration. The first box may be used as a practice or final demonstration, with the evaluator placing **S for Satisfactory** or **U for Unsatisfactory** if that is the grading criteria. The second box may be used as a final demonstration with a **grade point** written in the box.

| STEPS | POSSIBLE POINTS | S/U | POINTS EARNED |
|---|---|---|---|
| 1. Compare the items that arrived with the packing slip. | 20 | | |
| 2. Compare the packing slip with the original requisition to assure the proper items in the proper amounts were received. | 20 | | |
| 3. Determine if an invoice is also included in the package or if the packing slip has a notation that it also functions as an invoice (bill). | 10 | | |
| 4. If items are back-ordered, you may be charged at this time. Make a notation on the invoice that the items were charged but not received. | 20 | | |
| 5. File the invoice for payment, or transport to the person responsible for payment. | 10 | | |
| 6. Indicate on the inventory form the date and quantity of the items received or back-ordered. | 20 | | |
| **Total Points (if applicable)** | 100 | | |

**Comments:** _____

_____

_____

**Final Evaluator's Signature:** _____

**Date:** _____

## CAAHEP Competencies Achieved

V. C (12) Identify types of records common to the health-care setting

V. P (10) Perform an office inventory

## ABHES Competencies Achieved

2. d. Have knowledge of the general responsibilities of the medical assistant

8. a. Perform basic clerical functions

8. d. Apply concepts for office procedures

8. z. Maintain inventory equipment and supplies

## Procedure 8–3: Managing the Petty Cash Fund

**GOAL:** To provide the availability of petty cash for incidental expenses and a system to ensure accountability

**MATERIALS:** Pen, paper, receipts, money, cash box or cash drawer

**METHOD:** To pass this procedure the minimum required score is _____% or all elements must meet "satisfactory" ability on the final demonstration. The first box may be used as a practice or final demonstration, with the evaluator placing **S for Satisfactory** or **U for Unsatisfactory** if that is the grading criteria. The second box may be used as a final demonstration with a **grade point** written in the box.

| STEPS | POSSIBLE POINTS | S/U | POINTS EARNED |
|---|:---:|:---:|:---:|
| 1. Establish a predetermined amount to be kept in petty cash (usually $50 to $100). | 10 | | |
| 2. Complete a voucher for the person requesting the cash, which includes the date, person's name, amount, and the expense such as Band-Aids. A slip of paper or pad may be used as a voucher. The person receiving the cash should sign the voucher. | 20 | | |
| 3. Dispense the money and place the voucher in the petty cash container. | 15 | | |
| 4. Attach the voucher to the receipt that should be requested when the item is purchased. If change is returned, the amount is noted on the voucher. | 15 | | |
| 5. Count the money in the petty cash container daily at the close of business. The remaining cash and the receipts should equal the predetermined amount. Often a log or sheet is signed or initialed to indicate the cash balanced on that day. If the amount and receipts do not correspond, the issue should be reported to the physician or practice manager. | 20 | | |
| 6. Request additional cash as the remaining level decreases. The drawer should never have a higher or lower total than the sum of the cash on hand and the receipts indicating what was purchased. | 10 | | |
| 7. Keep the petty cash container locked and secure. | 10 | | |
| **Total Points (if applicable)** | 100 | | |

Comments: _____

_____

_____

**Final Evaluator's Signature:** _____

**Date:** _____

## CAAHEP Competencies Achieved

V. C (12) Identify types of records common to the health care setting

## ABHES Competencies Achieved

3. d. Have knowledge of the general responsibilities of the medical assistant

8. d. Apply concepts for office procedures

8. l. Establish and maintain a petty cash fund

Student Name: _____

## Procedure 8–4: Opening and Closing the Office

**GOAL:** To ensure readiness to receive and care for patients in an efficient, organized, and safe manner

**MATERIALS:** Forms for opening and closing the office (see Tables 8–2 and 8–3), pen, telephone, pad, school-simulated medical office or laboratory if available
*Note:* Tables 8–2 and 8–3 are available at the end of this study guide.

**METHOD:** To pass this procedure the minimum required score is _____% or all elements must meet "satisfactory" ability on the final demonstration. The first box may be used as a practice or final demonstration, with the evaluator placing **S for Satisfactory** or **U for Unsatisfactory** if that is the grading criteria. The second box may be used as a final demonstration with a **grade point** written in the box.

| STEPS | POSSIBLE POINTS | S/U | POINTS EARNED |
|---|---|---|---|
| 1. Using Table 8–2: Daily Checklist for Opening the Office, simulate the functions for opening the office. | | | |
| a. Begin with disarming the security system. | 10 | | |
| b. Telephone the answering service, write any messages on the pad, and notify appropriate person. | 20 | | |
| c. Conduct each task on the form and initial as you complete it. | 20 | | |
| 2. Using Table 8–3: Daily Checklist for Closing the Office, simulate the functions for closing the office. | | | |
| a. Begin with logging out and turning off the computers. | 15 | | |
| b. Use the telephone to notify the answering service that the office is closing. | 15 | | |
| c. Conduct each task on the form and initial as you complete it. | 20 | | |
| **Total Points (if applicable)** | 100 | | |

Comments: _____

_____

_____

**Final Evaluator's Signature:** _____

**Date:** _____

## CAAHEP Competencies Achieved

XI. C (2) Identify safety techniques that can be used to prevent accidents and maintain a safe work environment

## ABHES Competencies Achieved

8. d. Apply concepts for office procedures

8. x. Maintain medical facility

# 9 Asepsis for Administrative Areas

## Test Your Knowledge

### Vocabulary Review

Match the key terms in the right column with the definitions in the left column by placing the letter of each correct answer in the space provided.

_____ 1. stopping the spread of or reducing or eliminating pathogens through use of aseptic techniques

_____ 2. the study of the transmission and control of diseases

_____ 3. a disease-causing organism

_____ 4. the symptoms of a disease are so slight that they may go unnoticed

_____ 5. techniques for health-care personnel to minimize the risk of catching or spreading an infection

_____ 6. a person who is a reservoir host and does not exhibit symptoms yet spreads the disease to others

_____ 7. the inability to effectively fight off an infectious disease

_____ 8. a living organism too small to see with the naked eye

_____ 9. utilizing techniques to prevent the spread of, reduce, or eliminate pathogens

_____ 10. an individual who has little or no immunity to a specific organism

_____ 11. also known as the chain of infection; the manner in which pathogens are spread

**a.** alcohol hand disinfectant (AHD) **[LO9.5]**

**b.** asepsis **[LO9.2]**

**c.** carrier **[LO9.1]**

**d.** cycle of infection **[LO 9.1]**

**e.** epidemiology **[LO 9.1]**

**f.** fomite **[LO9.1]**

**g.** health-care acquired infections (HAI) **[LO9.2]**

**h.** immunocompromised **[LO9.2]**

**i.** infection control **[LO9.2]**

**j.** microbe **[LO9.1]**

**k.** pandemic **[LO9.3]**

**l.** pathogen **[LO9.1]**

**m.** personal protective equipment (PPE) **[LO9.5]**

**n.** reservoir host **[LO9.1]**

**o.** subclinical case **[LO9.2]**

_____ **12.** gels, foams, and liquid rubs that are used when running water is not readily available

_____ **13.** widespread disease or outbreak that affects populations throughout the world

_____ **14.** inanimate objects that transmit diseases

_____ **15.** an insect, animal, or human that has been invaded by a pathogen and is capable of sustaining its growth

_____ **16.** diseases that are a result of exposure in a health-care setting

_____ **17.** disposable gloves, mask, eye shields, and gowns worn to protect health-care personnel from contamination with blood and body fluids

**p.** susceptible host [LO9.1]

**q.** standard precautions [LO9.3]

## Multiple-Choice Certification Questions

There may be more than one answer; circle the letter of the choice that best completes each statement or answers each question.

**1.** [LO9.1] An insect, animal, or human whose body is capable of sustaining the growth of an organism is called the
a. fomite.
b. carrier.
c. reservoir host.
d. pathogen.
e. microbe.

**2.** [LO9.2] When the symptoms of infection are so slight that they may go unnoticed, it is referred to as a
a. cycle of infection.
b. subclinical case.
c. bloodborne pathogenic infection.
d. vector-borne infection.
e. slight infection.

**3.** [LO9.2] Conjunctivitis is typically spread through
a. the air.
b. sweat.
c. vector transmission.
d. blood transfusions.
e. direct contact.

**4.** [LO9.6] *Escherichia coli* and *Salmonella* are pathogens associated with
a. airborne illnesses.
b. bloodborne illnesses.
c. vector-borne illnesses.
d. food-borne illnesses.
e. None of the above.

**5.** [LO9.2] MRSA is a disease caused by
   a. *Staphylococcus aureus.*
   b. chlamydia.
   c. *E. coli.*
   d. rubella.
   e. varicella.

**6.** [LO9.1] The placenta may be a source of transmission of
   a. tuberculosis.
   b. varicella.
   c. rubella.
   d. spotted fever.
   e. typhoid.

**7.** [LO9.1] Increased susceptibility to contracting an illness is determined by all of the following factors *except*
   a. an increased stress level.
   b. a healthy immune system.
   c. poor hygiene habits.
   d. existence of comorbidities.
   e. genetic predisposition.

**8.** [LO9.1] Hepatitis B is an example of
   a. a food-borne pathogen.
   b. a health-care acquired pathogen.
   c. an airborne pathogen.
   d. a vector-borne infection.
   e. a bloodborne pathogen.

**9.** [LO9.1] A reservoir host who is unaware of the presence of a pathogen and therefore spreads disease is called a
   a. portal of exit.
   b. point of entry.
   c. susceptible host.
   d. carrier.
   e. fomite.

**10.** [LO9.1] The chain of infection consists of
   a. an infectious agent.
   b. a reservoir host.
   c. a mode of transmission.
   d. a portal of entry.
   e. All of the above.

**11.** [LO9.1] An insect that carries microorganisms from one infected person to another is a
   a. fomite.
   b. pathogen.
   c. vector.
   d. host.
   e. microbe.

**12.** [LO9.6] Influenza is commonly transmitted through
   a. the air.
   b. food contamination.
   c. fecal contamination.
   d. contact with open wounds.
   e. All of the above.

**13.** [LO9.2] Infection control regulations that must be followed in administrative areas include
   a. training of all employees about infection control.
   b. providing hepatitis B vaccinations to employees when appropriate.
   c. implementing an exposure control plan.
   d. having safety manuals available.
   e. All of the above.

**14.** [LO9.4] In administrative areas, general hand washing should take place
   a. before handling money.
   b. after handling laboratory specimens.
   c. before using the restroom.
   d. after filing charts.
   e. after each telephone call.

**15.** [LO9.5] Good aseptic practices in administrative areas include
   a. posting signs for visitors requesting that they not sneeze or cough when in the office.
   b. not scheduling appointments for patients who have a visible rash.
   c. asking all patients to wear a mask during flu season.
   d. wearing disposable gloves when answering the phone.
   e. placing patients who are coughing in an isolated waiting area.

**16.** [LO9.4] Which of the following is *not* proper technique for general hand washing?
   a. Using soap and warm water
   b. Rubbing hands vigorously for at least 20 seconds
   c. Turning off the water faucet with your bare hands
   d. Not touching the trash receptacle when disposing of the towel
   e. Using a disposable towel to dry your hands

**17.** [LO9.1] West Nile virus is transmitted through
   a. contact with contaminated food.
   b. contact with dust particles.
   c. blood transfusions.
   d. bites from mosquitoes.
   e. None of the above.

**18.** [LO9.1] A person who has an immunocompromised immune system is considered to be a
   a. susceptible host.
   b. reservoir host.
   c. viable vector.
   d. subclinical case.
   e. carrier.

**19.** [LO9.2] The principles of asepsis are designed to
   a. reduce the number of patients that arrive at a medical office with an infection.
   b. break the cycle of infection.
   c. treat infections.
   d. transmit pathogens.
   e. maintain the chain of infection.

**20.** [LO9.3] The branch of medical science that serves as the foundation for determining effective interventions for the public's health is
   a. clinical microbiology.
   b. the Occupational Safety and Health Administration.
   c. the health administration.
   d. bacteriology.
   e. epidemiology.

**21.** [LO9.5] Techniques that are designed to minimize the risk of catching or spreading an infection are referred to as
a. principles of epidemiology.
b. health-care acquired policies.
c. standard precautions.
d. employer regulations.
e. public health principles.

**22.** [LO9.3] Governmental agencies that are primarily responsible for the guidelines and regulations affecting the prevention of infection are the
a. HAI and CDC.
b. CDC and OSHA.
c. AHD and CDC.
d. HAI and AHD.
e. OSHA and HAI.

**23.** [LO9.5] Ideally, alcohol hand disinfecting products should be used when
a. you are in a hurry.
b. you have no running water.
c. you are handling laboratory specimens.
d. there is only warm water available.
e. there is a chance of running out of soap.

**24.** [LO9.1] Which of the following is *not* one of the five steps or requirements in the cycle of infection?
a. Reservoir host
b. Means of exit
c. Means of transmission
d. Means of entrance
e. Infection control principles

**25.** [LO9.1] Doorknobs in an office are examples of
a. carriers.
b. hosts.
c. fomites.
d. vectors.
e. helminths.

## True or False

Decide whether each statement is true or false. In the space at the left, write "T" for true or "F" for false. On the lines provided, rewrite the false statements to make them true.

_____ **1.** [LO9.1] After a pathogen exits the body of the reservoir host, it must find another host through transmission or travel.

_____

_____ **2.** [LO9.1] When a person sneezes and another person breathes in the droplets from the sneeze, it is a form of indirect transmission.

_____

_____ **3.** [LO9.2] Standard precautions only apply when dealing with vector-borne infections.

_____

_____ **4.** **[LO9.2]** HAI are infections or diseases acquired in health-care settings.

_____

_____ **5.** **[LO9.5]** Antimicrobial soaps are only recommended when dealing directly with body fluids.

_____

_____ **6.** **[LO9.5]** In administrative areas, it is recommended that you wash hands before leaving the medical office.

_____

_____ **7.** **[LO9.5]** It is recommended that used tissues are disposed of in red bags in biohazard containers.

_____

_____ **8.** **[LO9.5]** It is not necessary to wear disposable gloves when carrying a laboratory specimen that a patient brought from home.

_____

_____ **9.** **[LO9.5]** All employees in a medical office are required to receive the seasonal influenza vaccines or risk termination from their position.

_____

_____ **10.** **[LO9.1]** One break in the chain of infection can nullify all other efforts to promote disease prevention.

_____

## Sentence Completion

In the space provided, write the word or phrase that best completes each sentence.

1. **[LO9.5]** If gross amounts of blood or body fluids are present on gloves, a _____ trash receptacle should be used to dispose the gloves.

2. **[LO9.1]** A human _____ is a person who is a reservoir host and does not exhibit any symptoms, yet unknowingly or knowingly spreads the disease to others.

3. **[LO9.5]** In the health-care setting, asepsis is important to protect the _____, the _____, and _____ workers.

4. **[LO9.1]** All susceptible hosts are considered _____ or _____, which means their immune system does not have the ability to effectively fight off that infectious disease.

1. _____
   _____

2. _____
   _____

3. _____
   _____

4. _____
   _____

**5. [LO9.5]** In administrative areas, Hazardous Communication Standards include the use of MSDS, which are _____ _____ _____ Sheets.

**6. [LO9.4]** _____ _____ hand washing is appropriate for procedures requiring sterility such as surgeries.

**7. [LO9.5]** Wear gloves when contact with blood or other _____-_____ materials are a probability such as a patient presenting with a laceration.

**8. [LO9.1]** The infection cycle begins when the pathogen finds a place to live and _____.

**9. [LO9.1]** Two general means of transmission of pathogens include _____ and _____.

**10. [LO9.2]** The principles of asepsis are designed to _____ the cycle of infection or _____ it from starting.

5. _____

6. _____

7. _____

8. _____

9. _____

10. _____

# Apply Your Knowledge
## Short Answer

Write the answer to each question on the lines provided.

1. **[LO9.1]** Give two examples of direct transmission and two examples of indirect transmission.

_____

_____

_____

2. **[LO9.2]** List four reasons why it is important to maintain asepsis in health-care settings.

_____

_____

_____

3. **[LO9.5]** What are two methods of implementing occupational exposure to bloodborne pathogens standards in administrative areas?

_____

_____

_____

4. [LO9.5] Give four policies that should be followed when purchasing, cleaning, and managing toys in a pediatric practice.

_____

_____

_____

5. [LO9.1] Cite three ways to break the chain of infection.

_____

_____

_____

## Problem-Solving Activities

Follow the directions for each activity.

1. [LO9.6] Patient Education
   a. Using the Internet, access at least five items of information on the prevention of food-borne illness or food poisoning in children.
   b. Develop a patient education pamphlet or brochure using the information from the Web site(s) accessed.
   c. The brochure should provide information for the parents of children in a family practice or pediatric medical practice.

2. [LO9.5, 9.6] Control of Disease and Infections
   a. Refer to Table 9–1: Transmission of Pathogens

**Table 9–1 Transmission of Pathogens**

| MEANS OF TRANSMISSION | EXAMPLES | COMMON DISEASES |
|---|---|---|
| **Airborne** | Dust and soil particles Droplets—sneezing, coughing, respirations | Influenza, varicella (chickenpox), measles, tuberculosis, RSV |
| **Bloodborne: direct or indirect blood** | Blood transfusions, puncture wounds, broken skin or mucous membranes | Hepatitis B, hepatitis C, HIV/AIDS |
| **Pregnancy and childbirth** | Placenta<br><br>Birth canal | Rubella (German measles), HIV, hepatitis B<br>Syphilis, gonorrhea, _Chlamydia pneumoniae_ |
| **Food-borne** | Contaminated foods and liquids | _Escherichia coli_ and _Salmonella_ food poisoning, typhoid |
| **Vector-borne (vector is a living organism that carries disease from one infected organism to another)** | Fleas, flies, mosquitoes, ticks (Figure 9–2) | Plague, West Nile virus, malaria, Rocky Mountain spotted fever |
| **Touch: direct or indirect** | Hands, mouth, eyes, sexual organs | Conjunctivitis, herpes, Methicillin-resistant _Staphylococcus aureus_ (MRSA) |

b. For each of the six "means of transmission" listed, provide one way a person might prevent acquiring or transmitting a disease or infection.

# Thinking Critically

Write your response to each case study question on the lines provided.

## Case 1 [LO9.5]

You are working as an administrative medical assistant in a general medical practice. A 7-year-old patient, accompanied by her mother, arrives to see the doctor for a persistent, nonproductive cough. When you ask the mother to have her daughter wear a mask you have provided, the mother becomes very upset stating that "my daughter is not contagious, and I am not going to ask her to wear this silly mask in here."

**1.** What is the main problem in this scenario? Explain why this is a problem.

_____

_____

_____

**2.** How will you handle this situation if the mother refuses to have her daughter wear a mask while waiting to see the doctor?

_____

_____

_____

## Case 2 [LO9.4, 9.5]

An administrative medical assistant always shows up for work in wrinkled scrubs that don't smell clean and dirty sneakers. She also has dirty fingernails most of the time. Many of the fellow employees have given her hints about her unprofessional appearance. Two of these employees come to you and ask if you will talk with her about her personal appearance.

**1.** Why is it important to talk with this employee about her personal appearance?

_____

_____

_____

**2.** What should you specifically tell this employee that she needs to change about her appearance? Why?

_____

_____

_____

## Case 3 [LO9.5, 9.6]

Prior to the onset of seasonal flu, you are asked to contact patients who are recommended to come to the office to receive the flu vaccine. There are several elderly patients that are contacted, who are immunocompromised and should definitely have the flu shot. One of these patients says that he is not going to receive the flu shot because every time he gets this shot he gets sick.

**1.** What can you tell this patient to convince him that it is wise to come in and receive his flu shot?

_____

_____

_____

**2.** What are some of the consequences if this patient decides not to receive the flu shot?

_____

_____

_____

# Demonstrate Your Knowledge

**Student Name:** _____

## Procedure 9–1: General Hand Washing

**GOAL:** To use a general hand washing technique reducing pathogens on the hand surfaces and preventing recontamination in the process

**MATERIALS:** Sink with running water, soap as determined appropriate by the facility, paper towels, plastic-lined trash receptacle

**METHOD:** To pass this procedure the minimum required score is _____% or all elements must meet "satisfactory" ability on the final demonstration. The first box may be used as a practice or final demonstration, with the evaluator placing **S for Satisfactory** or **U for Unsatisfactory** if that is the grading criteria. The second box may be used as a final demonstration with a **grade point** written in the box.

| STEPS | POSSIBLE POINTS | S/U | POINTS EARNED |
|---|---|---|---|
| 1. Turn on the water faucet and wet hands using warm water. | 10 | | |
| 2. Apply soap. | 10 | | |
| 3. Lather well. | 15 | | |
| 4. Rub your hands vigorously for at least 20 seconds, scrubbing all surfaces, including the back of your hands, wrists, and between your fingers and your fingernails. | 25 | | |
| 5. Rinse well. | 10 | | |
| 6. Dry your hands with a disposable towel or air dryer. | 10 | | |
| 7. Use a disposable towel to turn off the faucet without touching your hands to any of its surfaces. | 10 | | |
| 8. Place the towel in the trash receptacle without touching your hands to any of its surfaces. | 10 | | |
| **Total Points (if applicable)** | 100 | | |

**Comments:** _____

_____

_____

**Final Evaluator's Signature:** _____

**Date:** _____

## CAAHEP Competencies Achieved

III. C (1) Describe the infection cycle, including the infectious agent, reservoir, susceptible host, means of transmission, portals of entry, and portals of exit

III. C (2) Define asepsis

III. C (3) Discuss infection control procedures

III. C (4) Identify personal safety precautions as established by the Occupational Safety and Health Administration (OSHA)

III. C (13) Identify the role of the Center for Disease Control (CDC) regulations in healthcare settings

III. P (2) Practice Standard Precautions

III. P (4) Perform hand washing

## ABHES Competencies Achieved

1. d. Have knowledge of the general responsibilities of the medical assistant

9. b. Apply principles of aseptic technique and infection control

9. i. Use standard precautions

## Procedure 9–2: Hand Cleansing with Alcohol Hand Disinfectant (AHD)

**GOAL:** To use a hand cleansing substance to reduce pathogens on the hand surfaces and prevent recontamination in the process when soap and water are not readily available

**MATERIALS:** 60–95% alcohol-based foam, gel, or liquid rub

**METHOD:** To pass this procedure the minimum required score is _____% or all elements must meet "satisfactory" ability on the final demonstration. The first box may be used as a practice or final demonstration, with the evaluator placing **S for Satisfactory** or **U for Unsatisfactory** if that is the grading criteria. The second box may be used as a final demonstration with a **grade point** written in the box.

| STEPS | POSSIBLE POINTS | S/U | POINTS EARNED |
|---|---|---|---|
| 1. Pump the AHD onto the palm of the hand. | 10 | | |
| 2. Rub the hands together vigorously ensuring that alcohol comes in contact with all surfaces including backs of hands, between fingers, and fingernails. | 30 | | |
| 3. Continue to rub the solution until it is evaporated and the hands are dry (10–15 seconds). Do not wave hands to hasten drying. | 40 | | |
| 4. Do not use an AHD cleansing procedure in the following circumstances: | | | |
| • When hands are visibly dirty | 5 | | |
| • When hands are contaminated with proteinaceous material | 5 | | |
| • Before or after eating | 5 | | |
| • After toileting activities | 5 | | |
| **Total Points (if applicable)** | 100 | | |

**Comments:** _____

_____

_____

**Final Evaluator's Signature:** _____

**Date:** _____

### CAAHEP Competencies Achieved

III. P (4) Perform hand washing

### ABHES Competencies Achieved

9. b. Apply principles of aseptic technique and infection control

## Procedure 9–3: Removing Contaminated Gloves

**GOAL:** To remove gloves contaminated with blood or body fluids, dirt, disinfectants or other materials while avoiding the transfer of the substance to your hands or other areas

**MATERIALS:** Contaminated gloves, plastic-lined trash receptacle (if gross amounts of blood or body fluids are present on the gloves, a biohazard trash receptacle should be used)

**METHOD:** To pass this procedure the minimum required score is _____% or all elements must meet "satisfactory" ability on the final demonstration. The first box may be used as a practice or final demonstration, with the evaluator placing **S for Satisfactory** or **U for Unsatisfactory** if that is the grading criteria. The second box may be used as a final demonstration with a **grade point** written in the box.

| STEPS | POSSIBLE POINTS | S/U | POINTS EARNED |
|---|---|---|---|
| 1. Grasp the palm of the glove of your nondominant hand with your gloved dominant hand without touching bare skin. | 15 | | |
| 2. Remove the glove, turning it inside out. | 15 | | |
| 3. Continue to hold the glove in your dominant hand. | 10 | | |
| 4. Slide the thumb into the inside of the glove of the dominant hand without touching the outside of the glove. | 15 | | |
| 5. Continue to use the thumb to pull the glove over the fingers, removing the glove inside out and over the first glove, which is now inside the second glove with no outside areas exposed. | 15 | | |
| 6. Toss the gloves in the appropriate trash container. | 10 | | |
| 7. Wash your hands. | 20 | | |
| **Total Points (if applicable)** | 100 | | |

**Comments:** _____

_____

_____

**Final Evaluator's Signature:** _____

**Date:** _____

## CAAHEP Competencies Achieved

III. P (2) Practice standard precautions

III. P (4) Perform hand washing

## ABHES Competencies Achieved

9. b. Apply principles of aseptic techniques and infection control

9. i. Use standard precautions

## Test Your Knowledge
### Vocabulary Review

Match the key terms in the right column with the definitions in the left column by placing the letter of each correct answer in the space provided.

_____ **1.** a computer program designed to increase access speed by rearranging files stored on a disk to occupy contiguous storage locations, a technique commonly known as defragmenting

_____ **2.** a high-resolution printer that uses a technology similar to that of a photocopier; the fastest type of computer printer and produces the highest-quality output

_____ **3.** a pointing device with a ball that is rolled to position a pointer or cursor on a computer screen; can be directly attached to the computer or wireless

_____ **4.** a microprocessor, the primary computer chip responsible for interpreting and executing programs

_____ **5.** a system that links several computers together

_____ **6.** a pictorial image; on a computer screen, a graphic symbol that identifies a menu choice

_____ **7.** a roll of film stored on a reel and imprinted with information on a reduced scale to minimize storage space requirements

**a.** abuse [LO10.6]

**b.** antivirus software [LO10.4]

**c.** CD-ROM [LO10.4]

**d.** central processing unit (CPU) [LO10.2]

**e.** cover sheet [LO10.10]

**f.** covered entity [LO10.6]

**g.** cursor [LO10.1]

**h.** database [LO10.4]

**i.** disclaimer [LO10.6]

**j.** disk cleanup [LO10.4]

**k.** disk defragmentation [LO10.4]

**l.** dot-matrix printer [LO10.2]

**m.** digital subscriber line (DSL) [LO10.4]

**n.** electronic mail [LO10.4]

**o.** electronic media [LO10.4]

_____ **8.** a practice or behavior that is not indicative of, or in line with, sound medical or fiscal practices

_____ **9.** an optical device that converts printed matter into a format that can be read by the computer and inputs the converted information

_____ **10.** any information stored on a computer storage device

_____ **11.** a vertical housing for the system unit of a personal computer

_____ **12.** a blinking line or cube on a computer screen that shows where the next character that is keyed will appear

_____ **13.** a laptop or slate-shaped mobile computer, equipped with a touch screen or graphics table to operate the computer with a digital pen, or a fingertip instead of a keyboard or mouse

_____ **14.** more than one medium, such as in graphics, sound, and text, used to convey information

_____ **15.** a global network of computers

_____ **16.** an impact printer that creates characters by placing a series of tiny dots next to one another

_____ **17.** to rent an item or piece of equipment

_____ **18.** trying to determine and correct a problem without having to call a service supplier

_____ **19.** the process or technology of reading data in printed form by a device that scans and identifies characters

_____ **20.** a nonimpact printer that forms characters by using a series of dots created by tiny drops of ink

_____ **21.** a device used to transfer information from one computer to another through telephone lines

_____ **22.** software that prevents and removes computer viruses; may also detect and remove adware and spyware

_____ **23.** a program that automatically changes the monitor display at short intervals or constantly shows moving images

**p.** firewall [LO10.4]

**q.** hard copy [LO10.10]

**r.** hardware [LO10.2]

**s.** icon [LO10.4]

**t.** ink-jet printer [LO10.2]

**u.** interactive pager [LO10.10]

**v.** Internet [LO10.2]

**w.** LAN [LO10.8]

**x.** laser printer [LO10.2]

**y.** lease [LO10.5]

**z.** maintenance contract [LO10.5]

**aa.** microfiche [LO10.8]

**bb.** microfilm [LO10.8]

**cc.** modem [LO10.2]

**dd.** motherboard [LO10.2]

**ee.** mouse [LO10.2]

**ff.** multimedia [LO10.8]

**gg.** multitasking [LO10.8]

**hh.** network [LO10.4]

**ii.** optical character recognition (OCR) [LO10.8]

**jj.** random access memory (RAM) [LO10.4]

**kk.** read-only memory [LO10.4]

**ll.** scanner [LO10.2]

**mm.** screen saver [LO10.4]

**nn.** service contract [LO10.5]

**oo.** software [LO10.4]

**pp.** tablet PC [LO10.2]

to prevent burn-in of images on the computer screen

___ **24.** a system that protects a computer network from unauthorized access by users on its own network or another network such as the Internet

___ **25.** a small program included in a software package designed to give users an overall picture of the product and its functions

___ **26.** a collection of records created and stored on a computer

___ **27.** A type of pointing device common to laptop and notebook computers that directs activity on the computer screen by positioning a pointer or cursor on the screen; a small, flat device, or surface that is highly sensitive to touch

___ **28.** running two or more computer software programs simultaneously

___ **29.** abbreviation for local-area network

___ **30.** a type of modem that operates over telephone lines but uses a different frequency than a telephone, allowing a computer to access the Internet at the same time that a telephone is being used

___ **31.** a contract that specifies when a piece of equipment will be cleaned, checked for worn parts, and repaired

___ **32.** abbreviation for virtual private network; used to connect two or more computer systems

___ **33.** a form sent with faxed information providing details about the transmission and a disclaimer regarding faxes received in error

___ **34.** the temporary, or programmable, memory in a computer

___ **35.** the main circuit board of a computer that controls the other components in the system

___ **36.** a contract that covers services for equipment that are not included in a standard maintenance contract

___ **37.** a readable paper copy or printout of information

**qq.** touchpad [LO10.2]

**rr.** touch screen [LO10.2]

**ss.** tower case [LO10.2]

**tt.** trackball [LO10.2]

**uu.** troubleshooting [LO10.7]

**vv.** tutorial [LO10.4]

**ww.** voice mail [LO10.8]

**xx.** VPN [LO10.9]

**yy.** WAN [LO10.8]

**zz.** warranty [LO10.5]

**aaa.** zip drive [LO10.4]

_____ **38.** a digital answering service provided by the phone company that allows a caller to leave a message if the phone line or person requested is busy

_____ **39.** a statement of denial of legal liability or that refutes the authenticity of a claim

_____ **40.** a type of computer monitor that acts as an intake device, receiving information through the touch of a pen, wand, or hand directly to the screen

_____ **41.** a contract that specifies free service and replacement of parts for a piece of equipment during a specified period of time, often a year

_____ **42.** a method of sending and receiving messages through a computer network; commonly known as e-mail

_____ **43.** microfilm in rectangular sheets

_____ **44.** a high-capacity, removable disk drive developed by Iomega

_____ **45.** any organization that transmits health information in an electronic form that is related in any way with a HIPAA-covered entity

_____ **46.** a computer's permanent memory, which can be read by the computer but not changed; provides the computer with the basic operating instructions it needs to function

_____ **47.** a pager designed for two-way communication; a screen displays a printed message and allows the receiver to respond by way of a mini keyboard

_____ **48.** a pointing device that can be added to a computer that directs activity on the computer screen by positioning a pointer or cursor on the screen; can be directly attached to the computer or can be wireless

_____ **49.** a compact disc that contains software programs; an abbreviation for compact disc read-only memory

_____ **50.** the physical components of a computer system, including the monitor, keyboard, and printer

_____ **51.** abbreviation for wide area network

_____ **52.** a computer maintenance utility designed to free up disk space on a computer hard drive

# Multiple-Choice Certification Questions

There may be more than one answer; circle the letter of the choice that best completes each statement or answers each question.

1. **[LO10.2]** Computer hardware devices are connected by cables such as
   a. extension cables.
   b. hardware and software bands.
   c. USB or serial cables.
   d. monitor connectors.
   e. None of the above.

2. **[LO10.2]** Carpal tunnel syndrome is associated with
   a. repetitive hand and finger motions.
   b. hand disorders from excessive computer use.
   c. tingling in the hands.
   d. weakness of the fingers.
   e. All of the above.

3. **[LO10.8]** A major reason that a scanner is so important in a medical office is that it
   a. can eliminate the need for word processing.
   b. makes it possible for an office to move to a paperless medical system.
   c. transcribes handwritten information to a word-processed format.
   d. can eliminate the need for fax machines.
   e. can merge software files into one folder.

4. **[LO10.8]** Which of the following devices will probably become obsolete because the storage capacity is not as great as other devices?
   a. Diskette
   b. Jump drive
   c. Zip drive
   d. DVD
   e. CD

5. **[LO10.3]** Which of the following is *not* a software program?
   a. Word
   b. Excel
   c. MediSoft
   d. Dot matrix
   e. PowerPoint

6. **[LO10.10]** Principles of managing e-mail include
   a. checking e-mail once a day just prior to leaving the office.
   b. not opening e-mail when you cannot identify the sender.
   c. discarding all e-mail that contains health information.
   d. keeping all e-mail for at least six months.
   e. not allowing any subfolders in the e-mail system.

7. **[LO10.6]** When sending e-mail within a medical practice, which of the following practices would *not* be compliant with HIPAA regulations?
   a. Maintain virus protection to guard your computer system.
   b. Always check the patient's medical record and computer for any special instructions for contacting the patient through e-mail.
   c. When in doubt, always send an e-mail with the patient information.
   d. Obtain authorization from the patient to send protected health information via e-mail.
   e. Even though it is more convenient, always follow patient requests not to send information via e-mail transmission.

**8.** [LO10.5] Which of the following is *not* a consideration when choosing an online service?
   a. The rate of speed and accessibility of services
   b. A free trial membership
   c. A local-access telephone number
   d. Good availability to medical information
   e. The monthly billing cycle of the service

**9.** [LO10.7] Which of the following is sound advice for using the technical support of an online service?
   a. Allow adequate uninterrupted time to spend on the phone with the technical support person.
   b. Contact the technical support before you try to check the system for errors that you might be able to fix.
   c. Call the technical support office to inquire about problems before you discuss it with your supervisor.
   d. Call the technical support center from a private area away from the computer.
   e. Do not use the technical support for questions regarding new software, only for hardware questions.

**10.** [LO10.7] The purpose of disk cleanup is to
   a. test antivirus software.
   b. check the status of the hard drive.
   c. free up space on the computer.
   d. add files to a jump drive.
   e. merge several documents into one.

**11.** [LO10.7] Which of the following is the main function of a screen saver?
   a. It eliminates the need to clean and dust the monitor screen.
   b. It provides a shield or cover to protect the software programs.
   c. It is a means to display personal pictures of the employee's family.
   d. When the computer is not in use, it automatically changes the monitor display at short intervals to hide private information.
   e. None of the above.

**12.** [LO10.7] When setting up a computer disaster recovery plan it is important to
   a. minimize damage to computer equipment.
   b. back up computer systems once a month.
   c. disregard HIPAA regulations in order to recover protected health information.
   d. not store any information on a hard drive but always use floppy disks to ensure there is always a back-up of information.
   e. develop a plan in-house and don't rely on any purchased software application or service.

**13.** [LO10.8] New technology that will allow physicians to provide better care for patients in rural areas is the use of
   a. diskettes with medical information loaded on them.
   b. telemedicine using video images of patient information.
   c. jump drives to load medical information patients can read.
   d. speech recognition to interpret spoken word into print.
   e. random access to provide more immediate care to patients.

**14.** [LO10.8] The advantage to utilizing an automated voice response unit in a medical practice is that it
   a. enhances the service provided to the patient.
   b. is an alternative to requiring multiple receptionists answering the phones.
   c. provides greater flexibility for the medical staff.
   d. gives the caller various options for immediate routing of their call.
   e. does all of the above.

**15.** [LO10.9] Which of the following is *not* a benefit to using a cell phone within a medical practice?
   a. The physician can respond quickly to a message from the staff.
   b. Key employees who conduct business for the practice outside the office can utilize a business cell phone.

c. Office staff can use cell phones in case of emergency when the traditional phone system fails.

d. Cell phones can interfere with electronic equipment that may be functioning inside the medical practice.

e. Physicians are able to respond more quickly to hospital calls.

**16.** [LO10.6] Which of the following is an appropriate message for an administrative medical assistant to leave on an answering machine?

a. "Please call this office immediately at 555-601-2345."

b. "This is your gynecologist's office calling with your test results. Please call us at 555-601-2345."

c. "This is Mary with Dr. Miller's office. Please contact us between 9:00 A.M. and 4:00 P.M. at 555-601-2345."

d. "This is Dr. Miller's office calling with your Pap results. Please call us."

e. "Dr. Miller's office calling with your pregnancy results. Call me at 555-601-2345."

**17.** [LO10.9] Which of the following is important when utilizing a fax machine?

a. Faxing documents should only be done in case of emergency since faxing documents is more expensive than using a telephone.

b. Overnight mail service is a better method than faxing when you need to get medical information to a referring physician by the next day.

c. A fax machine in a medical office should have its own telephone line so it does not tie up other telephone lines.

d. Faxed documents do not have the same information as the original document so some information may be lost.

e. None of the above.

**18.** [LO10.10] A cover sheet should always be used when faxing because

a. it is office policy.

b. it provides information about the transmission.

c. it is the law in all states.

d. HIPAA requires the use of cover sheets.

e. it ensures the fax will always be delivered to the correct person.

**19.** [LO10.8] A postage meter is ideal to use in a medical practice because it

a. provides the exact amount of postage needed for each item.

b. saves frequent trips to the post office.

c. can be refilled by a postage meter service.

d. applies the postage directly to the letter.

e. does all of the above.

**20.** [LO10.5] A benefit of leasing office equipment is

a. the office owns the equipment after the first few payments.

b. the office is never responsible for equipment maintenance.

c. the office staff does not have to negotiate leasing prices.

d. the equipment is a higher grade product than what the office could afford if purchased outright.

e. in most cases, businesses are able to take lease payments as a tax deduction each year.

**21.** [LO10.12] Which of the following is *not* considered information that is needed on an equipment inventory list?

a. The brand name of the equipment

b. A brief description of the equipment

c. The date the piece of equipment was purchased

d. How the piece of equipment is used

e. The model and registration number

**22.** [LO10.2] Which of the following devices is *not* a pointing device used with computers?

a. Modem

b. Mouse

c. Trackball

d. Touchpad

e. Touch screen

**23.** [LO10.10] In order to avoid physical strain when using a computer, you should
  a. keep your arms straight and not bent at the elbows.
  b. use a great amount of pressure to push on the keys so you don't have to repeat the key strikes.
  c. work for longer time periods in order to get the job completed sooner.
  d. use two hands to strike keys simultaneously such as "control" and "F1".
  e. keep your feet crossed at the ankles in order to relax your legs.

**24.** [LO10.1] The primary computer chip or microprocessor responsible for interpreting and executing programs is called the
  a. CPU.
  b. RAM.
  c. ROM.
  d. DVD.
  e. CD-ROM.

**25.** [LO10.5] The fastest and highest quality printer is a/an
  a. ink-jet printer.
  b. laser printer.
  c. dot-matrix printer.
  d. modem printer.
  e. scan printer.

## True or False

Decide whether each statement is true or false. In the space at the left, write "T" for true or "F" for false. On the lines provided, rewrite the false statements to make them true.

_____ **1.** [LO10.9] A scanner is a device that can be used to transport a document from one medical practice to another through a telephone line.

_____

_____ **2.** [LO10.3] Windows is an operating system that is not very beneficial because it cannot multitask very well.

_____

_____ **3.** [LO10.3] Software is a program or set of instructions that tells the computer what to do.

_____

_____ **4.** [LO10.10] Good e-mail management requires that you check your mailbox frequently and empty any unwanted e-mails.

_____

_____ **5.** [LO10.3] A database is a collection of records that can be created but not stored on a computer.

_____

_____ **6.** [LO10.12] A computer virus protection application on the computer will guard your system against infections that enter through the e-mail system.

_____

**7.** [LO10.9] A cable modem or DSL through a phone line is not desirable because it interferes with the regular telephone service at the facility.

_____

**8.** [LO10.7] When there is a computer problem requiring assistance from technical support, it is best to follow what the manual says instead of what the technical support representative tells you on the phone.

_____

**9.** [LO10.1] A disadvantage of using a computer network in a medical practice is that only one person can view and work on a patient file at one time.

_____

**10.** [LO10.6] Access codes or passwords only allow the user into approved areas according to the individual's job description.

_____

## Sentence Completion

In the space provided, write the word or phrase that best completes each sentence.

**1.** [LO10.1] Hardware comprises the physical components of a computer system, including the _____, _____ and _____.

**2.** [LO10.10] When you use the keyboard, it is important to position your hands properly to _____ _____.

**3.** [LO10.3] Computer software is generally divided into two categories, _____ system and _____ software.

**4.** [LO10.4] Accounting and billing software is useful in an office because it enables you to perform tasks including tracking patients' accounts, creating _____ _____, preparing _____ _____, and maintaining _____ records.

**5.** [LO10.6] HIPAA law requires that all transactions containing personal health information be _____.

**6.** [LO10.8] _____ _____ are specialized Web sites that search other Web sites for information.

**7.** [LO10.6] Great care must be taken to safeguard confidential files, make _____ copies on a regular basis, and prevent system _____.

**1.** _____
   _____

**2.** _____
   _____

**3.** _____
   _____

**4.** _____
   _____

**5.** _____
   _____

**6.** _____
   _____

**7.** _____
   _____

**8.** **[LO10.4]** Antivirus software responds to _____, persons that abuse e-mails by sending them en masse without permission.

**9.** **[LO10.6]** All computers should automatically log the user off after a period of no activity. The computer should require that all users must _____ their _____ to regain access after an idle period.

**10.** **[LO10.6]** Firewalls are helpful in putting a stop to offensive Internet sites and potential _____ _____.

**8.** _____
_____

**9.** _____
_____

**10.** _____
_____

# Apply Your Knowledge

## Short Answer

Write the answer to each question on the lines provided.

**1.** **[LO10.7]** List three steps in troubleshooting a problem with a piece of equipment.

_____

_____

_____

**2.** **[LO10.11]** List five items found on an equipment inventory document and why each is required.

_____

_____

_____

**3.** **[LO10.5]** Provide two reasons why leasing office equipment might be better than purchasing equipment.

_____

_____

_____

**4.** **[LO10.6]** Give three practices that should be followed when working with personal health information in order to comply with HIPAA laws.

_____

_____

_____

**5.** [LO10.8] List two areas of advancement in the use of computer equipment that have led to more efficiency in the medical office.

_____

_____

_____

## Problem-Solving Activities

Follow the directions for each activity.

**1.** [LO10.6] Medical Office Sign—Patient Cell Phone Use
   a. Using a word processing application, develop an 8½ × 11 inch sign that would be posted at the reception area of a medical office.
   b. The sign is notifying patients about the office's policy about no cell phone use.
   c. The sign should reflect a friendly attitude but also disclose why cell phones are not allowed in the office.
   d. The sign should be developed using a font size that is easy to read by patients in the immediate reception area.

**2.** [LO10.10] Internet Research—Carpal Tunnel Syndrome
   a. Go to the eMedicineHealth Web site at www.emedicinehealth.com.
   b. Type in the words "carpal tunnel syndrome" in the search box.
   c. Research the information provided about carpal tunnel syndrome and find at least five symptoms associated with this condition.
   d. From the information provided at this Web site, list three suggested treatment methods for this condition.
   e. Word process the information you researched and print out your document.

## Thinking Critically

Write your response to each case study question on the lines provided.

### Case 1 [LO10.4]

A coworker in your medical office is not comfortable operating the new appointment scheduling software that has been added to the computers. The vendor that supplied the software provided an in-service training for the office staff; however, this employee called in sick on the day of the training. She always seems to be busy or volunteers to do other things in order to avoid having to do the appointment scheduling. Every time you try to talk with her she says, "I'm not a computer techie like you are." You believe she is not willing to accept the change to the new application and is trying to avoid learning how to use it.

**1.** What do you think are some of the reasons why an employee would not want to learn how to perform his or her job and understand the operation of a new software application?

_____

_____

_____

**2.** How would you approach this employee and try to convince her to do the training?

_____

_____

_____

## Case 2 [LO10.10]

You are employed in a medical office that uses a postage meter to apply postage to letters that are mailed out during the billing cycle. You overhear a conversation between two coworkers who are operating the machine. One of the employees says that she forgot to pick up postage stamps for a couple of bills she needs to mail out today. The other employee says to just run them through the postage meter, that no one will even know.

**1.** What is the main problem or issue in this scenario? If the employee does use postage from the meter, what are the consequences she may face?

_____

_____

_____

**2.** As a coworker, what is your responsibility to intervene in this situation?

_____

_____

_____

## Case 3 [LO10.4]

A coworker has been asked by the physician to compose a letter that will be mailed to all the patients notifying them of the addition of a new physician to the practice. The employee completes the letter and asks if you will quickly read it and see if it looks all right before she hands it the physician to sign. As you start to read the letter you realize that there are numerous grammatical errors and misspelled words. If you don't point out the errors to her, it would be very embarrassing for her to give it to the physician the way it is. You also believe that if you assist her in making the corrections, she could take the corrected letter to the physician and present it as her own work.

**1.** What is the best way for you to handle this situation?

_____

_____

_____

**2.** How can you help this employee in the future to improve her skills?

_____

_____

_____

# Demonstrate Your Knowledge

**Student Name:** _____

## Procedure 10-1: Creating a Letter Using Word Processing Software

**GOAL:** To use a word processing program to create a form letter document

**MATERIALS:** Computer equipped with a word processing program, printer, form letter document to be created, 8½ × 11 inch paper

**METHOD:** To pass this procedure the minimum required score is _____% or all elements must meet "satisfactory" ability on the final demonstration. The first box may be used as a practice or final demonstration, with the evaluator placing **S for Satisfactory** or **U for Unsatisfactory** if that is the grading criteria. The second box may be used as a final demonstration with a **grade point** written in the box.

| STEPS | POSSIBLE POINTS | S/U | POINTS EARNED |
|---|---|---|---|
| 1. Turn on the computer. Select the word processing program. | 10 | | |
| 2. Use the keyboard to begin entering text into a new document. | 15 | | |
| 3. To edit text, press the arrow keys to move the cursor to the position at which you want to insert or delete characters, and enter the text. Either type directly or use the "Insert" mode to type over and replace existing text. | 15 | | |
| 4. To delete text, position the cursor to the left of the characters to be deleted and press the "Delete" key. Alternately, place the cursor to the right of the characters to be deleted and press the "Backspace" key (the left-pointing arrow usually found at the top right corner of the keyboard). | 15 | | |
| 5. If you need to move an entire block of text, you must begin by highlighting it. In most Windows-based programs, you first click the mouse at the beginning of the text to be highlighted. Then you hold down the left mouse button, drag the mouse to the end of the block of text, and release your finger from the mouse. The text should now be highlighted. Right-click the mouse and choose the button or command for cutting text. Then move the cursor to the place where you want to insert the text, right-click the mouse again, and select the button or command for retrieving or pasting text. | 15 | | |

*(Continued)*

| STEPS | POSSIBLE POINTS | S/U | POINTS EARNED |
|---|---|---|---|
| 6. As you input the letter document, it is important to save your work every 15 minutes or so. Some programs do this automatically. If yours does not, use the "Save" command or button to save the file. Be sure to save the file again when you have completed the letter. | 10 | | |
| 7. Carefully proofread the document and use the spell-checker, correcting any errors in spelling, grammar, or formatting. | 15 | | |
| 8. Print the letter using the "Print" command or button. | 5 | | |
| **Total Points (if applicable)** | 100 | | |

Comments: _____

_____

_____


Final Evaluator's Signature: _____


Date: _____

## CAAHEP Competencies Achieved

IV. C (8) Recognize elements of fundamental writing skills

IV. C (9) Discuss applications of electronic technology in effective communication

IV. C (12) Organize technical information and summaries

IV. P (2) Report relevant information to others succinctly and accurately

IV. P (10) Compose professional business letters

IV. A (8) Analyze communications in providing appropriate responses/feedback

## ABHES Competencies Achieved

7. a. Perform basic keyboarding skills including:

    (1) Locating the keys on a keyboard

    (2) Typing medical correspondence and basic reports

7. b. Identify and properly utilize office machines, computerized systems, and medical software such as:

    (1) Efficiently maintain and understand different types of medical correspondence and medical reports

    (2) Apply computer application skills using a variety of different electronic programs including both practice management software and EMR software

8. gg. Use pertinent medical terminology

8. hh. Receive, organize, prioritize, and transmit information expediently

8. jj. Perform fundamental writing skills, including correct grammar, spelling, and formatting

8. ll. Apply electronic technology

## Procedure 10–2: Using a Facsimile (Fax) Machine

**GOAL:** To correctly prepare and send a fax document, while following all HIPAA guidelines to guard patient confidentiality

**MATERIALS:** Fax machine, fax line, cover sheet with statement of disclaimer, area code and phone number of fax recipient, document to be faxed, telephone line, telephone

**METHOD:** To pass this procedure the minimum required score is _____ % or all elements must meet "satisfactory" ability on the final demonstration. The first box may be used as a practice or final demonstration, with the evaluator placing **S for Satisfactory** or **U for Unsatisfactory** if that is the grading criteria. The second box may be used as a final demonstration with a **grade point** written in the box.

| STEPS | POSSIBLE POINTS | S/U | POINTS EARNED |
|---|---|---|---|
| 1. Prepare a cover sheet, which provides information about the transmission. Cover sheets can vary in appearance but usually include the name, telephone number, and fax number of the sender and the receiver; the number of pages being transmitted; and the data of the transmission. Preprinted cover sheets can be used. | 15 | | |
| 2. All cover sheets must carry a statement of disclaimer to guard the privacy of the patient. A disclaimer is a statement of denial of legal liability. A disclaimer should be included on the cover sheet and may read something like the following: *This fax contains confidential or proprietary information that may be legally privileged. It is intended only for the named recipient(s). If an addressing or transmission error has misdirected the fax, please notify the author by replying to this message. If you are not the named recipient, you are not authorized to use, disclose, distribute, copy, print, or rely on this fax and should immediately shred it.* | 15 | | |
| 3. Place all pages of the document, including the cover sheet, either facedown or face up in the fax machine's sending tray, depending on the directions stamped on the sending tray. | 10 | | |
| 4. If the documents are placed facedown, write the area code and fax number on the back of the last page. | 5 | | |
| 5. Dial the telephone number of the receiving fax machine, using either the telephone attached to the fax machine or the numbers on the fax keyboard. Include the area code for long-distance calls. | 15 | | |

*(Continued)*

| STEPS | POSSIBLE POINTS | S/U | POINTS EARNED |
|---|---|---|---|
| 6. When using a fax telephone, listen for a high-pitched tone. Then press the "Send" or "Start" button, and hang up the telephone. This step completes the call circuit in older model fax machines. Your fax is now being sent. Newer fax machines do not require this step. | 10 | | |
| 7. If you use the fax keyboard, press the "Send" or "Start" button after dialing the telephone number. This button will start the call. | 5 | | |
| 8. Watch for the fax machine to make a connection. Often a green light appears as the document feeds through the machine. | 0 | | |
| 9. If the fax machine is not able to make a connection, as when the receiving fax line is busy, it may have a feature that automatically redials the number every few minutes for a specified number of attempts. | 5 | | |
| 10. When a fax has been successfully sent, most fax machines print a confirmation message. When a fax has not been sent, the machine either prints an error message or indicates on the screen that the transmission was unsuccessful. | 0 | | |
| 11. Attach the confirmation or error message to the documents faxed. File appropriately. | 10 | | |
| 12. If required by office policy, the sender should call the recipient to confirm the fax was received. | 10 | | |
| **Total Points (if applicable)** | 100 | | |

**Comments:** _____

_____

_____

**Final Evaluator's Signature:** _____

**Date:** _____

## CAAHEP Competencies Achieved

IV. C (9) Discuss applications of electronic technology in effective communication

V. P (6) Use office hardware and software to maintain office systems

## ABHES Competencies Achieved

7. b. Identify and properly utilize office machines, computerized systems, and medical software

8. ll. Apply electronic technology

**Student Name:** _____

## Procedure 10–3: Using a Photocopier Machine

**GOAL:** To produce copies of documents

**MATERIALS:** Copier machine, copy paper, documents to be copied

**METHOD:** To pass this procedure the minimum required score is _____% or all elements must meet "satisfactory" ability on the final demonstration. The first box may be used as a practice or final demonstration, with the evaluator placing **S for Satisfactory** or **U for Unsatisfactory** if that is the grading criteria. The second box may be used as a final demonstration with a **grade point** written in the box.

| STEPS | POSSIBLE POINTS | S/U | POINTS EARNED |
|---|---|---|---|
| 1. Make sure the machine is turned on and warmed up. It will display a signal when it is ready for copying. | 10 | | |
| 2. Assemble and prepare your materials, removing paper clips, staples, and self-adhesive flags. | 15 | | |
| 3. Place the document to be copied in the automatic feeder tray as directed, or upside down directly on the glass. The feeder tray can accommodate many pages; you may place only one page at a time on the glass. Automatic feeding is a faster process, and you should use it when you wish to collate stapled packets. Page-by-page copying is best if you need to copy a single sheet or to enlarge or reduce the image. To use any special features, such as making double-sided copies or stapling the copies, press the designated button on the machine. | 25 | | |
| 4. Set the machine for the desired paper size. | 10 | | |
| 5. Key in the number of copies you want to make, and press the "Start" button. The copies are made automatically. | 10 | | |
| 6. Press the "Clear" or "Reset" button when your job is finished. | 10 | | |
| 7. If the copier becomes jammed, follow the directions on the machine to locate the problem (for example, there may be multiple pieces of paper stuck inside the printer), and dislodge the jammed paper. Most copy machines will show a diagram of the printer and the location of the problem. | 20 | | |
| **Total Points (if applicable)** | 100 | | |

**Comments:** _____

_____

_____

**Final Evaluator's Signature:** _____

**Date:** _____

## CAAHEP Competencies Achieved

IV. C (9) Discuss applications of electronic technology in effective communication

V. P (6) Use office hardware and software to maintain office systems

## ABHES Competencies Achieved

7. b. Identify and properly utilize office machines, computerized systems, and medical software

8. kk. Adapt to individualized needs

8. ll. Apply electronic technology

## Procedure 10–4: Using a Postage Meter

**GOAL:** To correctly apply postage to an envelope or package for mailing, according to U.S. Postal Service guidelines

**MATERIALS:** Postage meter, addressed envelope or package, postal scale

**METHOD:** To pass this procedure the minimum required score is _____ % or all elements must meet "satisfactory" ability on the final demonstration. The first box may be used as a practice or final demonstration, with the evaluator placing **S for Satisfactory** or **U for Unsatisfactory** if that is the grading criteria. The second box may be used as a final demonstration with a **grade point** written in the box.

| STEPS | POSSIBLE POINTS | S/U | POINTS EARNED |
|---|:---:|:---:|:---:|
| 1. Check that there is postage available in the postage meter. | 5 | | |
| 2. Verify the day's date. | 5 | | |
| 3. Check that the postage meter is plugged in and switched on before you proceed. | 5 | | |
| 4. Locate the area where the meter registers the date. Many machines have a lid that can be flipped up, with rows of numbers underneath. Months are represented numerically, with the number "1" indicating the month of January, "2" indicating February, and so on. Check that the date is correct. If it is incorrect, change the number to the correct date. | 10 | | |
| 5. Make sure that all materials have been included in the envelope or package. Weigh the envelope or package on a postal scale. Standard business envelopes weighing up to 1 oz. require the minimum postage (the equivalent of one first-class stamp). Oversize envelopes and packages require additional postage. A postal scale will indicate the amount of postage required. | 15 | | |
| 6. Key in the postage amount on the meter, and press the button that enters the amount. For amounts over $1, press the $ sign or the "Enter" button twice. | 15 | | |
| 7. Check that the amount you typed is the correct amount. Envelopes and packages with too little postage will be returned by the U.S. Postal Service. Sending an envelope or package with too much postage is wasteful to the practice. | 10 | | |

*(Continued)*

| STEPS | POSSIBLE POINTS | S/U | POINTS EARNED |
|---|---|---|---|
| 8. While applying postage to an envelope, hold it flat and right side up (so that you can read the address). Seal the envelope (unless the meter seals it for you). Locate the plate or area where the envelope slides through. This feature is usually near the bottom of the meter. Place the envelope on the left side, and give it a gentle push toward the right. Some models hold the envelope in a stationary position. (If the meter seals the envelope for you, it is especially important that you insert it correctly to allow for sealing.) The meter will grab the envelope and pull it through quickly. | 15 | | |
| 9. For packages, create a postage label to affix to the package. Follow the same procedure for a label as for an envelope. Affix the postmarked label on the package in the upper right corner. | 10 | | |
| 10. Check that the printed postmark has the correct date and amount and that everything written or stamped on the envelope or package is legible. | 10 | | |
| **Total Points (if applicable)** | 100 | | |

**Comments:** _____

_____

_____

**Final Evaluator's Signature:** _____

**Date:** _____

### CAAHEP Competencies Achieved

IV. C (9) Discuss applications of electronic technology in effective communication

V. P (6) Use office hardware and software to maintain office systems

### ABHES Competencies Achieved

7. b. Identify and properly utilize office machines, computerized systems, and medical software

8. kk. Adapt to individualized needs

8. ll. Apply electronic technology

## Procedure 10–5: Using a Dictation-Transcription Machine

**GOAL:** To correctly use a dictation-transcription machine to convert verbal communication into the written word

**MATERIALS:** Dictation-transcription machine, audiocassette or magnetic tape or disk with the recorded dictation, word processor or computer, and printer

**METHOD:** To pass this procedure the minimum required score is _____% or all elements must meet "satisfactory" ability on the final demonstration. The first box may be used as a practice or final demonstration, with the evaluator placing **S for Satisfactory** or **U for Unsatisfactory** if that is the grading criteria. The second box may be used as a final demonstration with a **grade point** written in the box.

| STEPS | POSSIBLE POINTS | S/U | POINTS EARNED |
|---|---|---|---|
| 1. Assemble all the necessary equipment. | 0 | | |
| 2. Select a transcription tape, cassette, or disk for dictation. Select any transcriptions marked "Urgent" first. If there are none, select the oldest-dated transcription first. | 5 | | |
| 3. Turn on all equipment and adjust it according to personal preference. | 5 | | |
| 4. Prepare the format and style for the selected letter or form. | 15 | | |
| 5. Insert the tape or cassette and rewind. | 5 | | |
| 6. While listening to the transcription tape, cassette, or disk, key in the text. | 20 | | |
| 7. Adjust the speed and volume controls as needed. | 15 | | |
| 8. Proofread and spell-check the final document, making any corrections. | 20 | | |
| 9. Print the document for approval and signature. | 10 | | |
| 10. Turn off all equipment. Place the transcription tape, cassette, or disk in the proper storage area. | 5 | | |
| **Total Points (if applicable)** | 100 | | |

Comments: _____

_____

_____

Final Evaluator's Signature: _____

Date: _____

## CAAHEP Competencies Achieved

IV. C (9) Discuss applications of electronic technology in effective communication

V. P (6) Use office hardware and software to maintain office systems

V. P (7) Use the Internet to access information related to the medical office

## ABHES Competencies Achieved

7. b. Identify and properly utilize office machines, computerized systems, and medical software

8. kk. Adapt to individualized needs

8. ll. Apply electronic technology

Student Name: _____

## Procedure 10–6: Using a Check-Writing Machine

**GOAL:** To produce a check using a check-writing machine

**MATERIALS:** Check-writing machine, blank checks, office checkbook or accounting system

**METHOD:** To pass this procedure the minimum required score is _____ % or all elements must meet "satisfactory" ability on the final demonstration. The first box may be used as a practice or final demonstration, with the evaluator placing **S for Satisfactory** or **U for Unsatisfactory** if that is the grading criteria. The second box may be used as a final demonstration with a **grade point** written in the box.

| STEPS | POSSIBLE POINTS | S/U | POINTS EARNED |
|---|---|---|---|
| 1. Assemble all equipment. | 10 | | |
| 2. Turn on the check-writing machine. | 5 | | |
| 3. Place a blank check or a sheet of blank checks into the machine. | 15 | | |
| 4. Key in the date, the payee's name, and the payment amount. The check-writing machine imprints the check with this information, perforating it with the payee's name. The perforations are actual little holes in the paper, which prevent anyone from changing the name on the check. | 25 | | |
| 5. Turn off the check-writing machine. | 5 | | |
| 6. Have a doctor or another authorized person then sign the check. | 20 | | |
| 7. To complete the process, record the check in the office checkbook or accounting system. | 20 | | |
| **Total Points (if applicable)** | 100 | | |

Comments: _____

Final Evaluator's Signature: _____

Date: _____

### CAAHEP Competencies Achieved

IV. C (9) Discuss applications of electronic technology in effective communication

V. P (6) Use office hardware and software to maintain office systems

V. P (7) Use the Internet to access information related to the medical office

### ABHES Competencies Achieved

7. b. Identify and properly utilize office machines, computerized systems, and medical software

8. kk. Adapt to individualized needs

8. ll. Apply electronic technology

# 11

# Telecommunications in the Health-Care Setting

## Test Your Knowledge

### Vocabulary Review

Match the key terms in the right column with the definitions in the left column by placing the letter of each correct answer in the space provided.

| | | |
|---|---|---|
| _____ | **1.** the sounding out of words | **a.** enunciation [LO11.1] |
| _____ | **2.** the high or low quality in the sound of a person's speaking voice | **b.** etiquette [LO11.2] |
| _____ | **3.** a process of determining the level of urgency of each incoming telephone call and how it should be handled | **c.** pitch [LO11.1] |
| _____ | **4.** clear and distinct speaking | **d.** pronunciation [LO11.1] |
| _____ | **5.** a specially designed telephone, which looks very much like a laptop with a cradle for the telephone receiver, used for communicating with the deaf; they may type their responses, which appear on a screen | **e.** telephone triage [LO11.6] |
| | | **f.** telecommunication device for the deaf [LO11.1] |
| _____ | **6.** good manners | |

### Multiple-Choice Certification Questions

There may be more than one answer; circle the letter of the choice that best completes each statement or answers each question.

**1.** [LO11.2] When checking for understanding during a call, the administrative medical assistant should
   a. watch the caller for visual signals.
   b. periodically ask the caller if there are any questions about the conversation.
   c. repeat everything at least twice.
   d. ask the caller to explain the information to another person.
   e. speak louder into the phone.

**2.** [LO11.3] If the caller refuses to discuss her symptoms with anyone but the physician, you should
   a. ask the patient to make an appointment immediately.
   b. try to talk the patient into talking with you.
   c. tell the patient that you are authorized to answer her questions.
   d. call the patient the next day to see whether she still needs to talk with the physician.
   e. have the physician return the call to the patient.

**3.** [LO11.1] Pronunciation is
   a. the high or low level of speech.
   b. the pitch of the voice.
   c. the tone of the voice.
   d. saying words correctly.
   e. speaking without any accent.

**4.** [LO11.6] Telephone triage is
   a. the screening and sorting of emergency incidents over the phone.
   b. a procedure that should only be assigned to registered nurses.
   c. an automatic message that is routed through a programmed automatic router.
   d. a means of diagnosing the patient over the phone.
   e. a method that the administrative medical assistant can use to recommend treatment over the phone.

**5.** [LO11.1] A TDD allows patients to
   a. hear the caller on the phone much louder.
   b. make phone calls using an amplifier.
   c. view a written message on their device.
   d. better access the office's automated phone system.
   e. amplify the message the caller is sending.

**6.** [LO11.2] When telecommunicating, HIPAA guidelines require that you
   a. utilize proper triage techniques to sort out calls.
   b. provide telecommunication devices for the deaf with all patients that are hard of hearing.
   c. route all calls to the physician to maintain confidentiality of private information.
   d. secure computer monitors so others do not have access to personal medical information.
   e. keep all telephone logs in a locked cabinet when not in use.

**7.** [LO11.4] Calls that can be handled by the administrative medical assistant include all of the following *except*
   a. prescribing medications for a patient when his pharmacy calls.
   b. scheduling appointments.
   c. taking laboratory reports from the hospital laboratory.
   d. arranging referrals to other physicians.
   e. answering insurance-related questions for a patient.

**8.** [LO11.4] A call that should be referred immediately to the physician is a call from a
   a. patient who is complaining about his recent bill.
   b. referring physician.
   c. pharmaceutical salesperson who is a close friend of the physician.
   d. pharmacy inquiring about the number of refills a patient has remaining.
   e. patient who is hysterical on the phone and appears to have a medical emergency.

**9.** [LO11.3] When a patient calls inquiring about an error on her bill, the administrative medical assistant should
   a. refer the caller to the physician.
   b. tell the patient to call back when the office is not busy hoping she will not call back.
   c. give the patient the phone number of the practice's accountant.
   d. tell the patient that the error will be investigated and that a return call will be made as soon as possible.
   e. tell the patient that the office billing system does not make errors and that she needs to put the patient's request in writing.

**10.** [LO11.3] When a caller will not identify himself the administrative medical assistant should
   a. hang up immediately.
   b. transfer the call to the answering machine.
   c. put the caller on hold until he hangs up.
   d. tell the caller that you will call the police.
   e. ask the caller to identify himself and ask for the phone number he is calling from.

**11.** [LO11.6] Which of the following would be a recommended action when a caller describes symptoms that need immediate or emergency medical intervention?
   a. Ask the caller to stay on the phone and have another staff member call 911.
   b. Immediately transfer the call to the physician.
   c. Get the caller's phone number and transfer the call to the office nurse.
   d. Keep the caller on the phone and ask for the caller's phone number.
   e. All of the above.

**12.** [LO11.3] Which of the following is appropriate action for an administrative medical assistant regarding prescription refills?
   a. Authorize all refills as long as they are for a current patient of the practice.
   b. Authorize a refill if it is within the time frame stated in the patient's medical record.
   c. Make a note of all refills on the telephone log.
   d. Do not authorize any phoned prescription refill requests.
   e. Refer all prescription refills to the physician.

**13.** [LO11.3] Which of the following responses is appropriate when dealing with a patient who is calling with a complaint?
   a. During the conversation, do not apologize to the caller since this is an admission of wrongdoing.
   b. Tell the caller that everyone makes mistakes and that she should forgive the error.
   c. Take careful notes with all the details and read them back to the caller to ensure you have written them correctly.
   d. Ask the caller to contact the attorney for the medical practice.
   e. Tell the caller that you cannot help her but that someone in the office will call them back sometime.

**14.** [LO11.2] Which of the following statements represents proper telephone etiquette?
   a. You should make the caller feel important.
   b. You must rely on body language and facial expressions to interpret the patient's demeanor.
   c. If available, use the speakerphone so the caller is able to hear you more clearly.
   d. Use technical medical words so the caller will believe what you are telling her or him.
   e. If the call comes during a very busy time of day, speak very quickly to better facilitate the call.

**15.** [LO11.3] When a caller just keeps talking and the conversation is not ending, you should
   a. hang up on the caller.
   b. ask the patient to call back later to finish the conversation.
   c. place the caller on hold.
   d. summarize the important points of the call, thank the caller for calling, and then let the caller hang up first.
   e. tell the caller that you don't have time to spend on the phone and others need more attention.

**16.** [LO11.5] When documenting a phone call, all of the following information is important to obtain *except*
   a. the date and time of the call.
   b. the caller's e-mail address.
   c. the name of the person calling.
   d. the caller's phone number.
   e. the name or initials of the person taking the call.

**17.** [LO11.5] Which of the following is *not* a good tip when you are responsible for taking phone messages?
   a. Keep a pen and paper on hand close to the phone.
   b. When the call is over, write down the important points from the call.
   c. Verify the correct callback phone number.
   d. Never make a commitment on behalf of the physician.
   e. Ask for the correct spelling of the caller's name and medications if a refill is being requested.

**18.** [LO11.8] Which of the following is improper telephone etiquette for outgoing calls?
   a. Ensure that the time zone and time of day is appropriate to make the call.
   b. Make sure you have the correct telephone number.
   c. When the person you are calling picks up the phone, decide what you are going to say.
   d. Ask the person you are calling if it is a convenient time to call.
   e. Identify yourself when the person answers the phone.

**19.** [LO11.6] Telephone triage requires
   a. that there is proper training of office staff before assigning the responsibility to them.
   b. that the office has guidelines for handling common questions.
   c. that appropriate questions should be asked, such as when the patient's symptoms began.
   d. that the staff understands when to involve the physician or the office nurse or refer the patient to the emergency room.
   e. All of the above.

**20.** [LO11.3] When you manage incoming calls in a medical practice, it is important to remember to
   a. answer each call within 8–10 rings.
   b. be calm and courteous even if the caller appears to be in a hurry.
   c. wait until the caller identifies himself before you tell him who you are.
   d. hang up on the caller if he has a complaint about being put on hold.
   e. put the caller on hold when you are busy without identifying him first.

**21.** [LO11.2] When communicating on the phone, the administrative medical assistant should be concise, which means that the message
   a. is brief and direct.
   b. contains all the necessary information.
   c. is legible.
   d. is organized and free from ambiguity.
   e. is respectful of others.

**22.** [LO11.3] Which of the following statements is *false* regarding the disclosure of patient information?
   a. HIPAA guidelines apply to phone conversations and e-mail messages.
   b. When written authorization is provided from the patient, you can release the approved information.
   c. Information can be released for emergencies or when required by governmental agencies for compliance.
   d. No information can be released to other health-care providers when treatment is necessary.
   e. Confidentiality must be maintained when working with patient financial forms and reports.

**23.** [LO11.3] An appropriate greeting for the administrative medical assistant to use when initially answering the phone in a medical practice is
   a. "This is Mary, the doctor's assistant. May I help you?"
   b. "Doctor's office, who do you wish to speak with?"
   c. "Dr. Grey's office, this is Mary speaking. How may I help you?"
   d. "Doctor's office, will you please hold?"
   e. "This is 601-556-4444. Do you have the correct number?"

**24.** [LO11.8] Which of the following methods may be used to locate the correct phone number prior to placing an outgoing call?
   a. Consult a telephone directory such as the White or Yellow Pages
   b. Use an Internet phone directory
   c. Consult the company Web site for contact information
   d. Call directory assistance to locate the phone number
   e. All of the above methods may be used.

**25.** [LO11.1] Telephone communication skills involve being cohesive with messages, which means that they are
   a. free of spelling errors.
   b. short and to the point.
   c. respectful of the sender.
   d. organized and logical.
   e. printed, not written.

## True or False

Decide whether each statement is true or false. In the space at the left, write "T" for true or "F" for false. On the lines provided, rewrite the false statements to make them true.

_____ **1.** [LO11.2] Even if you are rushed, you should remain calm, courteous, and pleasant on the telephone.

_____

_____ **2.** [LO11.1] Good communication skills project a positive image and satisfy the needs and expectations of the patient.

_____

_____ **3.** [LO11.1] Clarity is a quality of communication that means the caller must briefly state the purpose of his call.

_____

_____ **4.** [LO11.3] If approval for a prescription renewal is not noted in the patient's chart, you should not authorize the refill.

_____

_____ **5.** [LO11.2] It is not important to use the caller's name at the end of the call prior to hanging up.

_____

_____ **6.** [LO11.3] If a patient is unwilling to discuss the purpose of her call but only wants to speak with the physician, you should tell the patient that the physician will only call her back if she discloses the nature of the problem.

_____

_____ **7.** [LO11.4] The physician is legally responsible for the actions of the administrative medical assistant including information relayed to patients over the telephone.

_____

_____ **8.** [LO11.3] If you need to transfer a call, ask for the caller's permission to place them on hold while you transfer the call.

_____

_____ **9.** [LO11.4] When a patient calls the office to obtain laboratory results, if the results are abnormal, inform the patient of the results and schedule the patient for another appointment to see the physician.

_____

_____ **10.** [LO11.4] If a patient calls requesting a refill of a medication that was prescribed for a previous condition that has now returned, the administrative medical assistant may authorize this refill.

_____

## Sentence Completion

In the space provided, write the word or phrase that best completes each sentence.

**1.** [LO11.1] The telephone is a _____ and _____ _____ tool that is essential to the operation of the medical office.

**2.** [LO11.2] Courtesy is expressed by projecting an attitude of _____.

**3.** [LO11.2] Using the caller's name during the conversation makes the caller feel _____.

**4.** [LO11.1] Excellent communication skills are necessary when using the _____ and other telecommunication devices such as _____ _____, _____, and _____.

**5.** [LO11.1] All e-mail messages to or from the patient regarding diagnosis or treatment will become a _____ part of the patient_____ _____.

**6.** [LO11.2] Telephone etiquette involves answering the phone promptly by the _____ or _____ ring.

**7.** [LO11.4] When a caller asks to speak with the physician, you should always ask the _____ of the call.

**8.** [LO11.4] Although a patient may ask you for your _____ opinion, do not give _____ advice of any kind.

**9.** [LO11.5] Guidelines for dealing with a complaint call include never making _____ you cannot keep.

**10.** [LO11.2] To make your voice pleasant and effective on the telephone, _____ directly into the receiver and to the person who is calling.

**1.** _____
_____

**2.** _____
_____

**3.** _____
_____

**4** _____
_____

**5.** _____
_____

**6.** _____
_____

**7.** _____
_____

**8.** _____
_____

**9.** _____
_____

**10.** _____
_____

# Apply Your Knowledge

## Short Answer

Write the answer to each question on the lines provided.

1. [LO11.1] List at least five features of good communication skills.

_____

_____

_____

2. [LO11.4] Give three examples of calls the administrative medical assistant can handle and three examples of those that will be transferred to someone else. Name the person that would receive the transferred call.

_____

_____

_____

3. [LO11.6] Explain how telephone triage is conducted. Be concise.

_____

_____

_____

4. [LO11.3] Explain the proper etiquette and steps used to place a caller on hold.

_____

_____

_____

5. [LO11.3] List at least five different incoming calls that would constitute a medical emergency.

_____

_____

_____

## Problem-Solving Activities

Follow the directions for each activity.

1. [LO11.3, 11.6] Medical Practice Training Manual
   a. You have been asked to assist in the development of materials for a training manual in a medical practice. You will list (1) the types of calls, (2) the action that should be taken by the administrative medical assistant when the call comes into the office, and (3) the person who will handle the call.

b. Using a chart or table similar to the example given here, provide the information for at least 10 types of incoming calls including the following examples:
- Referring physician to discuss the outcome of a patient's office visit
- Pharmacy requesting a refill on medication over one year
- Parent of a child who has an acute illness
- Friend of the physician

| TYPE OF CALL | ACTION/DISCUSSION (WHAT YOU WILL SAY OR DO) | PERSON TO HANDLE THE CALL |
|---|---|---|
|  |  |  |
|  |  |  |
|  |  |  |
|  |  |  |
|  |  |  |
|  |  |  |
|  |  |  |
|  |  |  |
|  |  |  |
|  |  |  |

2. **[LO11.3]** Practice Taking Telephone Messages. Work with a partner in your class to complete this assignment.
   a. Refer to Figure 11–6 in Chapter 11 of the text to create a mock telephone message form for a fictitious medical practice.

**TELEPHONE MESSAGE**

For: _Linda Wiley_ _____

_____

_Patient calling as requested with update. She is feeling much better after_

_3 days on Abx. Temperature is back to normal. No more sore throat; body aches_

_and pains are less._ _____

_____

_____

_____

Name of Caller: _Micha Ward_ _____

Name of Patient (if not caller): _____

Date/Time Called: _4/12/2012 @ 11:15 a.m._ _____

Message Taken by: _Kalisha Roberts_ _____

b. Develop at least 10 detailed phone messages that you will use in role-play with other students in your class. Write the data for each call on a separate index card or sheet of paper.

c. Select a fellow student to be the caller and another to be the administrative medical assistant.

d. Give the caller one of the mock telephone messages you developed and provide a copy of your telephone message form for the other student who will represent the administrative medical assistant.

e. In front of the class, have the caller place the mock call while the other student plays the role of an administrative medical assistant.

f. The other students will critique the call giving constructive feedback about how the call was received by the student who played the administrative medical assistant. The students should pay attention to the assistant's manner in answering the phone, questions asked, and the outcome of the call.

g. Each student in the class will have the opportunity to play both the caller and the assistant.

## Thinking Critically

Write your response to each case study question on the lines provided.

### Case 1 [LO11.3, 11.4]

A pharmaceutical representative calls to set up an appointment to see the physician about new products. He is only in town for the day and is demanding to see the physician for only a few minutes. You explain that the physician has a full appointment schedule and will be leaving the office at 5:00 P.M. today.

1. How should you handle this caller?

_____

_____

_____

2. What are alternatives for the representative to discuss new products with the physician?

_____

_____

_____

### Case 2 [LO11.3]

An unidentified caller requests to talk with the physician about another patient's laboratory results. The caller explains that he is the patient's husband. You try to explain your office telephone policy to the caller, but the caller is insistent on obtaining information.

1. How will you handle this call? What information should you attempt to get from the caller?

_____

_____

_____

**2.** What is the appropriate response to this caller's request?

_____

_____

_____

## Case 3 [LO11.2, 11.3]

A pharmacy calls the office to obtain authorization to refill a prescription for one of your patients. The refill is denied since it has been over a year since the patient has been in the office to see the physician. Later that day the patient calls the office very angry that the prescription refill was denied. The caller is becoming belligerent and aggressive on the call.

**1.** What can you say to this person in an attempt to calm her down?

_____

_____

_____

**2.** What are the solutions you can offer this patient?

_____

_____

_____

# Demonstrate Your Knowledge

**Student Name:** _____

## Procedure 11–1: Using a Telecommunication Device for the Deaf

**GOAL:** To properly communicate with the hearing impaired patient using a TDD

**MATERIALS:** Telephone, TDD (if available), patient chart for documentation, pen

**METHOD:** To pass this procedure the minimum required score is _____% or all elements must meet "satisfactory" ability on the final demonstration. The first box may be used as a practice or final demonstration, with the evaluator placing **S for Satisfactory** or **U for Unsatisfactory** if that is the grading criteria. The second box may be used as a final demonstration with a **grade point** written in the box.

| STEPS | POSSIBLE POINTS | S/U | POINTS EARNED |
|---|---|---|---|
| **Answering a TDD Call** | | | |
| 1. Answer the phone as usual. If you hear a rapid clinking sound you know you have a TDD call. You may hear no sound at all, but do not hang up; it may still be a TDD call. | 5 | | |
| 2. If you know (or believe) this is a TDD call, place your phone receiver on the TDD as directed. | 5 | | |
| 3. Type your normal office greeting: "Total Care Clinic, Denise Bagwell, How may I help you?" | 10 | | |
| 4. When you complete your message, type "GA," which stands for "go ahead." This tells the patient you have completed your message and it is his turn to respond. | 5 | | |
| 5. Give the patient time to type his response. When you see "GA" at the end of his message, it is your turn to respond. | 10 | | |
| 6. When the patient receives all of the information required, he will type "Bye, SK," which stands for "good bye, stop keying." | 5 | | |
| 7. If you agree that the call is completed, you may also reply "Bye, SK." This will give the patient the opportunity to be the one to end the call. | 5 | | |
| 8. When you receive a response of SKSK ("stop keying, stop keying"), the conversation is complete and you may hang up and turn off the TDD. | 5 | | |
| **Making a Call with TDD** | | | |
| 1. Turn on the TDD. | 5 | | |
| 2. Dial the patient's phone number on your standard telephone and listen for the phone to ring. | 10 | | |
| 3. When you hear the TDD-sound, place the phone receiver on the TDD as directed. | 5 | | |

*(Continued)*

| STEPS | POSSIBLE POINTS | S/U | POINTS EARNED |
|---|---|---|---|
| 4. After the patient types a greeting and "GA" appears on the TDD display, identify yourself and proceed with the conversation. | 10 | | |
| 5. Remember to type "GA" when you complete your message so that the patient knows it is his turn to respond. | 10 | | |
| 6. Even though you were the one to initiate the call, you should still allow the patient to make the decision that the call is completed by keying "SKSK." | 10 | | |
| **Total Points (if applicable)** | 100 | | |

**Comments:** _____

_____

_____


**Final Evaluator's Signature:** _____


**Date:** _____

## CAAHEP Competencies Achieved

IV. C (9) Discuss applications of electronic technology in effective communication

IV. P (7) Demonstrate telephone techniques

IV. A (2) Apply active listening skills

IV. A (8) Analyze communications in providing appropriate responses/feedback

## ABHES Competencies Achieved

8. aa. [Graduates] are attentive, listen, and learn

8. bb. [Graduates] are impartial and show empathy when dealing with patients

8. cc. Communicate on the recipient's level of comprehension

8. dd. Serve as liaison between physician and others

8. ee. Use proper telephone techniques

8. hh. Receive, organize, prioritize, and transmit information expediently

8. ii. Recognize and respond to verbal and nonverbal communication

8. kk. Adapt to individualized needs

8. ll. Apply electronic technology

**Student Name:** _____

## Procedure 11–2: Performing Telephone Screening and Call Routing

**GOAL:** To properly screen incoming telephone calls

**MATERIALS:** Telephone, telephone pad, pen or pencil, appointment book or computerized scheduling software (computer)

**METHOD:** To pass this procedure the minimum required score is _____ % or all elements must meet "satisfactory" ability on the final demonstration. The first box may be used as a practice or final demonstration, with the evaluator placing **S for Satisfactory** or **U for Unsatisfactory** if that is the grading criteria. The second box may be used as a final demonstration with a **grade point** written in the box.

| STEPS | POSSIBLE POINTS | S/U | POINTS EARNED |
|---|---|---|---|
| 1. Make sure all of the materials are within reach of the telephone equipment. | 5 | | |
| 2. Answer the telephone promptly within two to three rings. | 15 | | |
| 3. Identify the medical office and identify yourself. Make sure you know office procedure for answering the phone in your facility even if a telephone answering system is employed to route calls to you. For example: "Total Care Clinic, this is Denise Bagwell, how may I help you?" | 10 | | |
| 4. If the caller does not identify himself, ask him to do so and the number he is calling from, writing down this information. Get an idea what the call refers to. Listen carefully to what the caller has to say, listening for tone and feeling. Try to decide as soon as possible if this is a call that you can handle; if so, handle it. If this is a call that needs to be transferred to someone, tell the caller to whom and to what number you will be transferring the call. | 15 | | |
| 5. If you need to take a message, make sure you repeat the information that is given to you, especially the name of the person and his phone number. | 15 | | |
| 6. If you have to transfer a caller, ask permission to place him on hold. Make sure you write down the caller's name and phone number in case the call is dropped. Never place a caller on hold longer than 30 seconds. Come back to the caller and let him know that you are still waiting for the other individual to answer. If the other staff member does not answer promptly or the staff member is on another line, ask the caller if he would like to call back, be transferred to the staff member's voice mail (if available), or would like to leave a message. | 15 | | |

*(Continued)*

| STEPS | POSSIBLE POINTS | S/U | POINTS EARNED |
|---|---|---|---|
| 7. If the caller describes a symptom that is in need of immediate care, ask questions to assess the information (ask for his name and telephone number). If it is indeed an emergency call and the physician, PA, or nurse is in the office, transfer the call immediately. If the doctor, PA, or nurse is not in the building, do not let the caller hang up. Have another staff member dial 911 immediately with the name and address of the patient and his symptoms, while you stay on the phone with the patient, keeping him calm and aware that help is on the way. | 25 | | |
| **Total Points (if applicable)** | 100 | | |

**Comments:** _____

_____

_____


**Final Evaluator's Signature:** _____

**Date:** _____

## CAAHEP Competencies Achieved

IV. P (7) Demonstrate telephone techniques

VII. A (2) Demonstrate sensitivity in communicating with both providers and patients

## ABHES Competencies Achieved

8. ee. Use proper telephone techniques

8. hh. Receive, organize, prioritize, and transmit information expediently

11. b. Demonstrate professionalism by:

    (2) Exhibiting a positive attitude and a sense of responsibility

    (3) Maintaining confidentiality at all times

    (8) Being courteous and diplomatic

    (9) Conducting work within scope of education, training, and ability

**Student Name:** _____

## Procedure 11-3: Retrieving Messages from an Answering Service

**GOAL:** To follow standard procedures for retrieving messages from an answering service

**MATERIALS:** Telephone message pad, manual telephone log, or electronic telephone log

**METHOD:** To pass this procedure the minimum required score is _____% or all elements must meet "satisfactory" ability on the final demonstration. The first box may be used as a practice or final demonstration, with the evaluator placing **S for Satisfactory** or **U for Unsatisfactory** if that is the grading criteria. The second box may be used as a final demonstration with a **grade point** written in the box.

| STEPS | POSSIBLE POINTS | S/U | POINTS EARNED |
|---|---|---|---|
| 1. Set a regular schedule for calling the answering service to retrieve messages. | 10 | | |
| 2. Call at the regularly scheduled time(s) to see if there are any messages. | 5 | | |
| 3. Identify yourself and state that you are calling to obtain messages for the practice. | 10 | | |
| 4. For each message, write down all pertinent information on the telephone message pad or telephone log, or key it into the electronic telephone log. Be sure to include the caller's name and telephone number, time of call, message or description of the problem, and action taken, if any. | 25 | | |
| 5. Repeat the information, confirming that you have the correct spelling of all names. | 25 | | |
| 6. When you have retrieved all messages, route them according to the office policy. | 25 | | |
| **Total Points (if applicable)** | 100 | | |

**Comments:** _____

_____

_____

**Final Evaluator's Signature:** _____

**Date:** _____

## CAAHEP Competencies Achieved

IV. P (7) Demonstrate telephone techniques

## ABHES Competencies Achieved

8. ee. Use proper telephone techniques

8. hh. Receive, organize, prioritize, and transmit information expediently

8. ll. Apply electronic technology

11. b. Demonstrate professionalism by:

    (2) Exhibiting a positive attitude and a sense of responsibility

    (3) Maintaining confidentiality at all times

    (8) Being courteous and diplomatic

    (9) Conducting work within scope of education, training, and ability

**Student Name:** _____

## Procedure 11–4: Composing a Professional E-mail Message

**GOAL:** To compose a professional e-mail message

**MATERIALS:** Computer with e-mail (Internet) capabilities, e-mail message requiring response

**METHOD:** To pass thwis procedure the minimum required score is _____% or all elements must meet "satisfactory" ability on the final demonstration. The first box may be used as a practice or final demonstration, with the evaluator placing **S for Satisfactory** or **U for Unsatisfactory** if that is the grading criteria. The second box may be used as a final demonstration with a **grade point** written in the box.

| STEPS | POSSIBLE POINTS | S/U | POINTS EARNED |
|---|---|---|---|
| 1. Check the patient's medical record verifying that a "Consent to Use E-mail" form for communication with the office has been signed. | 15 | | |
| 2. Use a classic, easy-to-read font such as Times New Roman at 12 point (14 point is also acceptable). Keep a professional appearance in mind; use black ink only. | 5 | | |
| 3. If you are responding to a patient e-mail, open the e-mail and choose "Reply." If you are composing a new message, choose "New" to open a new e-mail document and carefully enter the patient's e-mail address. | 5 | | |
| 4. Add the e-mail address to the office address book for easy reference for later e-mails. | 5 | | |
| 5. If answering a patient e-mail, you may keep the subject line from the original message. If you are writing a new e-mail, enter a descriptive subject line. | 10 | | |
| 6. Insert a salutation, using the patient's surname as you would with an ordinary letter. | 5 | | |
| 7. Compose the body of the message, aligning the information with the left margin. | 15 | | |
| 8. Double-space at the end of the message and insert your name. Include a signature line with the practice information if available. | 10 | | |
| 9. Spell-check and proofread the message carefully for any errors. | 10 | | |
| 10. Click "Send" and wait for the message informing you the message has been sent. | 5 | | |
| 11. If the message is returned as undeliverable, verify the e-mail address was entered correctly. If necessary, correct the address and attempt delivery again. | 5 | | |
| 12. If the message is returned a second time as undeliverable, contact the patient by phone or by an alternate method to be sure he or she received the required information. | 10 | | |
| **Total Points (if applicable)** | 100 | | |

**Comments:** _____

_____

_____

**Final Evaluator's Signature:** _____

**Date:** _____

## CAAHEP Competencies Achieved

I. C (7) Identify resources and adaptations that are required based on individual needs, i.e., culture and environment, developmental life stage, language, and physical threats to communication

IV. C (9) Discuss applications of electronic technology in effective communication

IV. P (2) Report relevant information to others succinctly and accurately

IV. A (8) Analyze communications in providing appropriate responses/feedback

## ABHES Competencies Achieved

7. a. Perform basic keyboarding skills including:

  (1) Locating the keys on a keyboard

7. b. Identify and properly utilize office machines, computerized systems, and medical software such as:

  (1) Efficiently maintain and understand different types of medical correspondence and medical reports

  (2) Apply computer application skills using a variety of different electronic programs including both practice management software and EMR software

8. ii. Recognize and respond to verbal and nonverbal communication

8. kk. Adapt to individualized needs

8. ll. Apply electronic technology

## Test Your Knowledge

### Vocabulary Review

Match the key terms in the right column with the definitions in the left column by placing the letter of each correct answer in the space provided.

_____ **1.** the scheduling of similar appointments together at a certain time of the day or week

_____ **2.** a report of what happened and what was discussed and decided at a meeting

_____ **3.** a system of scheduling in which patients arrive at the doctor's office at their convenience and are seen on a first-come, first-served basis

_____ **4.** a patient who arrives without an appointment

_____ **5.** a substitute physician hired to see patients while the regular physician is away from the office

_____ **6.** a system of scheduling where patients arrive at regular, specified intervals, assuring the practice a steady stream of patients throughout the day

_____ **7.** a system of scheduling in which two or more patients are booked for the same appointment slot, with the assumption that both patients will be seen by the doctor within the scheduled period

_____ **8.** booking an appointment several weeks or even months in advance

**a.** advance scheduling [LO12.3]

**b.** agenda [LO12.7]

**c.** cluster scheduling [LO12.3]

**d.** double-booking system [LO12.3]

**e.** itinerary [LO12.7]

**f.** locum tenens [LO12.7]

**g.** matrix [LO12.1]

**h.** minutes [LO12.7]

**i.** modified-wave scheduling [LO12.3]

**j.** no-show [LO12.4]

**k.** open-hours scheduling [LO12.3]

**l.** overbooking [LO12.7]

**m.** time-specified scheduling [LO12.3]

**n.** underbooking [LO12.7]

_____ 9. a patient who does not call to cancel and does not come to an appointment

_____ 10. a system of scheduling in which the number of patients seen each hour is determined by dividing the hour by the length of the average visit and then giving that number of patients appointments with the doctor at the beginning of each hour

_____ 11. the basic format of an appointment book, established by blocking off times on the schedule during which the doctor is able to see patients

_____ 12. leaving large, unused gaps in the doctor's schedule; an approach that does not make the best use of the doctor's time

_____ 13. scheduling appointments for more patients than can reasonably be seen in the time allowed

_____ 14. a scheduling system similar to the wave system, with patients arriving at planned intervals during the hour, allowing time to catch up before the next hour begins

_____ 15. a detailed travel plan listing dates and times for specific transportation arrangements and events, the location of meetings and lodgings, and phone numbers

_____ 16. the list of topics discussed or presented at a meeting, in order of presentation

**o.** walk-in [LO12.5]

**p.** wave scheduling [LO12.3]

## Multiple-Choice Certification Questions

There may be more than one answer; circle the letter of the choice that best completes each statement or answers each question.

**1.** [LO12.4] When a patient has never been seen at the medical office for an appointment, the abbreviation _____ should be placed next to the patient's name.
a. US
b. RS
c. PT
d. NS
e. NP

**2.** [LO12.1] The typical length of a complete physical examination is
a. 10–15 minutes.
b. 15–20 minutes.
c. 20–30 minutes.
d. 60 minutes.
e. 90 minutes.

**3.** [LO12.1] Which of the following statements is *false* with regard to the physical appointment book?
a. The appointment book is considered a legal record.
b. Corrections should be made using an eraser or correction fluid.
c. All entries must be clear and easy to read.
d. The schedule should be written in blue or black ink.
e. The appointment book may be used as evidence in legal proceedings.

**4.** [LO12.4] When a patient cannot come in for his original scheduled appointment, the abbreviation used next to the patient's name in that time slot is
a. sig.
b. ref.
c. can.
d. cons.
e. resch.

**5.** [LO12.3] When patients are seen on a first-come, first-served basis, it is called
a. open-hours scheduling.
b. wave scheduling.
c. double-booking.
d. cluster scheduling.
e. advance scheduling.

**6.** [LO12.3] Which of the following represents wave scheduling?
a. Patient A 10:00 A.M., Patient B 10:15 A.M.
b. Patient A 10:00 A.M., Patient B 10:30 A.M.
c. Patient A 10:00 A.M., Patient B 10:00 A.M.
d. Patient A 10:00 A.M., Patient B 11:00 A.M.
e. Patient A 10:00 A.M., Patient B 11:30 A.M.

**7.** [LO12.3] Time-specified scheduling is also referred to as
a. open-hours scheduling.
b. physician preference scheduling.
c. stream scheduling.
d. cluster scheduling.
e. advance scheduling.

**8.** [LO12.4] Which of the following is an example of a new patient in the medical office?
a. A patient who had a medication refilled six months ago
b. A patient who comes into the office for an annual physical examination
c. A child who needs a school sports physical
d. A person who saw the physician four years ago for a physical
e. A patient who changed insurance companies after the first of the year

**9.** [LO12.4] Patients should be sent a reminder a few days prior to their scheduled appointment. Prior to mailing the reminder cards, they are stored in
a. a patient file.
b. a tickler file.
c. a reminder file.
d. a memory file.
e. None of the above.

**10.** [LO12.5] What is the best way to handle no-show patients?
a. Do not schedule future appointments for these patients.
b. Ask the physician to abandon these patients.
c. Refuse to give these patients the appointment when they want it.
d. Call these patients prior to their appointments to remind them of their day and time of the appointment.
e. Have the patient's employer remind the employee of the appointment.

**11.** [LO12.5] A patient who needs to be fasting for blood work prior to seeing the physician should be scheduled
  a. at the beginning of the day.
  b. during the noon hour.
  c. after lunch.
  d. before the end of the day.
  e. in the middle of the morning.

**12.** [LO12.5] Which of the following is appropriate for a patient that habitually arrives late for his appointments?
  a. The physician should send the patient a letter stating that if he arrives late for his appointments, then he will need to find another physician to care for him.
  b. The patient should be given the first appointment of the day so he can come in before going to work.
  c. Tell the patient to come in one hour prior to his actual appointment.
  d. Call the patient's family and explain the disturbance this causes in the office.
  e. Document each late arrival in the patient's chart.

**13.** [LO12.5] To schedule an emergency appointment, the administrative medical assistant should
  a. determine if the patient can wait until the next day and give medical advice about what the patient should do until she can be seen.
  b. ask the nature of the emergency and ask how soon before the patient can arrive at the office.
  c. tell the patient that the physician does not have any time left in his schedule for the day so the patient should go to the emergency room.
  d. cancel all the patients for the remainder of the day to accommodate the emergency.
  e. determine if the person is a patient of the practice and if her insurance covers emergency care in the private office.

**14.** [LO12.5] What is the best way to handle a cancellation?
  a. Reschedule the appointment while the patient is still on the phone.
  b. Call the patient the next day to see what time works best for a rescheduled appointment.
  c. Contact the patient's family to confirm that the patient needed to cancel the appointment.
  d. Notify the patient that the office policy only allows for two cancellations unless they can provide a note documenting the reason for the cancellation.
  e. None of the above.

**15.** [LO12.6] Scheduling outside appointments for patients includes the following events *except*
  a. prescription refills.
  b. laboratory work.
  c. x-rays.
  d. hospital stays.
  e. surgery.

**16.** [LO12.3] A type of scheduling that does not make the best use of the physician's time is
  a. wave scheduling.
  b. time-specific scheduling.
  c. underbooking.
  d. advance booking.
  e. modified scheduling.

**17.** [LO12.7] The term "locum tenens" refers to
  a. a subpoena for the physician to go to court.
  b. a multiple-physician practice.
  c. the abandoning of a patient.
  d. a substitute physician.
  e. a lawsuit for negligence.

18. **[LO12.5]** When the administrative medical assistant is planning a meeting for the physician, it is important to know
    a. when the meeting will be held.
    b. how many will be attending the meeting.
    c. how long the meeting will last.
    d. the purpose of the meeting.
    e. All of the above.

19. **[LO12.6]** The physician may give you the list of topics to be presented at a meeting. This list is referred to as the
    a. subjects for presentation.
    b. minutes of the meeting.
    c. agenda for the meeting.
    d. discussion for the members.
    e. report of findings.

20. **[LO12.4]** The abbreviation used to indicate that a patient is rescheduled for an appointment is
    a. RBS.
    b. RS.
    c. S/R.
    d. US.
    e. NS.

21. **[LO12.3]** The double-booking system of scheduling means
    a. one patient will be scheduled every 15 minutes.
    b. a patient will be scheduled for two follow-up appointments.
    c. the physician can see two patients at the same time.
    d. two or more patients are scheduled for the same appointment slot.
    e. None of the above.

22. **[LO12.3]** A patient booked two months prior to an annual gynecologic examination is a good example of the use of
    a. wave scheduling.
    b. open-hours scheduling.
    c. advance scheduling.
    d. time-specified scheduling.
    e. open-ended scheduling.

23. **[LO12.4]** When scheduling a new patient, it is important to
    a. obtain the patient's home address and daytime telephone number.
    b. ask the patient about insurance coverage.
    c. ask the patient the reason for the appointment.
    d. ask the patient to arrive 15 minutes ahead of the appointment time.
    e. Do all of the above.

24. **[LO12.5]** When making a return appointment, it is best to
    a. make the appointment while the patient is still in the office.
    b. have the patient go home and check his schedule to ensure there are no conflicts before setting the appointment time.
    c. have the patient call back at the end of the week after he has checked his agenda.
    d. call the patient in a day or two to set the return appointment.
    e. ask the physician if the patient can wait until he is feeling better.

25. **[LO12.5]** When scheduling patients for multiple return visits it is best to
    a. schedule the patient every other day, alternating morning and afternoon time slots.
    b. schedule the patient for the same time and day each week in order to keep a routine.
    c. ask the patient to come in at least once a week when she is available.
    d. have the patient call each Monday to set a new appointment for the week.
    e. schedule the patient only if she calls and needs to see the physician.

# True or False

Decide whether each statement is true or false. In the space at the left, write "T" for true or "F" for false. On the lines provided, rewrite the false statements to make them true.

_____ 1. [LO12.1] The appointment book is a legal record that should be held for at least three years.

_____

_____ 2. [LO12.3] Double-booking assumes that two patients will be seen at least 30 minutes apart.

_____

_____ 3. [LO12.3] Cluster scheduling is used to schedule patients with similar appointment needs.

_____

_____ 4. [LO12.5] Most minor medical problems, such as sore throats, earaches, or blood pressure follow-ups usually require only 10–15 minutes.

_____

_____ 5. [LO12.3] Medical offices are not allowed to schedule patients beyond 6 months.

_____

_____ 6. [LO12.5] Emergency patients should always be referred to the local emergency room for treatment.

_____

_____ 7. (LO12.5) Patients referred by another physician should be scheduled after all the regular patients since they are not regular patients and will probably never return.

_____

_____ 8. [LO12.5] You should avoid scheduling a diabetic patient in the late morning before lunch.

_____

_____ 9. [LO12.5] Patients who have a habit of arriving late for appointments should be scheduled toward the end of the day.

_____

_____ 10. [LO12.4] The abbreviation used to designate a patient who is returning to see the physician for a chronic condition is "cons."

_____

## Sentence Completion

In the space provided, write the word or phrase that best completes each sentence.

1. **[LO12.1]** The abbreviation CPE next to a patient's name in the appointment book indicates _____ _____ _____.

2. **[LO12.4]** The open-hours scheduling system is still used by _____ practices, _____ rooms, and _____ care centers.

3. **[LO12.3]** Online scheduling is relatively new. The patients schedule themselves via the _____ and _____.

4. **[LO12.1]** When a patient cancels an appointment, _____ the first appointment before entering the patient's _____ appointment.

5. **[LO12.7]** When a pharmaceutical representative who is unknown to you comes into the office, ask for a _____ _____ and check with the physician before scheduling an appointment.

6. **[LO12.7]** An _____ is a detailed travel plan, listing dates and times of _____ and _____.

7. **[LO12.3]** _____ means scheduling more patients than can reasonably be seen in the time allowed.

8. **[LO12.4]** Offices that routinely have long waiting times can end up with _____ patients.

9. **[LO12.3]** Wave scheduling works effectively in larger medical facilities that have enough _____ and _____ to provide services to _____ patients at the same time.

10. **[LO12.1]** To reduce the chance of error when using an appointment card, enter the appointment in the _____ _____ first, then fill out the card.

1. _____
   _____

2. _____
   _____

3. _____
   _____

4. _____
   _____

5. _____
   _____

6. _____
   _____

7. _____
   _____

8. _____
   _____

9. _____
   _____

10. _____
    _____

# Apply Your Knowledge

## Short Answer

Write the answer to each question on the lines provided.

1. [LO12.4] How can having a list of standard procedures and the time required for each procedure help you be an efficient scheduler?

_____

_____

_____

2. [LO12.3] How would you select a scheduling appointment system for a medical practice?

_____

_____

_____

3. [LO12.5] Explain the overall impact on the daily schedule when a patient is late for a scheduled appointment.

_____

_____

_____

4. [LO12.5] What is the advantage to scheduling new patients for the first morning appointments?

_____

_____

_____

5. [LO12.5] Why is it important to document a no-show in the appointment book and the patient chart?

_____

_____

_____

# Problem-Solving Activities

Follow the directions for each activity.

1. **[LO12.2]** Scheduling Appointments
   a. Refer to Figure 12–1 in Chapter 12 of the student text as an example and design a single-day appointment log for a physician using the appointment record below.

## APPOINTMENT RECORD

| | | | | |
|---|---|---|---|---|
| **12** November Tuesday | | | **13** November Wednesday | |
| | | **AM** | | |
| | | 8:00 | | |
| | | 8:15 | | |
| | | 8:30 | | |
| | | 8:45 | | |
| | | 9:00 | | |
| | | 9:15 | | |
| | | 9:30 | | |
| | | 9:45 | | |
| | | 10:00 | | |
| | | 10:15 | | |
| | | 10:30 | | |
| | | 10:45 | | |
| | | 11:00 | | |
| | | 11:15 | | |
| | | 11:30 | | |
| | | 11:45 | | |
| | | 12:00 | | |
| | | 12:15 | | |
| | | 12:30 | | |
| | | 12:45 | | |
| | | **PM** | | |
| | | 1:00 | | |
| | | 1:15 | | |
| | | 1:30 | | |
| | | 1:45 | | |
| | | 2:00 | | |
| | | 2:15 | | |
| | | 2:30 | | |
| | | 2:45 | | |
| | | 3:00 | | |
| | | 3:15 | | |
| | | 3:30 | | |
| | | 3:45 | | |
| | | 4:00 | | |
| | | 4:15 | | |
| | | 4:30 | | |
| | | 4:45 | | |
| | | 5:00 | | |
| | | 5:15 | | |
| | | 5:30 | | |
| | | 5:45 | | |

REMARKS & NOTES _____

b. Set up a matrix with the following information:
- Office hours: 8:30 A.M.–5:00 P.M.
- Lunch: 12:30 P.M.–1:30 P.M.
- Physician leaves office at 4:45 P.M. to visit hospital patients

c. Select at least six procedures performed at your mock office and determine the time allotment for each procedure.

d. Have the other students in your class select a procedure and schedule an appointment with you. Procedures may need to be duplicated for the number of students in the class.

e. Use appropriate scheduling techniques and information to schedule each student, including the abbreviations used in scheduling. You may have to use techniques such as double-booking and overbooking if you have a large class of students.

f. When all students have been scheduled, compare results of the project and see if you were able to accommodate the students with the appointments that they requested.

**2.** [LO12.5] Set Up a Staff Meeting.

a. Your physician has asked you to organize a staff meeting for the office. You need to prepare an agenda for the meeting.

b. The meeting will be held on Wednesday from 3:00 P.M.–5:00 P.M. in the office conference room. Snacks and beverages will be provided for the staff.

c. The practice manager will preside over the meeting and will present the following topics:
- New office vacation schedule
- Introduction of new employees
- 30 minutes in-service on new HIPAA guidelines
- New office hours

d. Develop the agenda for distribution at the meeting, placing the topics in the order that they should be presented.

## Thinking Critically

Write your response to each case study question on the lines provided.

### Case 1 [LO12.7]

You are a new employee in the medical office and are observing the office practices as part of your new employee orientation. When you observe the scheduling practices of the front-office administrative medical assistant, she appears to be turning away patients that day who want to schedule an appointment. She is telling the patients that the schedule is full and the physician cannot see any more patients that day. You look at the appointment log and see that there are several openings at the end of the day. When you ask the assistant why she isn't scheduling any more patients, she says, "I have plans tonight, and if I fill up the time, we won't be out of here until after 5:00 P.M., and besides, those patients don't have emergencies so I scheduled them later this week."

**1.** Is there a problem with this scenario? If so, what is it?

_____

_____

_____

**2.** As a new employee, how should you handle this situation?

_____

_____

_____

## Case 2 [LO12.5]

Your office has just opened for the day, and upon review of the appointment log for the day you see that the schedule is completely full. There are two new referral patients and four follow-up post-op exams. Also, a patient just called complaining of severe abdominal pain and was directed to come immediately to the office to be the first patient the physician will see. Five minutes after that call was received, the physician called the office to inform the staff that he has a personal emergency and cannot be at the office until mid-afternoon.

**1.** How should the scheduled appointments be handled?

_____

_____

_____

**2.** How will you specifically handle the patient with abdominal pain?

_____

_____

_____

## Case 3 [LO12.5]

A patient has been under the care of your physician for the past 10 years. Over the past year he has developed a chronic condition that requires him to see the physician once a month to regulate medication. In the past 6 months he has not showed up or called four times and the other two times he was late by 1 hour for his appointment. Since you have a good rapport with this patient, the physician has asked you to discuss his irresponsible behavior with him.

**1.** What method should you use to communicate with this patient? Why?

_____

_____

_____

**2.** What will you tell this patient about his behavior? Explain.

_____

_____

_____

# Demonstrate Your Knowledge

**Student Name:** _____

## Procedure 12–1: Creating an Appointment Matrix

**GOAL:** To create an appointment matrix to indicate the days and the hours the physician is not scheduling patients

**MATERIALS:** Appointment book; pencil or pen; physician schedule of meetings, conferences, vacations, and other times of unavailability, including staff meetings and hours when patients are not seen (*Note:* A blank appointment page is available at the end of this study guide.)

**METHOD:** To pass this procedure the minimum required score is _____ % or all elements must meet "satisfactory" ability on the final demonstration. The first box may be used as a practice or final demonstration, with the evaluator placing **S for Satisfactory** or **U for Unsatisfactory** if that is the grading criteria. The second box may be used as a final demonstration with a **grade point** written in the box.

| STEPS | POSSIBLE POINTS | S/U | POINTS EARNED |
|---|---|---|---|
| 1. Using the physician schedule of availability as the base for the matrix, confer with the physician or office manager to ensure that no additional schedule changes are planned. | 30 | | |
| 2. Indicate within each area the reason why the time is being closed to appointments, such as lunch, hospital rounds, AAMA meeting, etc., and place an "X" through the time frame. | 40 | | |
| 3. If the office utilizes cluster scheduling for certain appointments such as physical exams, blood sugar testing, etc., theses time frames must also be set apart. Following office policy, such as using brackets, note the appropriate appointment type to be scheduled during these time frames. | 30 | | |
| **Total Points (if applicable)** | 100 | | |

**Comments:** _____

_____

_____

**Final Evaluator's Signature:** _____

**Date:** _____

## CAAHEP Competencies Achieved

V. C (1) Discuss the pros and cons of various types of appointment management systems

V. C (2) Describe scheduling guidelines

V. C (3) Recognize office policies and protocols for handling appointments

V. C (13) Identify time management principles

V. P (1) Manage appointment schedules, using established priorities

V. A (2) Implement time management principles to maintain effective office function

## ABHES Competencies Achieved

8. c. Schedule and manage appointments

## Procedure 12–2: Creating an Appointment Matrix for an Electronic Scheduling System

**GOAL:** Using an electronic scheduling system, indicate the days and times when the office is not scheduling appointments

**MATERIALS:** Electronic scheduling program; physician schedule of meetings, conferences, vacations, and other times of unavailability, including staff meetings and hours when patients are not seen

**METHOD:** To pass this procedure the minimum required score is _____% or all elements must meet "satisfactory" ability on the final demonstration. The first box may be used as a practice or final demonstration, with the evaluator placing **S for Satisfactory** or **U for Unsatisfactory** if that is the grading criteria. The second box may be used as a final demonstration with a **grade point** written in the box.

| STEPS | POSSIBLE POINTS | S/U | POINTS EARNED |
|---|---|---|---|
| 1. Using the physician schedule of availability as the base for the matrix, confer with the physician or office manager to ensure that no additional schedule changes are planned. | 15 | | |
| 2. Open the office appointment scheduler per the program format. | 10 | | |
| 3. Block the dates and times when the general office or physician will not be available for patient appointments, using the physician and office schedules as guides. | 20 | | |
| 4. Choose the appropriate option if the time frame is repeatedly unavailable. | 10 | | |
| 5. Enter a reason that the time is not available for future reference. The office program may use color coding to assist with this process. | 15 | | |
| 6. If cluster scheduling is used for the office, most schedulers allow you to specify what types of appointments may be entered; again, color coding may be used by the scheduler to outline specific types of appointments. | 15 | | |
| 7. Many programs will allow you to specify specific time frames necessary for different types of appointments, and these also may be set up now. For instance, physical exams for new patients may require 45 minutes, and BP and typical sick visits are set up for 15 minutes. If the program allows, set up these matrixes now also. | 15 | | |
| **Total Points (if applicable)** | 100 | | |

**Comments:** _____

_____

_____

**Final Evaluator's Signature:** _____

**Date:** _____

## CAAHEP Competencies Achieved

V. C (1) Discuss the pros and cons of various types of appointment management systems

V. C (2) Describe scheduling guidelines

V. C (3) Recognize office policies and protocols for handling appointments

V. C (13) Identify time management principles

V. P (1) Manage appointment schedules, using established priorities

V. A (2) Implement time management principles to maintain effective office function.

## ABHES Competencies Achieved

8. c. Schedule and manage appointments

8. ll. Apply electronic technology

**Student Name:** _____

## Procedure 12–3: Scheduling Appointments

**GOAL:** Utilizing the previously created matrix, book patient appointments applying the correct amount of time for each appointment

**MATERIALS:** Appointment book and pen or electronic scheduler, template outlining time frames for patient appointment types
(*Note:* For paper scheduling, you may use the matrix created in Procedure 12–1.)

**METHOD:** To pass this procedure the minimum required score is _____% or all elements must meet "satisfactory" ability on the final demonstration. The first box may be used as a practice or final demonstration, with the evaluator placing **S for Satisfactory** or **U for Unsatisfactory** if that is the grading criteria. The second box may be used as a final demonstration with a **grade point** written in the box.

| STEPS | POSSIBLE POINTS | S/U | POINTS EARNED |
|---|---|---|---|
| 1. Establish the type of appointment required by a patient, particularly if this is a new or returning patient. | 15 | | |
| 2. If necessary, consult the template for the amount of time required for the patient appointment. Keep in mind the time reason for the appointment when scheduling (e.g., if the patient is required to be fasting) as that will affect the time frame for the appointment. | 15 | | |
| 3. When possible, schedule appointments earlier in the day first and then move to later time frames. Do ask the patient is he/she has a preferred time frame in mind and, if at all possible, accommodate the request. | 20 | | |
| 4. When using an appointment book, enter the patient name, phone number, and reason for the appointment in the appropriate space, blocking out additional blocks if necessary to accommodate a longer appointment time. | 20 | | |
| 5. If an electronic scheduler is used, use the search option to find the next available appointment for the time frame required for the appointment. Enter the patient name, phone number, and reason for the appointment. | 15 | | |
| 6. Repeat the appointment information to the patient, giving any necessary instructions to the patient regarding preparation for the appointment, such as early arrival for blood tests, completion of paperwork, etc. Also, this is a good time to remind patients about any copayments that will be due at the time of the appointment. | 15 | | |
| **Total Points (if applicable)** | 100 | | |

**Comments:** _____

_____

_____

**Final Evaluator's Signature:** _____

**Date:** _____

## CAAHEP Competencies Achieved

V. C (1) Discuss the pros and cons of various types of appointment management systems

V. C (2) Describe scheduling guidelines

V. C (3) Recognize office policies and protocols for handling appointments

V. C (13) Identify time management principles

V. P (1) Manage appointment schedules, using established priorities

V. A (2) Implement time management principles to maintain effective office function

## ABHES Competencies Achieved

8. c. Schedule and manage appointments

**Student Name:** _____

## Procedure 12–4: Completing a Patient Appointment Card

**GOAL:** To accurately complete a patient appointment card for the patient's next appointment

**MATERIALS:** Appointment book or electronic scheduler, pen, appointment card
(*Note:* A patient appointment card is available at the end of this study guide.)

**METHOD:** To pass this procedure the minimum required score is _____% or all elements must meet "satisfactory" ability on the final demonstration. The first box may be used as a practice or final demonstration, with the evaluator placing **S for Satisfactory** or **U for Unsatisfactory** if that is the grading criteria. The second box may be used as a final demonstration with a **grade point** written in the box.

| STEPS | POSSIBLE POINTS | S/U | POINTS EARNED |
|---|---|---|---|
| 1. After entering the patient's appointment in the appointment book or electronic scheduler, repeat the appointment date and time to the patient to verify accuracy. | 30 | | |
| 2. Complete the patient appointment card, entering the appointment date and time on the card. If the practice has multiple providers, there may also be a place for the appropriate physician name to be entered, and you should do so. | 40 | | |
| 3. Repeat the appointment information to the patient one more time when giving the card to him or her again, verifying the information. | 30 | | |
| **Total Points (if applicable)** | 100 | | |

**Comments:** _____

_____

_____

**Final Evaluator's Signature:** _____

**Date:** _____

### CAAHEP Competencies Achieved

V. C (1) Discuss the pros and cons of various types of appointment management systems

V. C (2) Describe scheduling guidelines

V. C (3) Recognize office policies and protocols for handling appointments

V. C (13) Identify time management principles

V. P (1) Manage appointment schedules, using established priorities

V. A (2) Implement time management principles to maintain effective office function

### ABHES Competencies Achieved

8. c. Schedule and manage appointments

## Procedure 12-5: Making Appointment Confirmation Calls

**GOAL:** To decrease the number of "no show" patients by making appointment confirmation calls 24–48 hours prior to the scheduled appointment

**MATERIALS:** Office appointment book, electronic scheduler or listing of patients scheduled to be seen tomorrow or the next day with their home phone numbers

**METHOD:** To pass this procedure the minimum required score is _____% or all elements must meet "satisfactory" ability on the final demonstration. The first box may be used as a practice or final demonstration, with the evaluator placing **S for Satisfactory** or **U for Unsatisfactory** if that is the grading criteria. The second box may be used as a final demonstration with a **grade point** written in the box.

| STEPS | POSSIBLE POINTS | S/U | POINTS EARNED |
|---|---|---|---|
| 1. Starting with the first appointment of the day, call the first patient listed. | 25 | | |
| 2. If the phone is answered, ask for the patient. If you reach the patient, give your name and the name of the practice and state that you are confirming the patient's appointment for the applicable date and time. | 25 | | |
| 3. Remind the patient about any special instructions regarding the appointment such as fasting, bringing in medical record or registration information, and copayments due. | 20 | | |
| 4. If the patient is not available, leave your name and phone number, asking that the patient return your call. | 0 | | |
| 5. If a voice mail or answering machine system is reached, follow the practice confidentiality rules unless you have permission from the patient to leave explicit information on voice mail. | 0 | | |
| 6. Thank the patient for his or her time, stating you will see them at the stated date and time. | 20 | | |
| 7. Allow the patient to hang up first, so if there are questions, you may answer them. | 10 | | |
| **Total Points (if applicable)** | 100 | | |

**Comments:** _____

_____

_____

**Final Evaluator's Signature:** _____

**Date:** _____

## CAAHEP Competencies Achieved

IV. P (7) Demonstrate telephone techniques

V. C (1) Discuss the pros and cons of various types of appointment management systems

V. C (2) Describe scheduling guidelines

V. C (3) Recognize office policies and protocols for handling appointments

V. C (13) Identify time management principles

V. P (1) Manage appointment schedules, using established priorities

V. A (2) Implement time management principles to maintain effective office function

## ABHES Competencies Achieved

8. c. Schedule and manage appointments

**Student Name:** _____

## Procedure 12–6: Scheduling Outpatient Surgical Appointments

**GOAL:** To schedule an outpatient surgical procedure

**MATERIALS:** Patient medical record, scheduling form, calendar, telephone, pen

**METHOD:** To pass this procedure the minimum required score is _____% or all elements must meet "satisfactory" ability on the final demonstration. The first box may be used as a practice or final demonstration, with the evaluator placing **S for Satisfactory** or **U for Unsatisfactory** if that is the grading criteria. The second box may be used as a final demonstration with a **grade point** written in the box.

| STEPS | POSSIBLE POINTS | S/U | POINTS EARNED |
|---|---|---|---|
| 1. From the physician and patient medical record, obtain detailed information regarding the name of procedure to be performed, the amount of the time the outpatient surgical suite will be needed, and the reason (diagnosis) for the procedure. | 15 | | |
| 2. Place a call to the appropriate surgery center or outpatient surgical unit at the requested facility. Have the name of the surgeon, assistant, or PA (if they will be used) available, as well as the patient and physician's preferred dates for the procedure. | 10 | | |
| 3. When the appointment scheduler answers the phone, identify yourself, the practice, and the procedure you need to schedule, as well as the preferred date for the procedure. | 10 | | |
| 4. When a date for the procedure is agreed upon by the patient, give the scheduler the patient's name, address, phone number, DOB, gender, and insurance information, including the prior authorization number if needed. Also give the patient's diagnosis as required for medical necessity. | 15 | | |
| 5. Inquire as to any preprocedure testing that may need to be done, as well as any patient preparation required prior to the procedure, including patient arrival time. | 10 | | |
| 6. Confirm the appointment date and time prior to hanging up. If necessary, book any preprocedure testing for the patient and document these appointments in the patient instructions and appropriate office form(s) such as the surgical checkoff sheet and/or within the patient's medical record. | 10 | | |
| 7. Provide the patient with written instructions from the physician as well as all information obtained while booking the appointment. The patient should also be informed that he should arrange for someone to drive him to and from this appointment. | 10 | | |

*(Continued)*

| STEPS | POSSIBLE POINTS | S/U | POINTS EARNED |
|---|---|---|---|
| 8. Go over the written dates and instructions with the patient, asking the patient if there are any questions, answering them if possible and if not, asking a clinical member of the team to do so. | 10 | | |
| 9. Give a copy of the instructions and information to the patient and keep a copy in the patient record. Remind the patient to feel free to call the office at any time with any questions or concerns. | 10 | | |
| **Total Points (if applicable)** | 100 | | |

**Comments:** _____

_____

_____

**Final Evaluator's Signature:** _____

**Date:** _____

**CAAHEP Competencies Achieved**

V. C (4) Identify critical information required for scheduling patient admissions and/or procedures

V. P (2) Schedule patient admissions and/or procedures

**AHBES Competencies Achieved**

8. c. Schedule and manage appointments

8. f. Schedule inpatient and outpatient admissions

8. s. Obtain managed care referrals and precertifications

**Student Name:** _____

## Procedure 12-7: Scheduling Inpatient Surgical Appointments

**GOAL:** To schedule an inpatient surgical procedure

**MATERIALS:** Patient medical record, scheduling form, calendar, telephone, pen

**METHOD:** To pass this procedure the minimum required score is _____ % or all elements must meet "satisfactory" ability on the final demonstration. The first box may be used as a practice or final demonstration, with the evaluator placing **S for Satisfactory** or **U for Unsatisfactory** if that is the grading criteria. The second box may be used as a final demonstration with a **grade point** written in the box.

| STEPS | POSSIBLE POINTS | S/U | POINTS EARNED |
|---|---|---|---|
| 1. From the physician and patient medical record, obtain detailed information regarding the name of the procedure to be performed, the amount of the time the operating room will be needed, and the reason (diagnosis) for the procedure. | 15 | | |
| 2. Place a call to the appropriate surgical unit at the requested hospital. Have the name of the surgeon, assistant, or PA (if they will be used) available, as well as the patient and physician's preferred dates for the procedure available. | 10 | | |
| 3. When the appointment scheduler answers the phone, identify yourself, the practice, and the procedure you need to schedule, as well as the preferred date for the procedure. | 10 | | |
| 4. When a date for the procedure is agreed upon by the patient, give the scheduler the patient's name, address, phone number, DOB, gender, and insurance information, including the prior authorization number if needed. Also give the patient's diagnosis as required for medical necessity. | 15 | | |
| 5. Inquire as to any preprocedure testing that may need to be done, as well as any patient preparation required prior to the procedure, including patient arrival time. | 10 | | |
| 6. Confirm the appointment date and time prior to hanging up. If necessary, book any preprocedure testing for the patient and document these appointments in the patient instructions and appropriate office form(s) such as the surgical checkoff sheet and/or within the patient's medical record. | 10 | | |
| 7. Provide the patient with written instructions from the physician, as well as all information obtained while booking the appointment. The patient should also be informed that she should arrange for someone to drive her to and from this appointment. | 10 | | |

*(Continued)*

| STEPS | POSSIBLE POINTS | S/U | POINTS EARNED |
|---|---|---|---|
| 8. Go over the written dates and instructions with the patient, asking the patient if there are any questions, answering them if possible and if not, asking a clinical member of the team to do so. | 10 | | |
| 9. Give a copy of instructions and information to the patient and keep a copy in the patient record. Remind the patient to feel free to call the office at any time with any questions or concerns. | 10 | | |
| **Total Points (if applicable)** | 100 | | |

**Comments:** _____

_____

_____

**Final Evaluator's Signature:** _____

**Date:** _____

### CAAHEP Competencies Achieved

V. C (4) Identify critical information required for scheduling patient admissions and/or procedures

V. P (2) Schedule patient admissions and/or procedures

### ABHES Competencies Achieved

8. c. Schedule and manage appointments

8. f. Schedule inpatient and outpatient admissions

8. s. Obtain managed care referrals and precertifications

## Test Your Knowledge

### Vocabulary Review

Match the key terms in the right column with the definitions in the left column by placing the letter of each correct answer in the space provided.

_____ **1.** the closing remark of a business letter found two spaces below the last line of the body of the letter

_____ **2.** a letter format in which all lines begin flush left; also called block style

_____ **3.** the act of inputting or entering information into a computer

_____ **4.** a title used before a person's name, such as "Dr.," "Mr.," or "Ms."

_____ **5.** a letter format in which the dateline, complimentary closing, signature block, and notations are aligned and begin at the center of the page or slightly to the right of center

_____ **6.** the process of ensuring that a document is accurate, clear, and complete; free of grammatical errors; organized logically; and written in the appropriate style

_____ **7.** the writer's name and business title found four lines below the complimentary closing in a business letter

_____ **8.** to underline or highlight key points of a document or to write reminders, make comments, and suggest actions in the margins

**a.** annotate [LO13.5]

**b.** body [LO13.3]

**c.** clarity [LO13.2]

**d.** complimentary closing [LO13.2]

**e.** concise [LO13.2]

**f.** courtesy title [LO13.3]

**g.** dateline [LO13.3]

**h.** editing [LO13.5]

**i.** enclosure [LO13.3]

**j.** full-block letter style [LO13.3]

**k.** identification line [LO13.3]

**l.** inside address [LO13.3]

**m.** key [LO13.5]

**n.** letterhead [LO13.3]

**o.** modified-block letter style [LO13.3]

_____ **9.** an electronic scanner that can "read" typed letters

_____ **10.** a guide that ensures consistency and accuracy

_____ **11.** optional line of two to three words that appears three lines below the inside address of a business letter

_____ **12.** clearness in writing or stating a message

_____ **13.** a written greeting, such as "Dear," used at the beginning of a letter

_____ **14.** formal business stationery, with the office name and address printed at the top, used for correspondence with patients, colleagues, and vendors

_____ **15.** checking a document for formatting, data, and mechanical errors

_____ **16.** materials that are included in the same envelope as the primary letter

_____ **17.** single-spaced lines of text that are the content of a business letter

_____ **18.** a line at the bottom of a letter containing the letter writer's initials and the typist's initials

_____ **19.** brevity; the use of no unnecessary words

_____ **20.** information found at the end of the business letter indicating enclosures included with the letter as well as the names of other people who will be receiving copies of the letter

_____ **21.** a modification of the letter format style in which the salutation and complimentary closing are omitted and a subject line typed in all capital letters is placed between the address and the body of the letter

_____ **22.** The name and address of the person to whom the letter is being sent; appears on a business letter two to four spaces down from the date and should be two, three, or four lines in length.

_____ **23.** the line at the top of a letter that contains the month, day, and year

**p.** notations [LO13.5]

**q.** optical character reader (OCR) [LO13.10]

**r.** proofreading [LO13.5]

**s.** salutation [LO13.3]

**t.** signature block [LO13.3]

**u.** simplified letter style [LO13.3]

**v.** subject line [LO13.3]

**w.** template [LO13.1]

# Multiple-Choice Certification Questions

There may be more than one answer; circle the letter of the choice that best completes each statement or answers each question.

1. **[LO13.1]** The size of standard letterhead paper is
   a. 8½ × 14 inches.
   b. 9 × 11 inches.
   c. 8½ × 11 inches.
   d. 9 × 12 inches.
   e. 9 × 13 inches.

2. **[LO13.1]** When ordering standard business envelopes for the office, you should order the most common size, which is
   a. No. 5.
   b. No. 7.
   c. No. 9.
   d. No. 10.
   e. None of the above.

3. **[LO13.3]** Which of the following is the correct order of the items appearing in a business letter?
   a. Dateline, inside address, letterhead
   b. Body, signature block, complimentary closing
   c. Inside address, salutation, dateline
   d. Salutation, subject line, inside address
   e. Salutation, subject line, body

4. **[LO13.3]** The subject line of a business letter is used to
   a. address the person that is to receive the letter.
   b. get the reader's attention.
   c. end the letter.
   d. state the number of enclosures in the letter.
   e. identify the sender of the letter.

5. **[LO13.2]** When you are trying to locate a synonym or similar word to use in professional writing, it is recommended to use a/an
   a. thesaurus.
   b. medical dictionary.
   c. English grammar and usage manual.
   d. word processing spell-checker.
   e. standard dictionary.

6. **[LO13.5]** One of the most important steps in proofreading is
   a. to use the spell-check feature on the computer.
   b. to check your document for grammar errors.
   c. to review your document for punctuation mistakes.
   d. to ask another person to proofread your work.
   e. None of the above.

7. **[LO13.3]** If you follow proper rules for writing, how are words divided in a document?
   a. Divide suffixes such as "–tial" and "–sion."
   b. Divide a word before a prefix.
   c. Divide according to pronunciation.
   d. Divide after a suffix.
   e. Divide hyphenated compound words after the first letter following the hyphen.

**8.** [LO13.5] Which of the following words is spelled correctly?
   a. Noticiable
   b. Necesary
   c. Mispelled
   d. Truely
   e. Recommend

**9.** [LO13.2] Which of the follow qualities is *not* part of a clean, concise letter?
   a. Discussing one topic at a time
   b. Stating the purpose of the letter in the last paragraph of the letter
   c. Listing events in chronological order
   d. Sticking to the subject
   e. Selecting words carefully

**10.** [LO13.5] Which of the following is a formatting type of error that can occur when preparing a document?
   a. A spelling error
   b. A mistyped monetary figure on a patient statement
   c. Words that are divided in the wrong place at the end of a line
   d. Improperly aligned paragraphs
   e. A punctuation error

**11.** [LO13.2] According to the rules of writing, when should a number be spelled out or written out?
   a. When the number is less than eleven
   b. When discussing a laboratory result
   c. When referring to specific sums of money
   d. When using a series of numbers in a sentence
   e. When citing statistics

**12.** [LO13.3] When you are writing a document, which of the following items should be capitalized?
   a. Proper names
   b. Days of the week
   c. Religious designations
   d. Titles of magazines
   e. All of the above

**13.** [LO13.3] Which of the following words is misspelled?
   a. Absence
   b. Associate
   c. Believe
   d. Counsil
   e. Discreet

**14.** [LO13.8] The main characteristic of first-class mail is that it
   a. must weigh at least 1 pound (16 ounces).
   b. cannot weigh over 11 ounces.
   c. is used for sending a minimum of 300 pieces such as promotional advertising.
   d. includes boxes at least 12 inches × 16 inches.
   e. is always delivered overnight.

**15.** [LO13.9] The first step in processing incoming mail is to
   a. read letters and underline or highlight key points.
   b. list all pieces of mail on the daily mail log.
   c. stamp all envelopes with the date received.
   d. discard junk mail.
   e. sort the mail by category.

**16.** [LO13.1] Which of the following is *not* considered a correspondence supply?
   a. Envelopes
   b. Labels

c. Staples

d. Statements

e. Letterhead

17. **[LO13.3]** Which of the following states is properly abbreviated for use in an address?
   a. Tennessee—TE
   b. Oklahoma—OL
   c. Montana—MN
   d. Maryland—MD
   e. Missouri—MI

18. **[LO13.3]** Which of the following would *not* be used in a complimentary closing of a letter?
   a. "Thank you and goodbye"
   b. " Sincerely"
   c. "Best regards"
   d. "Very truly yours"
   e. None of the above.

19. **[LO13.2]** A properly formatted letter should
   a. be double-spaced throughout the letter.
   b. have a 1 inch right and left margin for 8½ inch wide paper.
   c. have over 25 words in each sentence.
   d. include at least 10 sentences in each paragraph.
   e. be single-spaced between paragraphs.

20. **[LO13.3]** Which of the following is an example of a proper salutation?
   a. "Dear Mr. Laboratory Director;"
   b. "Dear Ms. Claims Representative,"
   c. "Dear Mr. James:"
   d. "Dear Doctor James, MD;"
   e. "Dear Miss Sally Jones;"

21. **[LO13.3]** Open punctuation style means that there is
   a. a colon after the salutation.
   b. a semicolon after the complimentary closing.
   c. no punctuation in the entire letter.
   d. a colon after the enclosure notation.
   e. no punctuation after the word "Attention" in the attention line.

22. **[LO13.4]** Which of the following is *not* part of an interoffice memo?
   a. The date of the memo
   b. A list of everyone who is receiving the memo
   c. A subject line indicating the general purpose of the memo
   d. A complimentary closing from the sender of the memo
   e. A "CC" line

23. **[LO13.3]** According to the basic rules of writing, when making a singular word plural
   a. a medical term ending in *-is* becomes plural by changing the *-is* to *-es*. For example, *metastasis* becomes *metastases*.
   b. add an *-es* to a word ending in "a"; for example, *vertebra* becomes *vertebraes*.
   c. add an *-s* to terms ending in *-um*. For example, *diverticulum* becomes *diverticulums*.
   d. do not change the word *virus*, which is both singular and plural.
   e. none of the above is correct.

24. **[LO13.3]** How many spaces are left between the complimentary closing and the signature line?
   a. 1–2 spaces
   b. 2–3 spaces
   c. 3–4 spaces
   d. 5–6 spaces
   e. 6–7 spaces

**25.** [LO13.8] Mail that is sent using registered mail includes
   a. first-class and Priority Mail.
   b. international and certified mail.
   c. parcel post and Priority Mail.
   d. bulk and parcel post mail.
   e. first-class and parcel post mail.

## True or False

Decide whether each statement is true or false. In the space at the left, write "T" for true or "F" for false. On the lines provided, rewrite the false statements to make them true.

_____ **1.** [LO13.3] The inside address of a letter is the preprinted portion of formal business stationery that includes the name and address of the medical office.

_____

_____ **2.** [LO13.3] A properly formatted letter is single-spaced in the body of the letter and double-spaced between paragraphs or parts of the letter.

_____

_____ **3.** [LO13.3] A full-block letter style is typed with all lines flush left, and no paragraphs are indented.

_____

_____ **4.** [LO13.2] An effectively written letter includes slang words or phrases if the recipient of the letter would understand slang language.

_____

_____ **5.** [LO13.3] If a physician has authorized you to sign a letter on his behalf, you should sign the physician's name, and the letter is ready for sending.

_____

_____ **6.** [LO13.8] The USPS guarantees delivery of Priority Mail items in 2 to 3 days.

_____

_____ **7.** [LO13.1] Legal-size paper is the same width but is shorter than standard or letter-size paper.

_____

_____ **8.** [LO13.3] A colon is used after the salutation, the complimentary closing, and the attention line.

_____

_____ **9.** [LO13.5] General formatting guidelines for all letters suggest dividing long paragraphs of 10 lines of type into shorter ones.

_____

_____ **10.** [LO13.4] Interoffice memorandums are used to communicate with employees of other medical practices and hospitals.

_____

## Sentence Completion

In the space provided, write the word or phrase that best completes each sentence.

1. [LO13.1] The two most common sizes of letterhead paper are _____ and _____.

2. [LO13.3] Letter styles include _____-_____ letter style, _____-_____ letter style, and _____ letter style.

3. [LO13.5] Editing involves checking a document for _____ _____, _____ _____, _____, _____, and _____.

4. [LO13.5] Proofreading involves checking a document for _____, _____, and _____ errors.

5. [LO13.8] Any first-class item that weighs between _____ ounces and _____ pounds requires Priority Mail service.

6. [LO13.8] Express delivery services are provided by companies such as _____ _____ and _____.

7. [LO13.6] The five steps to processing incoming mail include _____, _____, _____, _____, and _____.

8. [LO13.6] Incoming mail that is classified as urgent includes _____ mail, _____ mail, _____ mail, and _____ delivery.

9. [LO13.1] Preprinted _____ are used to send an original bill to a patient, and preprinted _____ are used to send a reminder that an account is 30 or more days past due.

10. [LO13.3] The signature block contains the letter writer's _____ on the first line and the letter writer's _____ _____ on the second line.

1. _____
   _____

2. _____
   _____

3. _____
   _____

4. _____
   _____

5. _____
   _____

6. _____
   _____

7. _____
   _____

8. _____
   _____

9. _____
   _____

10. _____
    _____

# Apply Your Knowledge

## Short Answer

Write the answer to each question on the lines provided.

1. [LO13.3] Explain the difference between open and mixed punctuation in a letter.

_____

_____

_____

2. [LO13.1, 13.3] Explain the structure and supplies used for a letter that is more than one page.

_____

_____

_____

3. [LO13.5] List at least five tools that can be used for editing and proofreading documents. Explain the purpose of each one.

_____

_____

_____

4. [LO13.2] List five items to consider when constructing a letter that will ensure that the content is clean and concise.

_____

_____

_____

5. [LO13.8] For each type of mail service listed, give an example of the type of mail that would be sent via this service: first-class mail, parcel post, Priority Mail.

_____

_____

_____

# Problem-Solving Activities

Follow the directions for each activity.

1. **[LO13.2]** What's the Difference?
   a. The following sets of words are pronounced the same or very similar but are spelled differently.
   b. Using a standard or medical dictionary, research the meaning of each set of words to see the difference in them.
      - Personal, Personnel
      - Principal, Principle
      - Stationary, Stationery
      - Humerus, Humorous
      - Ileum, Ilium
   c. Word-process the information you researched for each set of words into a document for submission to your instructor.

2. **[LO13.4]** Interoffice Memo to Staff
   a. Compose an interoffice memo that includes the following information:
      - Staff meeting
      - Monday, June 22
      - 1:00 P.M.—2:00 P.M.
      - A representative of the new employee benefits plan will discuss the new health insurance plans available to employees and the new 401(k) investment plan
   b. Word-process the interoffice memo, inserting a header with the name of the medical clinic and address so it appears to look like a letterhead. Print it out when you have completed the assignment.

# Thinking Critically

Write your response to each case study question on the lines provided.

## Case 1 [LO13.2]

Your physician asks you to write a letter for a patient to give to his employer requesting that the patient stay off work for one week and then return to light duty only for one week before resuming regular activities of his job. As the patient checks out at the reception desk after seeing the physician, you ask the patient for his employer's name and address for the letter. As you gather employer information from the patient, the patient asks if you will just write the letter to have him return to work immediately but to light duty for a week. The patient tells you that he forgot to tell the physician that he cannot afford to be off work that long and that he has no sick time left to take any more days off work.

1. How would you respond to this patient's request?

   _____

   _____

   _____

2. Is there anything you can offer or recommend for the patient to do at this time?

   _____

   _____

   _____

**Case 2** [LO13.3]

Your medical office manager is the only person the physician has authorized to sign the physician's signature to letters sent out of the office to patients. She signs his name and puts her initials next to it. You and a co-worker are responsible for composing these letters or to use templates to process new letters. When you complete them, you print them out and give them to the office manager to sign. One afternoon as you are doing other tasks in the reception area, you notice that your co-worker is signing patient letters and putting the office manager's initials next to the physician's name. The co-worker notices that you see her signing the name and initials. She explains to you that the office manager told her that it is alright to do this if the office manager is not available at the time.

**1.** Is there something that you should do in this situation?

_____

_____

_____

**2.** Is there any other action that should take place?

_____

_____

_____

**Case 3** [LO13.9]

The receptionist in your medical practice is responsible for sorting the mail as it arrives every day. Periodically packages arrive from pharmaceutical vendors with samples of prescription and nonprescription medications. The back-office medical assistant puts these samples in a storage area for the physicians to give to patients to try on a trial basis. One day when a package arrives, the receptionist opens it and finds that the prescription drug samples look like the ones that her mother takes. She tells you how expensive the drug is and that she sure wishes the company would send her mother some samples. Later that day, the back-office assistant is emptying the box of samples and discovers that the blood pressure pills that are listed on the packing slip are not included in the package.

**1.** What is the possible problem with this scenario?

_____

_____

_____

**2.** If the receptionist took the medication samples from the box, what are the consequences of this action?

_____

_____

_____

# Demonstrate Your Knowledge

**Student Name:** _____

## Procedure 13–1: Creating a Letter

**GOAL:** To follow standard procedure for constructing a business letter

**MATERIALS:** Word processor or personal computer, letterhead paper (refer to the blank letterhead located at the end of this study guide), dictionary or other reference sources

**METHOD:** To pass this procedure the minimum required score is _____% or all elements must meet "satisfactory" ability on the final demonstration. The first box may be used as a practice or final demonstration, with the evaluator placing **S for Satisfactory** or **U for Unsatisfactory** if that is the grading criteria. The second box may be used as a final demonstration with a **grade point** written in the box.

| STEPS | POSSIBLE POINTS | S/U | POINTS EARNED |
|---|---|---|---|
| 1. Format the letter according to the office's standard procedure. Use the same punctuation and style throughout. Refer to Figures 13–2 through 13–6 for spacing and formatting suggestions. | 10 | | |
| 2. Start the dateline three lines below the last line of the printed letterhead. (*Note:* Depending on the length of the letter, it is acceptable to start between two and six lines below the letterhead.) | 5 | | |
| 3. Two lines below the dateline, type in any special mailing instructions (such as REGISTERED MAIL, CERTIFIED MAIL, and so on). | 5 | | |
| 4. Three lines below any special instructions, begin the inside address. Type the addressee's courtesy title (Mr., Mrs., Ms.) and full name on the first line. If a professional title is given (MD, RN, PhD), type this title after the addressee's name instead of using a courtesy title. | 10 | | |
| 5. Type the addressee's business title, if applicable, on the second line. Type the company name on the third line. Type the street address on the fourth line including the apartment or suite number. Type the city, state, and zip code on the fifth line. Use the standard two-letter abbreviation for the state, followed by one space and the zip code. | 10 | | |
| 6. Two lines below the inside address, type the salutation, using the appropriate courtesy title (Mr., Mrs., Ms., Dr.) prior to typing the addressee's last name. | 5 | | |
| 7. Two lines below the salutation, type the subject line, if applicable. | 5 | | |
| 8. Two lines below the subject line, begin the body of the letter. Single-space between lines. Double-space between paragraphs. | 15 | | |

*(Continued)*

| STEPS | POSSIBLE POINTS | S/U | POINTS EARNED |
|---|---|---|---|
| 9. Two lines below the body of the letter, type the complimentary closing. | 5 | | |
| 10. Leave three blank lines (return four times), and begin the signature block. (Enough space must be left to allow for the signature.) Type the sender's name on the first line. Type the sender's title on the second line. | 5 | | |
| 11. Two lines below the sender's title, type the identification line. Type the sender's initials in all capitals and your initials in lowercase letters, separating the two sets of initials with a colon or a forward slash. | 5 | | |
| 12. One or two lines below the identification line, type the enclosure notation, if applicable. | 5 | | |
| 13. Two lines below the enclosure notation, type the copy notation, if applicable. | 5 | | |
| 14. Edit the letter. | 10 | | |
| 15. Proofread and spell-check the letter. | 0 | | |
| **Total Points (if applicable)** | 100 | | |

Comments: _____

_____

_____

**Final Evaluator's Signature:** _____

**Date:** _____

## CAAHEP Competencies Achieved

IV. C (8) Recognize elements of fundamental writing skills

IV. C (9) Discuss applications of electronic technology in effective communication

IV. P (10) Compose professional/business letters

IV. A (7) Analyze communications in providing appropriate responses/feedback

## ABHES Competencies Achieved

7. a. Perform basic keyboarding skills including:

    (1) Locating the keys on a keyboard

    (2) Typing medical correspondence and basic reports

7. b. Identify and properly utilize office machines, computerized systems, and medical software such as:

    (1) Efficiently maintain and understand different types of medical correspondence and medical reports

    (2) Apply computer application skills using a variety of different electronic programs including both practice management software and EMR software

8. gg. Use pertinent medical terminology

8. hh. Receive, organize, prioritize, and transmit information expediently

8. jj. Perform fundamental writing skills including correct grammar, spelling, and formatting techniques when writing prescriptions, documenting medical records, etc.

8. ll. Apply electronic technology

Student Name: _____

## Procedure 13–2: Sending an Electronic Patient Letter

**GOAL:** To create and send an electronic letter to a patient

**MATERIALS:** Information necessary to create required letter, EHR software program containing letter templates such as SpringCharts®

**METHOD:** To pass this procedure the minimum required score is _____% or all elements must meet "satisfactory" ability on the final demonstration. The first box may be used as a practice or final demonstration, with the evaluator placing **S for Satisfactory** or **U for Unsatisfactory** if that is the grading criteria. The second box may be used as a final demonstration with a **grade point** written in the box.

| STEPS | POSSIBLE POINTS | S/U | POINTS EARNED |
|---|---|---|---|
| 1. Access the "New" menu in the "Practice View" screen. Choose "New Template," then "New Letter Template." In the "Re:" window, key the subject line for the letter, such as "Welcome to Total Care Clinic, PC." | 15 | | |
| 2. In the text box, key the body of the letter. Begin the letter with an introductory welcoming statement, such as "Thank you for choosing Total Care Clinic for your healthcare needs. We look forward to working with you." Enter pertinent information that will be needed by a new patient such as the address, phone and fax number, and Web site information for the practice. It is also a good idea to include the names of the practitioners at Total Care Clinic, including the usual office hours for each. It may also be a good idea to include the paraprofessional personnel and their titles. | 20 | | |
| 3. When you complete the letter, give this new template a name, for example, "Welcome Patient Letter" and click the "Save" button. | 15 | | |
| 4. Open the new patient's chart. Click on the "New" menu and select "Welcome Patient Letter." Note that, because you are in the patient chart, the letter is already addressed to the patient and that the default greeting and disclosure are also present. Click the "Template" button at the bottom of the screen and highlight (select) "Welcome Patient Letter." | 20 | | |
| 5. Add a signature to the bottom of the letter by clicking on the "Sign" icon at the bottom of the window. Choose the correct provider to add his/her name to the closing of the letter. | 10 | | |

*(Continued)*

| STEPS | POSSIBLE POINTS | S/U | POINTS EARNED |
|---|---|---|---|
| 6. You can now choose to print the letter to send it via USPS mail, or use the e-mail option should you have a written permission from the patient to do so. | 10 | | |
| 7. Click the "Done" button and save the letter under the "Letters" category, saving the letter under "Welcome Patient Letter." | 10 | | |
| **Total Points (if applicable)** | 100 | | |

**Comments:** _____

_____

_____

**Final Evaluator's Signature:** _____

**Date:** _____

## CAAHEP Competencies Achieved

IV. C (8) Recognize elements of fundamental writing skills

IV. C (9) Discuss applications of electronic technology in effective communication

IV. P (10) Compose professional/business letters

IV. A (7) Analyze communications in providing appropriate responses/feedback

## ABHES Competencies Achieved

7. a. Perform basic keyboarding skills including:

(1) Locating the keys on a keyboard

(2) Typing medical correspondence and basic reports

7. b. Identify and properly utilize office machines, computerized systems, and medical software such as:

(1) Efficiently maintain and understand different types of medical correspondence and medical reports

(2) Apply computer application skills using a variety of different electronic programs including both practice management software and EMR software

8. gg. Use pertinent medical terminology

8. hh. Receive, organize, prioritize, and transmit information expediently

8. jj. Perform fundamental writing skills including correct grammar, spelling, and formatting techniques when writing prescriptions, documenting medical records, etc.

8. ll. Apply electronic technology

**Student Name:** _____

## Procedure 13–3: Writing a Memo

**GOAL:** To follow standard procedures to write a memo for interoffice use

**MATERIALS:** Word processor or personal computer, plain paper, dictionaries and other source texts such as the *PDR* or policies and procedures manuals as required

**METHOD:** To pass this procedure the minimum required score is _____% or all elements must meet "satisfactory" ability on the final demonstration. The first box may be used as a practice or final demonstration, with the evaluator placing **S for Satisfactory** or **U for Unsatisfactory** if that is the grading criteria. The second box may be used as a final demonstration with a **grade point** written in the box.

| STEPS | POSSIBLE POINTS | S/U | POINTS EARNED |
|---|---|---|---|
| 1. Gather all necessary documents to create the memo. | 10 | | |
| 2. Decide whether the memo will be created freehand or through the use of a template. | 20 | | |
| 3. If using a template, fill in the headings as listed with appropriate information. *If the memo is being created freehand, use the headings "DATE:", "TO:", "FROM:", and "SUBJECT:" and then complete the resulting blanks with appropriate information. | 0 | | |
| 4. Double- or triple-space after the memo headings or, if using a template, move to the body area of the memo and begin typing the information to be included in the memo. | 20 | | |
| 5. Single-space the information within the memo and double-space between paragraphs. Use either the block or indented paragraph format depending on office policy. | 20 | | |
| 6. At the end of the memo, if required by office policy, double-space after the last line of the memo and insert reference initials. | 10 | | |
| 7. Spell-check and proofread the document carefully, correcting errors as necessary. | 20 | | |
| **Total Points (if applicable)** | 100 | | |

**Comments:** _____

_____

_____

**Final Evaluator's Signature:** _____

**Date:** _____

## CAAHEP Competencies Achieved

IV. C (8) Recognize elements of fundamental writing skills

IV. C (9) Discuss applications of electronic technology in effective communication

IV. P (10) Compose professional/business letters

IV. A (7) Analyze communications in providing appropriate responses/feedback

## ABHES Competencies Achieved

7. a. Perform basic keyboarding skills including:

    (1) Locating the keys on a keyboard

    (2) Typing medical correspondence and basic reports

7. b. Identify and properly utilize office machines, computerized systems, and medical software such as:

    (1) Efficiently maintain and understand different types of medical correspondence and medical reports

    (2) Apply computer application skills using a variety of different electronic programs including both practice management software and EMR software

8. gg. Use pertinent medical terminology

8. hh. Receive, organize, prioritize, and transmit information expediently

8. jj. Perform fundamental writing skills including correct grammar, spelling, and formatting techniques when writing prescriptions, documenting medical records, etc.

8. ll. Apply electronic technology

**Student Name:** _____

## Procedure 13–4: Using the *PDR* as a Spelling Reference

**GOAL:** To use the *PDR* as a spelling reference

**MATERIALS:** Document, such as letter to a patient or physician including one or more references to specific medications; *PDR;* pen or word processing software package

**METHOD:** To pass this procedure the minimum required score is _____% or all elements must meet "satisfactory" ability on the final demonstration. The first box may be used as a practice or final demonstration, with the evaluator placing **S for Satisfactory** or **U for Unsatisfactory** if that is the grading criteria. The second box may be used as a final demonstration with a **grade point** written in the box.

| STEPS | POSSIBLE POINTS | S/U | POINTS EARNED |
|---|---|---|---|
| 1. After completing the document, use spell-check. | 10 | | |
| 2. Note any terms, including medication names, not recognized by the spell-checker. | 10 | | |
| 3. Open the *PDR* to Section 2 (pink section): Brand- and generic-name index. | 5 | | |
| 4. The index is in alphabetic order. Locate the alphabetic area where the drug in question is located. | 15 | | |
| 5. When you locate the medication name, note the spelling carefully and correct it within your document. | 15 | | |
| 6. If there are several medications listed that appear to be "possibilities" for the medication you are checking, it may be necessary to check with the physician so that you do not mistakenly list an incorrect drug. | 15 | | |
| 7. If the office word processing software contains a medical dictionary spell-checker, you may wish to carefully enter this new medical term into the dictionary for future reference. | 10 | | |
| 8. Carefully double-check the spelling of all other medications in the document, correcting spelling as necessary. | 10 | | |
| 9. Proofread and edit the rest of the document prior to sending it to the intended recipient. | 10 | | |
| **Total Points (if applicable)** | 100 | | |

**Comments:** _____

_____

_____

**Final Evaluator's Signature:** _____

**Date:** _____

## CAAHEP Competencies Achieved

I. C (11) Identify classifications of medications, including desired effects, side effects, and adverse reactions

IV. C (8) Recognize elements of fundamental writing skills

IV. P (10) Compose professional/business letters

## ABHES Competencies Achieved

6. b. Properly utilize *PDR,* drug handbook, and other drug references to identify a drug's classification, usual dosage, usual side effects, and contraindications

7. a. Perform basic keyboarding skills including:

   (2) Typing medical correspondence and reports

8. e. Locate resources and information for patients and employers

8. jj. Perform fundamental writing skills including correct grammar, spelling, and formatting techniques when writing prescriptions, documenting medical records, etc.

**Student Name:** _____

## Procedure 13–5: Managing Mail

**GOAL:** To follow a standard procedure for sorting, opening, and processing incoming office mail

**MATERIALS:** Letter opener, date and time stamp (manual or automatic), stapler, paper clips, adhesive notes

**METHOD:** To pass this procedure the minimum required score is _____% or all elements must meet "satisfactory" ability on the final demonstration. The first box may be used as a practice or final demonstration, with the evaluator placing **S for Satisfactory** or **U for Unsatisfactory** if that is the grading criteria. The second box may be used as a final demonstration with a **grade point** written in the box.

| STEPS | POSSIBLE POINTS | S/U | POINTS EARNED |
|---|---|---|---|
| 1. Check the address on each letter or package to be sure that it has been delivered to the correct location. | 5 | | |
| 2. Sort the mail into piles according to priority and type of mail. Your system may include the following:<br>• Top priority. This pile will contain any items that were sent by overnight mail delivery in addition to items sent by registered mail, certified mail, or special delivery. (Faxes and e-mail messages are also top priority.)<br>• Second priority. This pile will include personal or confidential mail.<br>• Third priority. This pile will contain all first-class mail, airmail, and Priority Mail items. These items should be divided into payments received, insurance forms, reports, and other correspondence.<br>• Fourth priority. This pile will consist of packages.<br>• Fifth priority. This pile will contain magazines and newspapers.<br>• Sixth priority. This last pile will include advertisements and catalogs. | 15 | | |
| 3. Set aside all letters labeled "Personal" or "Confidential." Unless you have permission to open these letters, only the addressee should open them. | 5 | | |
| 4. Arrange all the envelopes with the flaps facing up and away from you. | 5 | | |
| 5. Tap the lower edge of the envelope to shift the contents to the bottom. This step helps to prevent cutting any of the contents when you open the envelope. | 5 | | |
| 6. Open all the envelopes. | 5 | | |
| 7. Remove and unfold the contents, making sure that nothing remains in the envelope. | 10 | | |

*(Continued)*

| STEPS | POSSIBLE POINTS | S/U | POINTS EARNED |
|---|---|---|---|
| 8. Review each document, and check the sender's name and address.<br>• If the letter has no return address, save the envelope, or cut the address off the envelope and tape it to the letter.<br>• Check to see if the address matches the one on the envelope. *If* there is a difference, staple the envelope to the letter, and make a note to verify the correct address with the sender. | 10 | | |
| 9. Compare the enclosure notation on the letter with the actual enclosures to make sure that all items are included. Make a note to contact the sender if anything is missing. | 10 | | |
| 10. Clip together each letter and its enclosures. | 5 | | |
| 11. Check the date of the letter. If there is a significant delay between the date of the letter and the postmark, keep the envelope. | 5 | | |
| 12. If all contents appear to be in order, you can discard the envelope. | 5 | | |
| 13. Review all bills and statements.<br>• Make sure the amount enclosed is the same as the amount listed on the statement.<br>• Make a note of any discrepancies. | 5 | | |
| 14. Stamp each piece of correspondence with the date (and sometimes the time) to record its receipt. If possible, stamp each item in the same location, such as the upper-right corner. | 10 | | |
| **Total Points (if applicable)** | 100 | | |

Comments: _____

_____

_____

Final Evaluator's Signature: _____

Date: _____

## CAAHEP Competencies Achieved

None

## ABHES Competencies Achieved

7. b. Identify and properly utilize office machines, computerized systems, and medical software such as:

    (1) Efficiently maintain and understand different types of medical correspondence and medical reports

8. a. Perform basic clerical functions

8. d. Apply concepts for office procedures

8. hh. Receive, organize, prioritize, and transmit information expediently

## Test Your Knowledge

### Vocabulary Review

Match the key terms in the right column with the definitions in the left column by placing the letter of each correct answer in the space provided.

_____ **1.** a file used infrequently

_____ **2.** how patient records are created, filed, and maintained

_____ **3.** a small group of two or three numbers at the end of a patient number, used as an identifying unit in a filing system

_____ **4.** a file for a patient who has died, moved away, or for some other reason no longer consults the office for medical expertise

_____ **5.** a filing cabinet featuring pull-out drawers that usually contain a metal frame or bar equipped to handle letter- or legal-sized documents in hanging file folders

_____ **6.** files kept on rolling shelves that slide along permanent tracks in the floor and are stored close together or staked when not in use

_____ **7.** a schedule that details how long to keep different types of patient records in the office after they have become inactive or closed and how long the records should be stored

**a.** active file **[LO14.5]**

**b.** alphabetic filing system **[LO14.3]**

**c.** closed file **[LO14.5]**

**d.** compactible file **[LO14.3]**

**e.** cross-referenced **[LO14.3]**

**f.** file guide **[LO14.3]**

**g.** inactive file **[LO14.5]**

**h.** indexing **[LO14.3]**

**i.** indexing rules **[LO14.3]**

**j.** lateral file **[LO14.3]**

**k.** middle digit **[LO14.3]**

**l.** numeric filing system **[LO14.3]**

**m.** out guide **[LO14.3]**

**n.** records management system **[LO14.2]**

_____ **8.** a horizontal filing cabinet that features doors that flip up and a pull-out drawer, where files are arranged with sides facing out

_____ **9.** the naming of a file

_____ **10.** a marker made of stiff material and used as a placeholder when a file is taken out of a filing system

_____ **11.** a reminder file for keeping track of time-sensitive obligations

_____ **12.** a file used on a consistent basis

_____ **13.** a tapered rectangular or rounded extension at the top of a file folder

_____ **14.** filed in two or more places, with each place noted in each file; the exact contents of the file may be duplicated, or a cross-reference form can be created, listing all the places to find the file

_____ **15.** a filing system that organizes files by numbers instead of names; each patient is assigned a number in the order in which she comes to the practice

_____ **16.** rules used as guidelines for the sequencing of files based on current business practice

_____ **17.** a part of an individual's name or title, described in indexing rules

_____ **18.** a filing system in which the files are arranged in alphabetical order, with the patient's last name first, followed by the first name and middle initial

_____ **19.** one after another in a predictable pattern or sequence

_____ **20.** a small group of two to three numbers in the middle of a patient number that is used as an identifying unit in a filing system

_____ **21.** a heavy cardboard or plastic insert used to identify a group of file folders in a file drawer

**o.** retention schedule [LO14.5]

**p.** sequential order [LO14.3]

**q.** tab [LO14.3]

**r.** terminal digit [LO14.3]

**s.** tickler file [LO14.3]

**t.** unit [LO14.3]

**u.** vertical file [LO14.3]

# Multiple-Choice Certification Questions

There may be more than one answer; circle the letter of the choice that best completes each statement or answers each question.

1. [LO14.3] The medical record of a patient who moved out of state would be considered what kind of file?
   a. Active
   b. Inactive
   c. Opened
   d. Closed
   e. Electronic

2. [LO14.3] A specific pediatric office only sees patients until age 16. The medical record of a 17-year-old would be placed in what type of file?
   a. Active
   b. Inactive
   c. Opened
   d. Closed
   e. Electronic

3. [LO14.3] A medical record of a patient who was seen 1 year ago would be considered a(n)
   a. active file.
   b. inactive file.
   c. opened file.
   d. closed file.
   e. electronic file.

4. [LO14.4] The medical record of a patient first seen in a pediatrician's office as a newborn would most likely be kept
   a. 2 to 5 years.
   b. 7 to 10 years.
   c. until the patient is 18 years old.
   d. until the patient is 21 years old.
   e. 28 to 31 years.

5. [LO14.1] The purpose of the medical record is all the following *except*
   a. continuity of care.
   b. research.
   c. verification of insurance eligibility.
   d. education.
   e. documentation for legal purposes.

6. [LO14.3] The medical record filing system using the patient's last name, first name, and middle initial to file is referred to as
   a. numerical.
   b. alphabetical.
   c. terminal digit.
   d. color coding.
   e. indexing.

7. [LO14.2] Of the elements of medical record management, one of the final steps is
   a. assembling.
   b. retaining.
   c. maintaining.
   d. destroying.
   e. securing.

**8.** **[LO14.4]** A violation of HIPAA concerning a medical record would be to
   a. release the medical record of an adult to a parent.
   b. release a medical record to an attorney with the patient's consent.
   c. release the medical record to the medical assistant for the patient's appointment.
   d. omit placing the diagnostic test results in the medical record.
   e. omit filing the medical record in the correct area of the storage shelf.

**9.** **[LO14.3]** Which of the following is a true statement concerning alphabetical filing?
   a. Frank Smith, Jr., is filed after Frank Smith, Sr.
   b. Frank Smith, Sr., is filed after Frank Smith, Jr.
   c. Frank Smith III is filed after Frank Smith, Jr.
   d. Frank is the first unit in Frank Smith, Sr.
   e. Jr. is the second unit in Frank Smith, Jr.

**10.** **[LO14.3]** When you file alphabetically, which of the following patient names would come first?
   a. Williams, William
   b. Williams, William A.
   c. William, William
   d. William, Bill R.
   e. William, Bill W.

**11.** **[LO14.1]** If an insurance company auditor reviewed the medical records of all asthmatic patients seen within that week, the purpose would probably be
   a. quality of care.
   b. education.
   c. continuity of care.
   d. legal documentation.
   e. confidentiality.

**12.** **[LO14.2]** The order of the documents within a patient's record falls under what elements of medical records management?
   a. Filing
   b. Assembling
   c. Maintaining
   d. Retaining
   e. Securing

**13.** **[LO14.5]** Disposing of a medical record in a dumpster would be considered
   a. destroying the record.
   b. purging the record.
   c. a violation of HIPAA.
   d. standard practice.
   e. an alternative to shredding.

**14.** **[LO14.2]** The extension on a file that may be used to place identifying numbers is referred to as a(n)
   a. out guide.
   b. file guide.
   c. tab.
   d. terminal digit.
   e. placeholder.

**15.** **[LO14.4]** Medical offices that do not use an electronic health record by a specific date designated by the government may experience
   a. problems with submitting electronic claims.
   b. loss of Medicare contracts.
   c. computer problems.
   d. different levels of reimbursement from CMS.
   e. an increase in storage costs.

**16.** [LO14.2] An out guide for medical records is used as a
   a. file extension.
   b. file guide.
   c. tab.
   d. reminder.
   e. placeholder.

**17.** [LO14.2] One of the major concerns with the electronic health record is
   a. storage.
   b. maintenance.
   c. security.
   d. copying files.
   e. destroying files.

**18.** [LO14.2] A tickler file is used as a
   a. file extension.
   b. file guide.
   c. tab.
   d. reminder.
   e. placeholder.

**19.** [LO14.1] A *subpoena duces tecum* would involve what purpose of the medical record?
   a. Continuity of care
   b. Research
   c. Verification of insurance eligibility
   d. Education
   e. Documentation for legal purposes

**20.** [LO14.1] A governmental entity that may request a medical record is all the following *except* the
   a. IRS.
   b. CMS.
   c. CDC.
   d. AMA.
   e. VAERS.

**21.** A medical record specialist who has obtained a certification in that field is referred to as a(n)
   a. RHIT.
   b. RMRS.
   c. CMRS.
   d. CHIT.
   e. CMS.

**22.** [LO14.3] A medical record filed using terminal digits would be cross-referenced in a(n):
   a. alphabetical file.
   b. numerical file.
   c. tickler file.
   d. color-coded file.
   e. middle digit file.

**23.** [LO14.5] Security risks for the electronic health record include all the following *except*
   a. sharing passwords.
   b. leaving computer screens in view of others.
   c. using inadequate electronic firewalls.
   d. releasing records without consent.
   e. inadequately shredding documents.

**24.** [LO14.3] If two individuals have exactly the same names, the next identifying factor used is the
a. father's name.
b. mother's name.
c. birth date.
d. medical record number.
e. address.

**25.** [LO14.1] If a physician was seeing the patient of his partner, who is on vacation, an important function of the medical record would be
a. continuity of care.
b. research.
c. verifying insurance eligibility.
d. education.
e. documentation for legal purposes.

## True or False

Decide whether each statement is true or false. In the space at the left, write "T" for true or "F" for false. On the lines provided, rewrite the false statements to make them true.

_____ **1.** [LO14.3] Horizontal filing cabinets or lateral files are kept on rolling shelves that slide along permanent tracks in the floor.

_____ **2.** [LO14.3] The most basic filing supply is the file folder, often referred to as an active folder.

_____ **3.** [LO14.3] Numeric files are sequential by the order in which patients have come to the practice or randomly assigned by a computerized system.

_____ **4.** [LO14.5] Files of children must be kept for 7–10 years after the child reaches the age of majority, which is state dependent.

_____ **5.** [LO14.5] The medical practice should select a reputable commercial records company or center to manage its stored documents.

_____ **6.** [LO14.4] Due to HIPAA, most offices continue to use alphabetic filing on medical records labels.

_____ **7.** [LO14.4] In the hospital setting, the RHIT deals strictly with health information and has no patient contact.

_____ **8.** [LO14.3] The specific rules to follow when filing personal names alphabetically are called the rules of medical records maintenance.

_____ 9. **[LO14.3]** Rules for alphabetic filing of personal names treat hyphenated names as a single unit, disregarding the hyphen.

_____

_____ 10. **[LO14.3]** When you file a folder with the tab label Stephen Brent Jacobson, the word Brent is the third unit in the filing sequence.

_____

## Sentence Completion

In the space provided, write the word or phrase that best completes each sentence.

1. **[LO14.3]** When using terminal digit filing, numbers are assigned in small groups of _____ or _____ numbers and are read from _____ to _____.

2. **[LO14.3]** Frequently used files are called _____ files, and infrequently used ones are called _____ files.

3. **[LO14.5]** No matter where you store files, you must consider the issue of _____ as well as _____.

4. **[LO14.5]** A storage site should be equipped with a smoke alarm, sprinkler system, and _____ _____.

5. **[LO14.4]** In determining how long to retain medical records, if your state's retention requirements are more stringent than HIPAA, follow _____ _____ requirements.

6. **[LO14.5]** The Internal Revenue Service usually requires doctors to keep _____ records for up to _____ years.

7. **[LO14.3]** File folders come in two sizes: _____ size, which is 8½ by _____ inches; and _____ size, which is 8½ by _____ inches.

8. **[LO14.2]** One purpose of the medical record is to provide _____ protection to the patient and the physician by documenting what has _____ done or _____ done.

1. _____
   _____

2. _____
   _____

3. _____
   _____

4. _____
   _____

5. _____
   _____

6. _____

7. _____
   _____

8. _____
   _____

# Apply Your Knowledge

## Short Answer

Write the answer to each question on the lines provided.

**1.** **[LO14.3]** If you are responsible for setting up a medical practice with a new filing system, what are the considerations you need to keep in mind as you select the type of storage units you would purchase? Why?

_____

_____

_____

**2.** **[LO14.3]** Explain why the alphabetic filing system for patient records would not be the most desirable type of filing system to use in a large medical practice.

_____

_____

_____

**3.** **[LO14.5]** Why is it necessary to retain the medical practice's financial records for 10 years?

_____

_____

_____

**4.** **[LO14.3]** What are two safety concerns when using vertical filing cabinets?

_____

_____

_____

**5.** **[LO14.3]** Explain the use of an out guide. What are two types of out guides that are available?

_____

_____

_____

# Problem-Solving Activities

Follow the directions for each activity.

1. **[LO14.3]** Filing Cabinet Employee Safety
   a. Gather information from Chapter 14 and Internet Web sites about file cabinet safety.
   b. Using this information, develop a one-page safety sheet that could be posted in a file room or area of a medical office.
   c. The safety sheet should list information for employees to be aware of when accessing and returning files.

2. **[LO14.5]** Off-Site Storage of Files
   a. Access the Internet and type in your browser "off-site storage of medical records."
   b. Locate a company that provides storage of records off-site. Answer the following questions for the company you locate:
      - How much does the company charge per month or year for storing records?
      - How does the company comply with HIPAA regulations?
      - How are the records accessed when needed?

3. **[LO14.3]** Alphabetic Filing
   a. Place the patient names in Column A into alphabetical order in Column B.

| COLUMN A | COLUMN B |
|---|---|
| Peter St. Clair | |
| George B. Diaz | |
| Mark J. Middleton | |
| H. S. Werner | |
| Walter G. MacKay | |
| William Smith, Jr. | |
| Jill Thompson-Turner | |
| A. Fred Murray | |
| James R. Foster, Jr. | |
| Bruce H. Jacoby | |
| James J. Jones, Jr. | |
| D. R. Jones | |
| Mary Del Rosa | |
| P. S. St. Clair | |
| Hannah J. Werner | |
| Ivey McVeigh | |
| William S. Smith III | |
| Jillian Thompson | |
| Mark De La Rosa | |
| Mary J. Middleton | |
| James Thomas Jones, Jr. | |
| Irene J. Mackay | |
| Ivan MacVeigh | |
| David Russell Jones | |

# Thinking Critically

Write your response to each case study question on the lines provided.

## Case 1 [LO14.3]

You are responsible for pulling the patient charts each afternoon for the next day's appointments. Over the past couple of weeks you have been unable to locate several patient files. The files are those of patients that just recently had prescription medication refills authorized. Two other co-workers would have pulled those files to enter refill information. When you inquire about these files, the co-workers state that they don't know what happened to them. The practice utilizes an alphabetical filing system and as you continue to look for these files, you discover that they have been alphabetically misfiled.

**1.** What are the consequences of misfiled patient files?

_____

_____

_____

**2.** What can you do to help prevent this from happening again?

_____

_____

_____

## Case 2 [LO14.5]

Your office is running out of space to store medical records, and the physician asks the administrative staff to come up with solutions for this problem. There are three other co-workers assigned with you in the administrative area. They look to you to "fix" the problem. They don't believe it is their responsibility to help with this problem.

**1.** What will you do to get your co-workers to help with this problem?

_____

_____

_____

**2.** What are some of the ideas that may be used to resolve the problem of not having enough file space?

_____

_____

_____

## Case 3 [LO14.4]

Cindy is a new employee working in an office where there are three other administrative medical assistants. During her first few days on the job she notices that there is a huge stack of paper filing. It appears the other assistants do not like to do the necessary filing to keep the medical records up-to-date. The size of the stack of papers indicates that it may have been a month since filing has been done. The physicians have complained frequently about not being able to locate laboratory results, x-ray reports, and referral letters for their patients. The administrative staff spends a lot of time searching for the documents when the physicians ask for them.

**1.** Are there suggestions that Cindy can make to initially help with filing documents?

_____

_____

_____

**2.** How can the office staff ensure that the filing of documents is maintained so that it does not get behind?

_____

_____

_____

# Demonstrate Your Knowledge

**Student Name:** _____

## Procedure 14–1: Creating an Office Tickler File

**GOAL:** To create a comprehensive office tickler file designed for year-round use

**MATERIALS:** 12 manila file folders, 12 file labels, pen and paper or computer

**METHOD:** To pass this procedure the minimum required score is _____% or all elements must meet "satisfactory" ability on the final demonstration. The first box may be used as a practice or final demonstration, with the evaluator placing **S for Satisfactory** or **U for Unsatisfactory** if that is the grading criteria. The second box may be used as a final demonstration with a **grade point** written in the box.

| STEPS | POSSIBLE POINTS | S/U | POINTS EARNED |
|---|---|---|---|
| 1. Write or type 12 file labels, 1 for each month of the year. Abbreviations are acceptable. Do *not* include the current calendar year, just the month. | 10 | | |
| 2. Affix one label to the tab of each file folder. | 10 | | |
| 3. Arrange the folders so that the current month is first. Months should follow in chronological order. | 10 | | |
| 4. Write or type a list of upcoming responsibilities and activities. Next to each activity, indicate the date by which the activity should be completed. Leave a column after this date to indicate when the activity has been completed. Use a separate sheet of paper for each month and place one in the front of each of the 12 folders. | 20 points for step 4 or 5 | | |
| 5. In place of folders and files, an Excel-type spreadsheet may be used, listing each month with the corresponding activities. | 20 points for step 4 or 5 | | |
| 6. File the folders, with the current month on top, continuing to add documents, such as certificate renewals, to the appropriate months. | 10 | | |
| 7. Review the tickler file weekly on the same day, preferably Monday. | 10 | | |
| 8. Complete the activities as scheduled, recording date and name or initials of the person completing the task. If tasks are not completed on time, place a note with the reason, and report the delay to your supervisor or physician and document it. | 10 | | |
| 9. At the end of the month, place the file folder at the back of the file. If there are notes remaining in that month's folder that are not completed, report them to the supervisor or physician. If instructed, add them to the next month's activities. | 10 | | |
| 10. Continue to add new notes and activities to the appropriate month's files. | 10 | | |
| **Total Points (if applicable)** | 100 | | |

**Comments:** _____

_____

_____

**Final Evaluator's Signature:** _____

**Date:** _____

## CAAHEP Competencies Achieved

V. C (9) Describe indexing rules

V. C (10) Discuss filing procedures

V. P (8) Maintain organization by filing

V. A (1) Consider staff needs and limitations in establishing a filing system

## ABHES Competencies Achieved

8. a. Perform basic clerical functions

8. d. Apply concepts for office procedures

# 15 The Health Record

## Test Your Knowledge

### Vocabulary Review

Match the key terms in the right column with the definitions in the left column by placing the letter of each correct answer in the space provided.

_____ **1.** information such as patient SSN or insurance policy number that easily reveals patient identity

_____ **2.** problem-oriented medical record

_____ **3.** an acronym for a documentation method that includes these steps: subjective, objective, assessment, and plan

_____ **4.** subjective or internal condition felt by the patient (such as a headache) that generally cannot be seen or felt by the physician or measured by instruments

_____ **5.** document signed by the patient to verify that the patient understands the treatment offered and the possible outcomes or side effects of the treatment

_____ **6.** examining and reviewing a group of patients' records for completeness and coding correctness

_____ **7.** objective or external factor such as elevated BP, rash, or swelling that can be seen or felt by the physician or measured by an instrument

_____ **8.** an acronym for a documentation method that includes these items: chief

**a.** audit [LO15.1]

**b.** CHEDDAR [LO15.2]

**c.** documentation [LO15.3]

**d.** electronic health records (EHR) [LO15.6]

**e.** electronic medical records (EMR) [LO15.6]

**f.** individual identifiable health information (IIHI) [LO15.8]

**g.** informed consent form [LO15.3]

**h.** noncompliant [LO15.1]

**i.** objective [LO15.2]

**j.** patient record/chart [LO15.3]

**k.** POMR [LO15.2]

**l.** sign [LO15.2]

**m.** SOAP [LO15.2]

**n.** subjective [LO15.2]

complaint, history, examination, details of problems and complaints, drugs and dosages, assessment, and return

**o.** symptom [LO15.2]

**p.** transcription [LO15.6]

**q.** transfer [LO15.8]

_____ **9.** a medical term used to describe a patient who does not follow the medical advice he or she is given

_____ **10.** data from the patient describing history of symptoms; usually in his or her own words

_____ **11.** recording information in the medical record

_____ **12.** data from the physician examination and from test results

_____ **13.** transforming spoken notes into accurate written form

_____ **14.** medical records kept in an electronic format; available to providers outside the medical office that has ownership

_____ **15.** documentation of important information about a patient's medical history and present condition serving as both communication tool and legal record

_____ **16.** with patient consent, giving PHI to another party outside the treating physician's office

_____ **17.** medical records kept in an electronic format; generally not available to providers outside the medical office that has ownership

## Multiple-Choice Certification Questions

There may be more than one answer; circle the letter of the choice that best completes each statement or answers each question.

**1.** [LO15.1] All of the following would be found in the patient's health record *except*
   a. a referral to a specialist.
   b. the amount the patient owes.
   c. the medical treatment plan.
   d. a prescription refill.
   e. the name of the patient's insurance company.

**2.** [LO15.1] A noncompliant patient is one who
   a. the physician has abandoned.
   b. is unable to afford treatment.
   c. ignores medical advice.
   d. follows instructions.
   e. arrives on time for appointments.

**3.** [LO15.3] The medical record contains the
   a. implied consent.
   b. informed consent.
   c. privacy practices.
   d. next of kin.
   e. medical office policies.

**4.** [LO15.3] The type of history normally included in a patient's health record include all the following *except* the
   a. social history.
   b. family history.
   c. medical history.
   d. surgical history.
   e. employment history.

**5.** [LO15.4] The patient's own words are used when documenting the
   a. primary diagnosis.
   b. secondary diagnosis.
   c. signs and symptoms.
   d. patient history.
   e. chief complaint.

**6.** [LO15.4] The six Cs of charting include which of the following?
   a. Conciseness
   b. Chief complaint
   c. Consultations
   d. Conversations
   e. Complete physical exam

**7.** [LO15.2] The acronym SOAP used in charting refers to
   a. suggestive, objective, assessment, problem.
   b. subjective, objective, assessment, plan.
   c. suggestive, objective, accurate, problem.
   d. subject, object, aim, purpose.
   e. secondary, opinion, accommodation, plan.

**8.** [LO15.2] Documentation of a blood pressure is considered what kind of data?
   a. Primary
   b. Secondary
   c. Subjective
   d. Objective
   e. Electronic

**9.** [LO15.2] Documentation of a headache is considered what kind of data?
   a. Primary
   b. Secondary
   c. Subjective
   d. Objective
   e. Electronic

**10.** [LO15.2] The charting method that includes a problem list is
   a. POMR.
   b. SOAP.
   c. PRN.
   d. CHEDDAR.
   e. SOMR.

**11.** [LO15.6] To correct an error in a paper-based medical record, the mistake is
   a. covered with correction fluid.
   b. marked out with a dark pen.

c. stricken through with a single line.

d. crossed out.

e. erased.

12. **[LO15.5]** The process of transforming spoken notes into written form is called

a. transportation.

b. transcription.

c. subscription.

d. word processing.

e. prescription.

13. **[LO15.2]** The medical abbreviation that means twice a day is

a. b.i.d.

b. t.i.d.

c. q.i.d.

d. X2d.

e. A.M./P.M.

14. **[LO15.6]** Generally, once an electronic health record entry is locked, a correction is made by

a. adding an addendum.

b. highlighting the error and placing a comment.

c. deleting the error.

d. striking through the error and adding initials.

e. printing the page, correcting the error, and scanning in the page.

15. **[LO15.6]** When you correct a charting error, it is important to ensure that the original information is

a. removed.

b. still visible.

c. unable to be read.

d. kept in a separate file.

e. not available if the record is subpoenaed.

16. **[LO15.7]** The physical medical record belongs to the

a. medical practice.

b. patient.

c. court.

d. insurance company.

e. employer.

17. **[LO15.6]** Late entries in a medical record

a. are never permitted.

b. are illegal.

c. should be witnessed.

d. will not hold up in court.

e. are usually done to cover up a mistake.

18. **[LO15.7]** The information in the medial record belongs to the

a. medical practice.

b. patient.

c. court.

d. insurance company.

e. employer.

19. **[LO15.4]** Which of the following statements is inappropriate to document in a medical record?

a. "The patient is slurring his words."

b. "The patient has an odor of alcohol."

c. "The patient stated, 'I am not taking my medication.'"

d. "The patient was a no-call/no-show for his 2:15 P.M. appointment today."

e. "The patient is acting bizarre."

**20.** [LO15.8] Charging for a copy of a medical record is
  a. illegal.
  b. frowned upon.
  c. unusual.
  d. standard business practice.
  e. unprofessional.

**21.** [LO15.1] The medical record is updated
  a. only when the patient visits the office.
  b. only when the patient changes insurance plans.
  c. each time a payment is received.
  d. each time the patient has contact with the office.
  e. when an appointment is made.

**22.** [LO15.1] The general rule is that, if a procedure was not documented, it
  a. was most likely done.
  b. was not done.
  c. is exempt from subpoena.
  d. is not legal.
  e. cannot be billed.

**23.** [LO15.5] Passwords for the electronic health record system should
  a. be shared only with trusted co-workers.
  b. not be changed once set.
  c. never be shared.
  d. always be at least six digits.
  e. be reset each week.

**24.** [LO15.5, 15.7] When you electronically transmit a medical record,
  a. it is not necessary to obtain a signed release.
  b. HIPAA does not apply.
  c. faxing is prohibited.
  d. the same rules apply as with a paper record.
  e. a paper copy must be maintained in the office.

**25.** [LO15.5] Medical offices that do not implement the electronic medical record per the federal guidelines may
  a. experience a difference in reimbursement.
  b. continue with a paper-based system.
  c. not know the benefits.
  d. wait for updated technology.
  e. not see Medicare patients.

## True or False

Decide whether each statement is true or false. In the space at the left, write "T" for true or "F" for false. On the lines provided, rewrite the false statements to make them true.

_____ **1.** [LO15.1] The Joint Commission is an organization that is a type of auditing agency.

_____

_____ **2.** [LO15.8] A noncompliant patient is one who prefers to see a different physician.

_____

_____ **3.** [LO15.3] An informed consent form is used to ensure that a patient will pay her bill.

_____

_____ **4.** [LO15.3] A hospital discharge form will not include the admitting diagnosis since the patient is being released from the hospital.

_____

_____ **5.** [LO15.3] When an office receives a mailed copy of a document that was originally faxed to the office, the faxed copy of the document should be shredded and the mailed copy filed as part of the patient's record.

_____

_____ **6.** [LO15.8] The patient's rights under HIPAA law require the medical practice to allow the patient to review his records but not receive a copy of them.

_____

_____ **7.** [LO15.5] When you document in the patient's record, it is appropriate to chart that "The patient has pain" rather than "The patient says he has pain."

_____

_____ **8.** [LO15.5] When documents are chronologically filed in a patient's file, they are in order by date with the most recent documents first or on top.

_____

_____ **9.** [LO15.2] Subjective data is information that comes directly from the patient such as the patient's description of pain and location of the pain.

_____

_____ **10.** [LO15.6] One of the advantages of having electronic health records in a medical practice is that the entire staff can be retrained on the new software system therefore eliminating errors in charting and billing.

_____

## Sentence Completion

In the space provided, write the word or phrase that best completes each sentence.

**1.** [LO15.4] Prior to seeing the physician, a new patient will complete two forms, a _____ form and a medical _____ form.

**1.** _____
_____

**2.** [LO15.5] When charting, you need to be concise, which means to be _____ and to the _____.

**2.** _____
_____

**3.** [LO15.2] When documenting patient problems in a medical record, the objective or external factors such as blood pressure are called _____, while the subjective or internal factors such as pain are called _____.

**4.** [LO15.2] Two common types of medical records are _____ -oriented and _____ -oriented.

**5.** [LO15.8] All physical patient medical records are the property of the _____.

**6.** [LO15.1, 15.7] An audit of medical records performed by the medical staff of the practice is a(n) _____ audit and an audit performed by the government and private insurance carriers is a(n) _____ audit.

**7.** [LO15.6] The federal government recommends that all health records become electronic by the year _____.

**8.** [LO15.1] All written correspondence from the patient or other physicians and laboratories should be _____ with the _____ the doctor's office received the document.

**9.** [LO15.8] HIPAA law states that all patients have rights regarding their health information, which is known as _____ _____ _____.

**10.** [LO15.8] Never discuss a patient's records, forward them to another office, fax them, or show them to anyone but the physician unless you have the patient's _____ _____ to do so.

**3.** _____
   _____
   _____

**4.** _____
   _____

**5.** _____
   _____

**6.** _____
   _____

**7.** _____
   _____

**8.** _____
   _____

**9.** _____
   _____

**10.** _____
   _____

# Apply Your Knowledge

## Short Answer

Write the answer to each question on the lines provided.

**1.** [LO15.1] Explain the appropriate way for a physician to dismiss a noncompliant patient from care at a medical office.

_____

_____

_____

**2.** [LO15.8] List the six "rights" patients have under HIPAA law.

_____

_____

_____

**3.** [LO15.2] List and explain the components of the SOAP method of charting.

_____

_____

_____

**4.** [LO15.1] Give three examples of how the administrative medical assistant can ensure the accuracy of charting information.

_____

_____

_____

**5.** [LO15.8] Describe three procedural practices that should take place when releasing patient medical records.

_____

_____

_____

## Problem-Solving Activities

Follow the directions for each activity.

**1.** [LO15.1, 15.3, 15.4, 15.5, 15.7] Initiating a New Patient Medical Record
Work with two partners to complete this activity. Each of you will take turns being an administrative medical assistant, a patient, and an observer/evaluator. Assume that this is the patient's first visit to the medical office. Each person will need a copy of the Patient Registration Form (Figure 15–3 from your student text) and the Medical History Form (Figure 15–4 from your student text).
  a. Have one partner play the role of the administrative medical assistant and another partner play the role of a patient complaining of headaches. The third partner should act as the observer and evaluator. Have the administrative medical assistant help the patient complete the Patient Registration Form.
  b. Using the same partners and roles, interview the patient to complete the portions of the Medical History Form that are in the scope of responsibility of the administrative medical assistant. Use standard abbreviations where appropriate, ending with a description of the patient's reason for the visit. Any entry errors should be properly corrected in the documents. The administrative medical assistant should document any signs, symptoms, or other information the patient wishes to share.
  c. The evaluator will critique the interview and the documentation in the patient chart. The critique should take into account the accuracy of the documentation, the order in which the medical history was taken, and the history's completeness. The evaluator will also note the administrative medical assistant's ability to follow the six Cs of charting, including the correct use of medical abbreviations.
  d. Upon completion of the evaluation, the three partners will discuss the evaluator's comments, noting the strengths and weaknesses of the interview and the quality of the documentation.
  e. Exchange roles and repeat the activity with a new patient with a different medical problem.
  f. Exchange roles again so that each member of the team has an opportunity to play the interviewer, the patient, and the evaluator.

**Figure 15–3** The patient registration form.

## TOTAL CARE CLINIC, PC

342 East Park Blvd
Funton, XY   12345-6789
521-234-0001   Fax: 521-234-0002

# Patient Registration
## Patient Information

Name: _____   Today's Date: _____

Address: _____

City: _____   State: _____   Zip Code: _____

Telephone (Home): _____   (Work): _____   (Cell): _____

Birthdate: _____   Age: _____   Sex:  M   F   No. of Children _____   Marital Status:  M  S  W  D

Social Security Number: _____   Employer: _____   Occupation: _____

Primary Physician: _____

Referred by: _____

Person to Contact in Emergency: _____

Emergency Telephone: _____

Special Needs: _____

## Responsible Party

Party Responsible for Payment:        Self          Spouse          Parent          Other

Name (If Other Than Self): _____

Address: _____

City: _____   State: _____   Zip Code: _____

## Primary Insurance

Primary Medical Insurance: _____

Insured party:        Self        Spouse        Parent        Other

ID#/Social Security No.: _____   Group/Plan No.: _____

Name (If Other Than Self): _____

Address: _____

City: _____   State: _____   Zip Code: _____

## Secondary Insurance

Secondary Medical Insurance: _____

Insured party:        Self        Spouse        Parent        Other

ID#/Social Security No.: _____   Group/Plan No.: _____

Name (If Other Than Self): _____

Address: _____

City: _____   State: _____   Zip Code: _____

**Figure 15–4** The medical history form.

## Total Care Clinic, PC
### Medical History

| | | | |
|---|---|---|---|
| Name | Age | Sex | S M W D |
| Address | Phone | Date | |

Occupation _____ Ref. by _____

Chief Complaint _____

Present Illness _____

History —Military _____
    —Social _____
    —Family _____
    —Marital _____
    —Menstrual    Menarche _____ Para. _____ LMP _____

| —Illness | Measles | Pert. | Var. | Pneu. | Pleur. | Typh. | Mal. | Rh. Fev. | Sc. Fev. | Diphth. | Other |
|---|---|---|---|---|---|---|---|---|---|---|---|

    —Surgery _____
    —Allergies _____
    —Current Medications _____

### Physical Examination

| Temp. | Pulse | Resp. | BP | Ht. | Wt. |
|---|---|---|---|---|---|

| | | | |
|---|---|---|---|
| General Appearance | Skin | Mucous Membrane | |
| Eyes: | Vision | Pupil | Fundus |

Ears: _____
Nose: _____

| | | |
|---|---|---|
| Throat: | Pharynx | Tonsils |
| Chest: | Breasts | |

Heart: _____
Lungs: _____
Abdomen: _____
Genitalia: _____
Rectum: _____
Pelvic: _____

Extremities: _____ Pulses: _____

| Lymph Nodes: | Neck | Axilla | Inguinal | Abdominal |
|---|---|---|---|---|

Neurological: _____
Diagnosis: _____

Treatment: _____

Laboratory Findings:
Date _____ Blood _____

Date _____ Urine _____

# Thinking Critically

Write your response to each case study question on the lines provided.

## Case 1 [LO15.5]

A patient is seen in your medical clinic today following a minor office surgical procedure to remove an ingrown toenail a week ago. The patient was directed to keep the toe dry and to change the bandage daily. After the procedure, she was provided a written sheet of instructions and enough bandage materials to do the daily changes for a week. When she arrives at the clinic for her appointment she is noticeably limping and is complaining that her toe is not healing well and is causing severe pain. When you put her into an exam room to see the physician, she tells you that she didn't have time to change the bandage every day and that she got it wet when she showered. The toe is red and swollen where the toenail used to be and is probably infected. She states that "The doctor didn't do a good job and that is why it isn't healing."

**1.** How should you respond to the patient?

_____

_____

_____

**2.** Why is this patient considered a noncompliant patient?

_____

_____

_____

## Case 2 [LO15.5]

Cheryl, an administrative medical assistant, is asked to work with a new employee, Linda, who is a recent graduate. When Linda is finished rooming a patient and charting the chief complaint, Cheryl reviews Linda's entries before the physician sees the patient. Cheryl discovers several problems with the entries because they reflect Linda's interpretation of the patient's comments instead of stating the patient's exact words. For example, Linda entered a statement that "The patient is in a lot of pain in the lower back and needs stronger pain medication than what she is buying over the counter."

**1.** When you are charting, why is it important to clarify what the patient said instead of putting it in your own words?

_____

_____

_____

**2.** How should Linda's statement have been written to properly capture what the patient said?

_____

_____

_____

## Case 3 [LO15.8]

A patient contacts the clinic stating that he has moved out of state and is seeing his new physician tomorrow afternoon for a sore throat. He is asking you to fax all his medical records to the new physician by noon the next day when he has his first appointment. This patient has not been seen at your office for three years and his medical records are in storage and unable to be accessed and faxed by that time. Because the records are in storage, there is no possible way the records can be sent to the new office by the next day.

1. What should you tell the patient about the request to send his records to the new office?

_____

_____

_____

2. What are the guidelines established under HIPAA that give patients the right to request and receive a copy of their own medical records?

_____

_____

_____

# Demonstrate Your Knowledge

**Student Name:** _____

## Procedure 15–1: Initiating a Paper-Based Patient Medical Record/Chart

**GOAL:** To assemble a new paper-based patient medical record/chart

**MATERIALS:** File folder, labels as appropriate (alphabet, numbers, dates, insurance, allergies, etc.), forms (patient information, advance directives, physician progress notes, referrals, laboratory forms), hole punch (*Note*: A patient registration form and medical history and exam form can be found in the Problem-Solving Activities section of this chapter [Figures 15–3 and 15–4]. A progress note can be found at the end of this student study guide.)

**METHOD:** To pass this procedure the minimum required score is _____% or all elements must meet "satisfactory" ability on the final demonstration. The first box may be used as a practice or final demonstration, with the evaluator placing **S for Satisfactory** or **U for Unsatisfactory** if that is the grading criteria. The second box may be used as a final demonstration with a **grade point** written in the box.

| STEPS | POSSIBLE POINTS | S/U | POINTS EARNED |
|---|---|---|---|
| 1. Carefully create a chart label according to practice policy. This label may include the patient's last name followed by the first name, or it may be a medical record number for those offices that utilize numeric or alpha-numeric filing. | 15 | | |
| 2. Place the chart label on the right edge of the folder, extending the label the length of the tab on the folder. | 15 | | |
| 3. Place the date label on the top edge of the folder, updating the date according to the practice's policy. (The date is usually updated annually, provided the patient has come into the office within the last year.) | 15 | | |
| 4. If alpha or numeric filing labels are utilized, place a patient name label on the chart according to the practice's policy. | 15 | | |
| 5. Punch holes in the appropriate forms for placement within the patient's medical record/chart. Each paper form must also include patient identifying information on each sheet; both front and back. | 20 | | |
| 6. Place all the forms in appropriate sections of the patient's medical record/chart. | 20 | | |
| **Total Points (if applicable)** | 100 | | |

**Comments:** _____

_____

_____

**Final Evaluator's Signature:** _____

**Date:** _____

## CAAHEP Competencies Achieved

V. C (6) Describe various types of content maintained in a patient's medical record

V. P (3) Organize a patient's medical record

## ABHES Competencies Achieved

8. b. Prepare and maintain medical records

Student Name: _____

## Procedure 15–2: Creating a New Patient Record Using an EHR Program

**GOAL:** To create a new patient record in an EHR program

**MATERIALS:** Initial patient forms (patient information, advance directives, physician progress notes, referrals, laboratory orders)

**METHOD:** To pass this procedure the minimum required score is _____ % or all elements must meet "satisfactory" ability on the final demonstration. The first box may be used as a practice or final demonstration, with the evaluator placing **S for Satisfactory** or **U for Unsatisfactory** if that is the grading criteria. The second box may be used as a final demonstration with a **grade point** written in the box.

| STEPS | POSSIBLE POINTS | S/U | POINTS EARNED |
|---|---|---|---|
| 1. Open the "New Patient Window" of the EHR software as directed by the software vendor. | 5 | | |
| 2. Enter the patient's full name as directed, being careful to enter the name in the correct order (some software programs require first name, middle name, last name, and others start with the last name). | 5 | | |
| 3. If the patient has a family member who also comes to the office, you may be able to use a shortcut to copy the patient's address from the existing patient; otherwise, enter the patient's demographic information of address and phone number. Be sure to fill in each screen completely and accurately before moving on to the next screen. | 15 | | |
| 4. Follow the software directions for completing each screen, including the patient's insurance, guarantor, and employer information. | 20 | | |
| 5. Depending on the office policy, you may also enter the patient's medical history information. Open the medical history screen of the software program and carefully key in the information required for each screen. | 20 | | |
| 6. Carefully inspect all information for accuracy and save the new patient record as directed by the software program instructions. | 15 | | |
| 7. Depending on the office policy, you may be able to scan information from a hard copy medical record into the EHR or a manual file created to maintain it. | 20 | | |
| **Total Points (if applicable)** | 100 | | |

**Comments:** _____

_____

_____

**Final Evaluator's Signature:** _____

**Date:** _____

## CAAHEP Competencies Achieved

V. C (6) Describe various types of content maintained in a patient's medical record

V. C (11) Discuss the principles of using electronic medical records (EMR)

V. P (3) Organize a patient's medical record

V. P (5) Execute data management using electronic health-care records such as the EMR

## ABHES Competencies Achieved

7. b. Identify and properly utilize office machines, computerized systems, and medical software such as

    (2) Apply computer application skills using a variety of different electronic programs including EMR software

8. b. Prepare and maintain medical records

8. ll. Apply electronic technology

## Procedure 15–3: Correcting Paper Medical Records

**GOAL:** To follow standard procedures for correcting a paper medical record

**MATERIALS:** Patient file, other pertinent documents that contain the information to be used in making corrections (for example, transcribed notes, telephone notes, physician's comments, correspondence), good ballpoint pen

**METHOD:** To pass this procedure the minimum required score is _____% or all elements must meet "satisfactory" ability on the final demonstration. The first box may be used as a practice or final demonstration, with the evaluator placing **S for Satisfactory** or **U for Unsatisfactory** if that is the grading criteria. The second box may be used as a final demonstration with a **grade point** written in the box.

| STEPS | POSSIBLE POINTS | S/U | POINTS EARNED |
|---|---|---|---|
| 1. Always make the correction in a way that does not suggest any intention to deceive, cover up, alter, or add information to conceal a lack of proper medical care. | 20 | | |
| 2. When deleting information, never black it out, never use correction fluid to cover it up, and never in any other way erase or obliterate the original wording. Draw a line through the original information so that is still legible. | 20 | | |
| 3. Write or type in the correct information above or below the original line, or in the margin. The location on the chart for the new information should be clear. You may need to attach another sheet of paper or another document with the correction on it. Note in the record "See attached document A" or similar wording to indicate where the corrected information can be found. | 20 | | |
| 4. Place a note near the correction stating why it was made (for example, "error, wrong date" or "error, interrupted by phone call.") Make sure you initial and date the correction. This indication can be a brief note in the margin or an attachment to the record. As a general rule of thumb, do not make any changes without noting the reason for them. | 20 | | |
| 5. Enter the date and time, and initial the correction. | 20 | | |
| 6. If possible, have another staff member or the physician witness and initial the correction to the record when you make it. | 0 | | |
| **Total Points (if applicable)** | 100 | | |

**Comments:** _____

**Final Evaluator's Signature:** _____

**Date:** _____

## CAAHEP Competencies Achieved

V. C (6) Describe various types of content maintained in a patient's medical record

V. P (3) Organize a patient's medical record

## ABHES Competencies Achieved

8. b. Prepare and maintain medical records

8. jj. Perform fundamental writing skills including correct grammar, spelling, and formatting techniques when writing prescriptions, documenting medical records, etc.

## Procedure 15–4: Entering Information in Paper Medical Records

**GOAL:** To document continuity of care by creating a complete, accurate, timely record of the medical care provided at your facility

**MATERIALS:** Patient file, other pertinent documents (test results, x-rays, telephone notes, correspondence), blue ballpoint pen, notebook, keyboard, transcribing equipment

**METHOD:** To pass this procedure the minimum required score is _____ % or all elements must meet "satisfactory" ability on the final demonstration. The first box may be used as a practice or final demonstration, with the evaluator placing **S for Satisfactory** or **U for Unsatisfactory** if that is the grading criteria. The second box may be used as a final demonstration with a **grade point** written in the box.

| STEPS | POSSIBLE POINTS | S/U | POINTS EARNED |
|---|---|---|---|
| 1. Verify that you have the correct chart for the records to be filed. | 5 | | |
| 2. Transcribe dictated doctor's notes as soon as possible, and enter them into the patient record. | 10 | | |
| 3. Spell out the names of disorders, diseases, medications, and other terms the first time you enter them into the patient record, followed by the appropriate abbreviation (for example: "congestive heart failure (CHF)"). Thereafter, you may use the abbreviation alone. | 10 | | |
| 4. Enter only what the doctor has dictated. Do not add your own comments, observations, or evaluations. Use self-adhesive flags or other means to call the doctor's attention to something you have noticed that may be helpful to the patient's case. Date and initial each entry. | 10 | | |
| 5. Follow office procedure to record routine or special laboratory test results. They may be posted in a particular section of the file or on a separate test summary form. If you use the summary form, make a note in the file that the results were received and recorded. Place the original laboratory report in the patient's file if required to do so by office policy. Date and initial each entry. Always note in the chart the date of the test and the results, whether or not test result printouts are filed in the record. | 10 | | |

*(Continued)*

| STEPS | POSSIBLE POINTS | S/U | POINTS EARNED |
|---|---|---|---|
| 6. Make a note in the record of all telephone calls to and from the patient. Date and initial the entries. These entries also may include the doctor's comments, observations, changes in the patient's medication, new instructions to the patient, and so on. If calls are recorded in a separate telephone log, note in the patient's record the time and date of the call and refer to the log. It is particularly important to record such calls when the patient resists or refuses treatment, skips appointments, or has not made follow-up appointments. | 10 | | |
| 7. Make notations in the medical record of any immunizations and vaccines that have been given to the patient. Notations should be posted in the patient's immunization record inside the medical chart. Input them into your state's public health database as well. Immunization records are kept indefinitely. | 10 | | |
| 8. Read over the entries for omissions or mistakes. Ask the doctor to answer any questions you have. | 10 | | |
| 9. Make sure that you have dated and initialed each entry. | 5 | | |
| 10. Be sure that all documents are included in the file. | 10 | | |
| 11. Replace the patient's file in the filing system as soon as possible. | 10 | | |
| **Total Points (if applicable)** | 100 | | |

Comments: _____

_____

_____

**Final Evaluator's Signature:** _____

**Date:** _____

## CAAHEP Competencies Achieved

V. C (6) Describe various types of content maintained in a patient's medical record

V. P (3) Organize a patient's medical record

## ABHES Competencies Achieved

8. b. Prepare and maintain medical records

8. jj. Perform fundamental writing skills including correct grammar, spelling, and formatting techniques when writing prescriptions, documenting medical records, etc.

## Procedure 15–5: Making an Addition (Addendum) to the Electronic Health Record

**GOAL:** To follow standard procedures for correcting or making an addendum to an electronic health record

**MATERIALS:** Access to the patient's electronic health record, other pertinent documents that contain the information to be used in making corrections (for example, handwritten notes, telephone notes, physician's comments, correspondence, lab results)

**METHOD:** To pass this procedure the minimum required score is _____ % or all elements must meet "satisfactory" ability on the final demonstration. The first box may be used as a practice or final demonstration, with the evaluator placing **S for Satisfactory** or **U for Unsatisfactory** if that is the grading criteria. The second box may be used as a final demonstration with a **grade point** written in the box.

| STEPS | POSSIBLE POINTS | S/U | POINTS EARNED |
|---|---|---|---|
| 1. Open the patient record requiring the correction or addendum. | 20 | | |
| 2. Click the "Edit" button as directed by the software program. | 20 | | |
| 3. When the pop-up window appears stating the record is "not editable" (signed and locked), but asking if an addendum is desired, choose "Yes." | 20 | | |
| 4. The program will automatically date, time-stamp the entry with the current date and time, and initial-stamp the entry with the user's initials when the "Save" button is chosen, once the entry is written. | 40 | | |
| **Total Points (if applicable)** | 100 | | |

Comments: _____

_____

_____

Final Evaluator's Signature: _____

Date: _____

## CAAHEP Competencies Achieved

V. C (6) Describe various types of content maintained in a patient's medical record

V. C (11) Discuss principles of using electronic medical records (EMR)

V. P (3) Organize a patient's medical record

V. P (5) Execute data management using electronic health-care records such as the EMR

## ABHES Competencies Achieved

8. b. Prepare and maintain medical records

8. jj. Perform fundamental writing skills including correct grammar, spelling, and formatting techniques when writing prescriptions, documenting medical records, etc.

8. ll. Apply electronic technology

# 16 Prescriptions and Reports

## Test Your Knowledge

### Vocabulary Review

Match the key terms in the right column with the definitions in the left column by placing the letter of each correct answer in the space provided.

_____ **1.** an organization of the government that sets standards for all new drugs to be approved and sold

_____ **2.** drugs that can be bought without a prescription

_____ **3.** a health-care professional who is legally allowed to order prescription medications; includes physicians, nurse practitioners, and physician assistants

_____ **4.** a formal request from a staff member or doctor for the purchase of equipment or supplies

_____ **5.** a drug's brand or proprietary name

_____ **6.** a law enacted in 2008 that among other things provides positive incentives for physicians to use e-prescribing

_____ **7.** when a health-care professional evaluates a patient (consults) at the request of another health-care professional

_____ **8.** the national clearinghouse for e-prescribing; electronically connects physicians, pharmacists, and payers nationwide, enabling them to exchange health information and prescribe without paper; also collaborates with national EHR vendors, pharmacies,

**a.** authorized prescriber (AP) [LO16.3]

**b.** controlled substance [LO16.3]

**c.** consultation [LO16.5]

**d.** e-prescribing [LO16.4]

**e.** Food and Drug Administration (FDA) [LO16.2]

**f.** generic name [LO16.1]

**g.** Medicare Improvements for Patients and Providers Act of 2008 (MIPPA) [LO16.4]

**h.** over-the-counter (OTC) drugs [LO16.1]

**i.** prescription [LO16.1]

**j.** requisition [LO16.4]

**k.** Surescripts [LO16.4]

**l.** trade name [LO16.1]

and health plans to support physicians using EHR software

_____ **9.** a drug's official name

_____ **10.** a drug or drug product that is categorized as potentially dangerous and addictive and is strictly regulated by federal laws

_____ **11.** a physician's written order for medication

_____ **12.** when prescription medication orders are entered electronically and transmitted directly to a pharmacy to be filled

## Multiple-Choice Certification Questions

There may be more than one answer; circle the letter of the choice that best completes each statement or answers each question.

**1.** **[LO16.2]** To check the spelling of a drug using the *PDR*, you would look in Section
   a. 1.
   b. 2.
   c. 3.
   d. 4.
   e. 5.

**2.** **[LO16.2]** A package insert provided with prescription medications includes the
   a. patient's pharmacy information.
   b. patient's insurance member number.
   c. physician's practice name.
   d. product information.
   e. number of refills authorized.

**3.** **[LO16.2]** A pharmaceutical representative
   a. sells drug samples to the physicians.
   b. must be a licensed pharmacist.
   c. conducts all business via e-mail with the physician's office.
   d. is a nuisance to the physician.
   e. introduces physicians to new products.

**4.** **[LO16.2]** The FDA ensures
   a. drugs are accurately labeled.
   b. physicians use only prescription drugs.
   c. pharmaceutical representatives are licensed.
   d. fair prices are set for prescription drugs.
   e. none of the above.

**5.** **[LO16.3]** According to the schedule of controlled substances, which schedule of drugs is *not* obtained using a written prescription?
   a. Schedule V
   b. Schedule IV
   c. Schedule III
   d. Schedule II
   e. Schedule I

**6.** [LO16.3] The organization that acts to enforce drug laws is
   a. the CSA.
   b. the CDC.
   c. the DEA.
   d. the FDA.
   e. OSHA.

**7.** [LO16.3] In order to monitor dispensed controlled drugs and maintain compliance with laws, in a medical office the physician must keep
   a. patient files up-to-date.
   b. inventory records.
   c. drugs in a locked, safe place.
   d. only a small quantity of drugs on hand.
   e. a DEA license.

**8.** [LO16.4] Basic components of a prescription include all of the following items *except* the
   a. patient's full name.
   b. prescriber's address.
   c. patient's insurance information.
   d. date.
   e. generic or brand name of the drug.

**9.** [LO16.4] The abbreviation used in prescriptions that means "before meals" is
   a. A.M.
   b. a.
   c. ac.
   d. amp.
   e. bc.

**10.** [LO16.4] E-prescribing is recommended for ordering patient medications from a pharmacy because
   a. the actual prescription is not in the hands of the patient.
   b. it provides an automatic check for drug and allergy interaction.
   c. it eliminates medication errors due to poor handwriting.
   d. it provides greater efficiency.
   e. all of the above.

**11.** [LO16.2] Lipitor and Crestor are prescription medications that fall under the category of
   a. antilipidemic.
   b. antihypertensive.
   c. antidepressant.
   d. antiasthmatic.
   e. antidiabetic.

**12.** [LO16.2] Which of the following drugs is used to control seizures?
   a. Coumadin
   b. Nexium
   c. Dilantin
   d. Atropine
   e. Inderal

**13.** [LO16.3] If you wanted to contact a drug manufacturer for information not included in the package insert, you could use this section of the *PDR* for contact information:
   a. Section 1.
   b. Section 2.
   c. Section 3.
   d. Section 4.
   e. Section 5.

**14.** [LO16.4] The conditions under which a drug should not be used is called the
   a. indication.
   b. contraindication.
   c. adverse reaction.
   d. precautions.
   e. description.

**15.** [LO16.2] Epocrates is
   a. a format for electronically ordering drugs.
   b. an automated inventory system.
   c. a drug warehouse/mail-order company.
   d. an electronic informational drug software program.
   e. none of the above.

**16.** [LO16.1] The Durham-Humphrey Amendment of 1952 provided
   a. a set of rules describing the patient's rights for refills.
   b. a mechanism to ensure that drugs are pure and safe to use.
   c. for the distinction between prescription and nonprescription drugs.
   d. a way for physicians to obtain a DEA license.
   e. a clause stating that patients are required to use the same pharmacy for refills.

**17.** [LO16.3] Which of the following statements is true regarding the schedule of controlled substances?
   a. Schedules II and III can be authorized over the phone by the administrative medical assistant.
   b. Schedules I, III, and IV allow up to 5 refills in 6 months.
   c. Schedules I and II require a written prescription.
   d. Schedules II and III have the lowest potential for abuse.
   e. Schedules IV and V must be called in by the physician.

**18.** [LO16.1] Which of the following is *not* used as a name for drugs?
   a. Generic name
   b. Trade name
   c. Chemical name
   d. Brand name
   e. Category name

**19.** [LO16.3] One of the distinct characteristics of a Schedule V drug is
   a. it has very limited physical dependence.
   b. it includes opioids and morphine.
   c. the physician must call in these drugs to the pharmacy.
   d. there is a high possibility for abuse.
   e. the drug script must be filled within 7 days and cannot be refilled.

**20.** [LO16.4] MIPAA is a law that was enacted to
   a. prohibit the abuse of narcotics.
   b. ensure the purity of manufactured drugs.
   c. discipline physicians who overprescribe drugs to patients.
   d. provide incentives to physicians who use e-prescribing.
   e. require physicians to obtain a DEA license.

**21.** [LO16.2] The classification of drugs used to relieve allergic symptoms is
   a. steroid.
   b. antidote.
   c. antihistamine.
   d. MAO inhibitor.
   e. decongestant.

**22.** [LO16.5] Critical information that is included on the laboratory report is the
   a. patient's insurance provider name.
   b. cost of the laboratory exam.
   c. name of the person who collected the blood specimen.

d. patient's diagnosis.

e. normal values from the reference lab.

23. **[LO16.4]** An abbreviation that should not be used since it is prone to cause errors is
   a. H.S.
   b. mL.
   c. gtt.
   d. bid.
   e. dx.

24. **[LO16.5]** A consultation is a type of medical report that is
   a. faxed back to the referring physician.
   b. filed in a separate binder labeled "Referrals."
   c. sent to the insurance carrier as part of the authorization for payment of services.
   d. a permanent, legal document.
   e. typically three to four pages in length.

25. **[LO16.5]** Of the following, which one is not found on the laboratory requisition form?
   a. The patient's full name
   b. The test to be performed
   c. The patient's past diagnoses
   d. The patient's insurance information
   e. The physician's address and phone number

## True or False

Decide whether each statement is true or false. In the space at the left, write "T" for true or "F" for false. On the lines provided, rewrite the false statements to make them true.

_____ 1. **[LO16.3]** An authorized prescriber includes a licensed pharmacist.

_____

_____ 2. **[LO16.4]** The DEA number is required for prescriptions of Schedules II and III only.

_____

_____ 3. **[LO16.1]** An OTC drug is one that the FDA has approved for use without the supervision of an authorized prescriber.

_____

_____ 4. **[LO16.1]** When a new patient comes to a health-care facility, it is necessary to get a record of his or her prescription and nonprescription (OTC) drugs.

_____

_____ 5. **[LO16.2]** A generic name is also considered a drug's official name.

_____

_____ 6. **[LO16.1]** A drug's name is selected by the FDA.

_____

_____ 7. **[LO16.2]** Antibiotics are used to inhibit the growth of microorganisms.

_____

_____ **8.** [LO16.4] Administrative medical assistants cannot prescribe medications, but they can dispense medications.

_____

_____ **9.** [LO16.2] Section 6 of the *PDR* is used to obtain product information, including a full-color photo of the actual medications.

_____

_____ **10.** [LO16.2] The drug package insert includes information about adverse reactions, which are the possible reactions to the drug.

_____

## Sentence Completion

In the space provided, write the word or phrase that best completes each sentence.

**1.** [LO16.2] Drugs are categorized by their action on the _____, general _____ effect, or the body _____ affected.

**2.** [LO16.2] Drugs have three names: the _____ or "official name," the _____ name given by the company that manufactures the drug and the _____ name which indicates the chemical properties of the drug.

**3.** [LO16.3] All physicians must be registered with the DEA and follow the legal requirements of the CSA of 1970 to _____, _____, and _____ controlled drugs.

**4.** [LO16.3] Telephone refills may be done for all medications except Schedule _____ and _____ drugs.

**5.** [LO16.3] A prescription drug is one that can be used only by order of a(n) _____ prescriber such as a(n) _____, _____ _____, or _____ _____.

**6.** [LO16.4] By educating the patient about how to use a drug properly, you will not only help the patient improve medically but also increase the probability of patient _____ and _____.

**7.** [LO16.2] The FDA ensures that drugs are _____, labeled _____ and _____, and do not mislead _____ _____.

**8.** [LO16.3] A doctor who administers or dispenses controlled drugs to patients must maintain two types of records: _____ records and _____ records.

**1.** _____
_____

**2.** _____
_____

**3.** _____
_____

**4.** _____
_____

**5.** _____
_____

**6.** _____
_____

**7.** _____
_____

**8.** _____
_____

9. [LO16.2] When a practice disposes of medications, the DEA does not allow businesses to _____ any medications, and medications should not be placed in the _____.

9. _____
   _____

10. [LO16.5] If a specimen accompanies a requisition form, it should include the _____ of the specimen and the _____ and _____ the specimen was collected.

10. _____
    _____

# Apply Your Knowledge

## Short Answer

Write the answer to each question on the lines provided.

1. [LO16.2] Provide at least four sources, including print and electronic, where you can access drug information.

   _____

   _____

   _____

2. [LO16.3] What are the major factors that differentiate the five schedules of controlled substances?

   _____

   _____

   _____

3. [LO16.3] What is the difference between the role of the DEA and the FDA?

   _____

   _____

   _____

4. [LO16.1] What are the reasons a patient may receive a generic version of a drug instead of a trade brand?

   _____

   _____

   _____

**5.** **[LO16.2]** When a cardiovascular specialist wants to affect a patient's blood pressure and heart function, what are four classifications of drugs that the physician might choose from?

_____

_____

_____

## Problem-Solving Activities

Follow the directions for each activity.

**1.** **[LO16.4]** Charting Prescription Telephone Orders
   a. The physician has requested the administrative staff to call in the following new prescriptions to the patient's pharmacy.
   b. Using the chart sample provided, enter chart information for each of the prescriptions, which are telephoned to the Rx Pharmacy from the medical office.
   c. Use proper charting format, including appropriate abbreviations as listed in Chapter 16.

   - Patient: Mary Butcher, Amoxil 500 mg capsules, sig: one capsule three times a day before meals, dispense 30 capsules with no refills.

| TOTAL CARE CLINIC | |
| --- | --- |
| **PROGRESS NOTES** | |
| DATE | Patient Name: |
| | |

   - Patient: James Fischer, Benicar 20 mg tablets, sig: one tablet once a day in the morning with food, dispense 30 tablets with 3 refills.

| TOTAL CARE CLINIC | |
| --- | --- |
| **PROGRESS NOTES** | |
| DATE | Patient Name: |
| | |

   - Patient: Suzanne Metcalf, Celebrex 100 mg capsules, sig: one capsule two times a day, one in the morning and one at night, dispense 60 tablets with 6 refills.

| TOTAL CARE CLINIC | |
| --- | --- |
| **PROGRESS NOTES** | |
| DATE | Patient Name: |
| | |

   - Patient: William Barnes, Klonopin 0.25 mg, sig: one tablet two times a day with food, dispense 60 tablets with no refills.

| TOTAL CARE CLINIC | |
| --- | --- |
| **PROGRESS NOTES** | |
| DATE | Patient Name: |
| | |

- Patient: Cindy Ruhe, Glucophage 500 mg tablets, sig: one tablet once a day in the morning, dispense 90 tablets with 1 refill.

| TOTAL CARE CLINIC | |
|---|---|
| **PROGRESS NOTES** | |
| DATE | Patient Name: |
| | |

2. **[LO16.2]** Prescription Medication Identification
   a. Using the *PDR* or another source for medication information, describe the appearance of the following medications.
   b. Information should include what form the medication is available in (tablets, capsules), any identifying labeling on the tablet or capsule, and the strength(s) available.
   c. Next to each drug description, draw a picture of the tablet/capsule, showing the markings on the pill. Include both sides of the pill.
      - Flexeril 5 mg
      - Percocet 325 mg/5 mg
      - Lipitor 10 mg
      - Diazepam 5 mg
      - Zoloft 50 mg
      - Ambien 5 mg

# Thinking Critically

Write your response to each case study question on the lines provided.

## Case 1 [LO16.4]

In the medical practice where you are newly employed, the administrative staff receives numerous phone calls each day from patients or pharmacies requesting authorization for medication refills. Each time a call comes into the office, the person who takes the call retrieves the patient's chart and takes it to the physician for approval of the refill. This becomes time consuming, and the staff is getting frustrated with all the calls they receive and the interruption that they cause.

1. What might you recommend to the staff to help better manage the prescription calls?

_____

_____

_____

2. How will you implement your recommendations to improve the authorization of pharmacy refills?

_____

_____

_____

## Case 2 [LO16.5]

Brenda Nash, an administrative medical assistant, is assigned to the front desk. She receives an incoming call from a person who identifies herself as Jane Wise. Ms. Wise is inquiring about laboratory results from blood work she had performed at an outside laboratory several days ago. Brenda remembers seeing the laboratory report arrive in the mail and filing it in Ms. Wise's chart. She explains to Ms. Wise that the report did arrive and that most of the results were in the normal range according to the normal values listed on the report. She also tells Ms. Wise that the doctor wants to see her for an appointment to discuss the abnormal results.

**1.** Was this call handled properly? If not, why?

_____

_____

_____

**2.** What is the proper technique for handling patient calls regarding test results?

_____

_____

_____

## Case 3 [LO16.4]

Jeff Bass is a patient who was treated in your medical clinic on a Monday for minor muscle strain of the back. The injury was work related and the patient was released to return to light duty. He is scheduled for an appointment the following Monday when the physician will release him to full duty and close the worker's compensation claim. He was prescribed 30 tablets of Vicodin for the pain. The instructions were to take 1 tablet every 4 to 6 hours as needed for pain. The patient calls the office on Thursday (three days later) to get a medication refill, complaining that the pain is still there and he needs more Vicodin. The physician will not refill this type of medication without seeing the patient in the office. The patient refuses to come to the office until his follow-up appointment on Monday and insists that you call his pharmacy to refill the prescription, and then he abruptly hangs up. The patient calls back in a half-hour asking if you have called in his refill of medication.

**1.** Why does the physician have a policy about not refilling a medication such as Vicodin without seeing the patient in the office?

_____

_____

_____

**2.** When this patient calls back the second time to see if you have refilled the drug, what will you tell the patient?

_____

_____

_____

# Demonstrate Your Knowledge

**Student Name:** _____

## Procedure 16–1: Record Medications in a Patient's Chart

**GOAL:** To create and/or maintain a current list of medications in the patient's chart

**MATERIALS:** Medication list and electronic health record such as SpringCharts®
(*Note:* A patient record of medication list can be found at the end of this study guide.)

**METHOD:** To pass this procedure the minimum required score is _____% or all elements must meet "satisfactory" ability on the final demonstration. The first box may be used as a practice or final demonstration, with the evaluator placing **S for Satisfactory** or **U for Unsatisfactory** if that is the grading criteria. The second box may be used as a final demonstration with a **grade point** written in the box.

| STEPS | POSSIBLE POINTS | S/U | POINTS EARNED |
|---|---|---|---|
| 1. Obtain a list of current medications the patient is taking from the patient or from the written or electronic chart. | 10 | | |
| 2. Verify the spelling of each medication before adding it to the printed health record. This can be done while entering it into the electronic health record through an electronic resource. | 15 | | |
| 3. Identify the amount the patient takes of each medication, for example, "1 tablet." | 10 | | |
| 4. Include how often and/or when the patient takes the medication, for example, "daily" or "3 times a day with meals." | 10 | | |
| 5. Enter the patient electronic chart and select the medication link. | 10 | | |
| 6. Perform a search for the desired medication and select. Most programs have a data base or a direct link to a medication site such as Epocrates to check on drug interactions and formulary references. | 15 | | |
| 7. Enter new medications and edit any existing medications according to the directions for the EHR program you are using. | 15 | | |
| 8. Check and verify all medication entries before exiting the program. | 15 | | |
| **Total Points (if applicable)** | 100 | | |

Comments: _____

_____

_____

Final Evaluator's Signature: _____

Date: _____

## CAAHEP Competency Achieved

V. P (5) Execute data management using electronic health-care records such as the EMR

## ABHES Competency Achieved

9. g. Maintain medication and immunization records

## Procedure 16–2: Assist the Authorized Prescriber in Complying with the Controlled Substance Act of 1970

**GOAL:** To comply with the Controlled Substances Act of 1970

**MATERIALS:** Access to DEA Forms 224, 224a, 222, and 41 and ability to complete them with either pen or Internet access (*Note:* These forms are available at the end of this study guide.)

**METHOD:** To pass this procedure the minimum required score is _____ % or all elements must meet "satisfactory" ability on the final demonstration. The first box may be used as a practice or final demonstration, with the evaluator placing **S for Satisfactory** or **U for Unsatisfactory** if that is the grading criteria. The second box may be used as a final demonstration with a **grade point** written in the box.

| STEPS | POSSIBLE POINTS | S/U | POINTS EARNED |
|---|---|---|---|
| 1. Use DEA Form 224 (shown in Figure 16–8) to register the physician with the Drug Enforcement Administration. Be sure to register each office location at which the physician administers or dispenses drugs covered under Schedules II through V. | 0 | | |
| 2. Renew all registrations every 3 years using DEA Form 224a. | | | |
| a. Calculate a period of 3 years from the date of the original registration or the most recent renewal. Note that date as the expiration date of the physician's DEA registration. | 10 | | |
| b. Subtract 45 days from the expiration date, and mark this date on the calendar or create a reminder in your electronic calendar program. | 10 | | |
| c. Before the expiration deadline, complete the DEA form and have the physician sign it. Prepare or request a check for the fee. | 10 | | |
| d. For paper forms, submit the original and one copy of the completed form with the appropriate fee to the DEA so that it will arrive before the deadline. Keep one copy for the office records. | 10 for step "2.d." *or* "2.e." | | |
| e. Applicants are encouraged to use the online forms system for electronic renewal. Search the Internet for DEA Form 224A. (*Note:* The DEA form Web site is for renewals only, and Internet renewals should not be done if you have already sent a paper application or renewal.) Update and complete the areas of the form including Personal Information, Activity, State License(s), Background Information, Payment, and Confirmation. You will be able to print copies of the form once completed. | | | |
| 3. Order Schedule II drugs using DEA Form 222, shown in Figure 16–9, as instructed by the physician. (Stocks of these drugs should be kept to a minimum.) Accurate instruction from the physician is necessary to ensure safety. | 10 | | |

*(Continued)*

| STEPS | POSSIBLE POINTS | S/U | POINTS EARNED |
|---|---|---|---|
| 4. Include the physician's DEA registration number on every prescription for a drug in Schedules II through V or the prescriptions will not be accepted by the pharmacy. | 10 | | |
| 5. Complete an inventory of all drugs in Schedules II through V every 2 years (as permitted in your state; this task may be restricted to other health-care professionals). | 10 | | |
| 6. Store all drugs in Schedules II through V in a secure, locked safe or cabinet (as permitted in your state) to prevent theft. | 10 | | |
| 7. Keep accurate dispensing and inventory records for at least 2 years. | 10 | | |
| 8. Dispose of expired or unused drugs according to the DEA regulations. Always complete DEA Form 41 (shown in Figure 16–10) when disposing of controlled drugs. | 10 | | |
| **Total Points (if applicable)** | 100 | | |

**Comments:** _____

_____

_____

**Final Evaluator's Signature:** _____

**Date:** _____

**CAAHEP Competency Achieved**

IX. C (13) Discuss all levels of governmental legislation and regulation as they apply to medical assisting practice, including FDA and DEA regulations

**ABHES Competency Achieved**

6. e. Comply with federal, state, and local health laws and regulations

**Student Name:** _____

## Procedure 16–3: Interpret a Prescription

**GOAL:** To read and accurately interpret a prescription

**MATERIALS:** Prescription, Table 16–3 showing abbreviations used in prescriptions, method of recording (pen or electronic)

**METHOD:** To pass this procedure the minimum required score is _____% or all elements must meet "satisfactory" ability on the final demonstration. The first box may be used as a practice or final demonstration, with the evaluator placing **S for Satisfactory** or **U for Unsatisfactory** if that is the grading criteria. The second box may be used as a final demonstration with a **grade point** written in the box.

| STEPS | POSSIBLE POINTS | S/U | POINTS EARNED |
|---|---|---|---|
| 1. Verify the prescriber information. This is especially important in a multi-physician practice or electronic health record. | 15 | | |
| 2. Ensure patient information is accurate, including correct spelling of name, date of birth, and address. For written prescriptions, check legibility. | 15 | | |
| 3. Confirm the date of the prescription. | 15 | | |
| 4. Check the medication name and double-check spelling. | 15 | | |
| 5. Verify that instructions to the pharmacist are complete and include refill authorization and generic substitution. | 15 | | |
| 6. Translate the instructions to the patient using Table 16–4. | 15 | | |
| 7. Make sure that the prescription is signed in ink for handwritten prescriptions and digitally for electronic prescriptions. | 10 | | |
| **Total Points (if applicable)** | 100 | | |

**Comments:** _____

_____

_____

**Final Evaluator's Signature:** _____

**Date:** _____

## Table 16–3 Abbreviations Used in Prescriptions

| ABBREVIATION | MEANING | ABBREVIATION | MEANING |
|---|---|---|---|
| a | Before | min | Minute, minimum |
| aa | Of each | mL | Milliliters |
| ac | Before meals | mm | Millimeters |
| AM | Morning | neb | Nebulizer |
| amp | Ampule | noct | Night |
| apl | Applicatorful | NPO | Nothing by mouth |
| aq | Water | nr | No refills |
| bid | Twice daily | oz | Ounce |
| $\overline{c}$ | With | pc | After meals |
| cap | Capsule | per | By means of, through |
| cd | Cycle day (menstrual cycle) | PM | Evening or nighttime |
| cmpd | Compound | po, PO | By mouth |
| cr | Cream | PR, pr | Rectally |
| d | Daily or day | q | Every |
| DAW | Dispense as written (no generic) | qam | Every morning |
| disp | Dispense | q4h | Every 4 hours |
| ds | Double strength | qid | Four times daily |
| dx | Diagnosis | qs | Sufficient amount |
| elix | Elixir | r, rec | Rectally |
| eq | Equivalent | rept | Repeat |
| g, gm | Gram | rf | Refill(s) |
| gen | Generic | s | Without |
| gr | Grain (60 to 65 mg) | stat | Immediately |
| gtt | Drop(s) | subcut | Subcutaneously |
| h, hr | Hour | sup | Suppository |
| $H_2O$ | Water | susp | Suspension |
| IM | Intramuscularly | sx | Symptoms |
| inj | Inject, injection | syr | Syrup |
| IV | Intravenously | tab | Tablet(s) |
| kg | Kilogram | tsp | Teaspoon |
| L | Liter | tbsp | Tablespoon |
| liq | Liquid | tx | Treatment |
| lot | Lotion | ud, utd | As directed |
| MDI | Metered dose inhaler | ung | Ointment |
| mEq | Milliequivalent | vag | Vaginally, into vagina |
| mg | Milligram(s) | YO | Years old |
| mg | Milligram | | |

## CAAHEP Competencies Achieved

IV. P (2) Report relevant information to others succinctly and accurately

IV. P (3) Use medical terminology, pronouncing medical terms correctly, to communicate information, patient history, data, and observations

## ABHES Competencies Achieved

6. b. Properly utilize the *PDR*, drug handbook, and other drug references to identify a drug's classification, usual dosage, usual side effects, and contraindications

6. c. Identify and define common abbreviations that are accepted in prescription writing

6. d. Understand legal aspects of writing prescriptions, including federal and state laws

## Procedure 16–4: Manage a Prescription Refill

**GOAL:** To ensure the patient receives a complete and accurate prescription

**MATERIALS:** Telephone, appropriate phone numbers, message pad or prescription refill request form, pen, patient chart with prescription order *(Note: A progress note can be found at the end of this study guide.)*

**METHOD:** To pass this procedure the minimum required score is _____ % or all elements must meet "satisfactory" ability on the final demonstration. The first box may be used as a practice or final demonstration, with the evaluator placing **S for Satisfactory** or **U for Unsatisfactory** if that is the grading criteria. The second box may be used as a final demonstration with a **grade point** written in the box.

| STEPS | POSSIBLE POINTS | S/U | POINTS EARNED |
|---|---|---|---|
| 1. Take the message from the call or the message system. For the prescription to be complete, you must obtain the patient's name, date of birth, phone number, pharmacy name and/or phone number, medication, and dosage. | 10 | | |
| 2. Follow your facility policy regarding prescription renewals. Typically, the prescription is usually called into the pharmacy the day it is requested. An example policy may be posted at the facility and may state, "Non-emergency prescription refill requests must be made during regular business hours. Please allow 24 hours for processing." | 0 | | |
| 3. Communicate the policy to the patient. You should know the policy and let the patient know the policy and the time when the refills will be reviewed. For example, you might state, "Dr. Alexander will review the prescription between patients, and it will be telephoned within 1 hour to the pharmacy. I will call you back if there is a problem." | 5 | | |
| 4. Obtain the patient's chart or reference the electronic chart to verify you have the correct patient and that the patient is currently taking the medication. Check the patient's list of medications, which is usually part of the chart. | 10 | | |
| 5. Give the prescription refill request and the chart to the physician or prescriber. Do not give a prescription refill request to the physician without the chart or chart access information. Wait for an authorization from the physician before you proceed. | 5 | | |
| 6. Once the physician authorizes the prescription, prepare to call the pharmacy with the renewal information. You cannot call in Schedule II or III medications. However, renewals can be called in for Schedule IV and V medications. Be certain to have the physician order, the patient's chart, and the refill request in front of you when you make the call. The request should include the name of the drug, the drug dosage, the frequency and mode of administration, the number of refills authorized, and the name and phone number of the pharmacy. | 10 | | |

*(Continued)*

| STEPS | POSSIBLE POINTS | S/U | POINTS EARNED |
|---|---|---|---|
| 7. Telephone the pharmacy. Since only an identified representative from a medical practice can authorize a refill, you must identify yourself by name, the practice name, and the doctor's name. | 5 | | |
| 8. State the purpose of the call. (Example: "I am calling to request a prescription refill for a patient.") | 5 | | |
| 9. Identify the patient. Include the patient's name, date of birth, address, and phone number. It is essential that the correct drug be prescribed for the correct patient according to doctor's order. | 10 | | |
| 10. Identify the drug, including the strength of the drug (spelling the name when necessary), the dosage, the frequency and mode of administration, and any other special instructions or changes for administration (such as "take at bedtime"). | 10 | | |
| 11. State the number of refills authorized. | 5 | | |
| 12. If leaving a message on a pharmacy voice mail system set up for physicians, state your name, the name of the doctor you represent, and your phone number before you hang up. If the pharmacist has any questions, he must be able to reach the physician. | 10 | | |
| 13. Document the prescription renewal in the chart after the medication has been called into the pharmacy. Include the date, the time, the name of pharmacy, the person taking your call, the medication, dose, amount, directions, and number of refills. Sign your first initial, last name, and title. An example of charting is as follows: 5/03/11 Rx telephoned to Beth Stone at Noname Pharmacy: Zyrtec 10 mg, one tablet daily at bedtime, #30, 6 refills. —K. Buckwalter, RMA (AMT). | 15 | | |
| **Total Points (if applicable)** | 100 | | |

**Comments:** _____

_____

_____


**Final Evaluator's Signature:** _____


**Date:** _____

## CAAHEP Competencies Achieved

IV. P (2) Report relevant information to others succinctly and accurately.

IV. P (7) Demonstrate telephone techniques

## ABHES Competencies Achieved

8. ee. Use proper telephone techniques

8. jj. Perform fundamental writing skills including correct grammar, spelling, and formatting techniques when writing prescriptions, documenting medical records, etc.

## Procedure 16–5: Electronically Order and Track Medical Test Results

**GOAL:** To order and track medical tests electronically

**MATERIALS:** Electronic patient chart (for this example SpringCharts® is used) and the medical test ordered (*Note:* A referral form and requisition form can be found at the end of this study guide.)

**METHOD:** To pass this procedure the minimum required score is _____% or all elements must meet "satisfactory" ability on the final demonstration. The first box may be used as a practice or final demonstration, with the evaluator placing **S for Satisfactory** or **U for Unsatisfactory** if that is the grading criteria. The second box may be used as a final demonstration with a **grade point** written in the box.

| STEPS | POSSIBLE POINTS | S/U | POINTS EARNED |
|---|---|---|---|
| 1. Access the patient's electronic chart. For example, in SpringCharts® the electronic chart can be accessed from many different places: in the "Practice View" screen by clicking on the patient's name in the "Scheduler," via the patient's name in the "Patient Tracker," or by selecting a "ToDo" or "Message" associated with a patient. | 15 | | |
| 2. Access the test menu within the electronic chart. In SpringCharts®, use the "Actions" menu (Figure 16–15). For example, in SpringCharts®, the term "tests" includes lab tests, imaging tests, and medical tests. | 20 | | |
| 3. Search and then select the test to be ordered. Double-check that you have the right test before making your final selection. For example, in SpringCharts®, use the "Order Test" window (Figure 16–16). In EHR, actions can be completed by selecting different items. You should be familiar with the EHR you are using. | 20 | | |
| 4. When results are received, locate and store the results in the pending tests area of the EHR. For example, in SpringCharts®, once the test is ordered it is stored in the "Pending Tests" area. | 20 | | |
| 5. Enter the results in the patient chart and notify the physician. For example, in SpringCharts® when data is entered manually into "Pending Tests," it is sent to the "Completed Tests" area of the program for the physician's viewing. Once the tests have been viewed by the physician, they are permanently filed in the patient's chart. | 25 | | |
| **Total Points (if applicable)** | 100 | | |

**Comments:** _____

_____

_____

**Final Evaluator's Signature:** _____

**Date:** _____

## CAAHEP Competencies Achieved

V. P (3) Organize a patient's medical record

V. P (5) Execute data management using electronic health-care records such as the EMR

## ABHES Competencies Achieved

8. b. Prepare and maintain medical records

8. hh. Receive, organize, prioritize, and transmit information expediently

8. ll. Apply electronic technology

# 17

# Insurance and Billing

## Test Your Knowledge

### Vocabulary Review

Match the key terms in the right column with the definitions in the left column by placing the letter of each correct answer in the space provided.

_____ **1.** care that provides comfort only; not meant to be curative in nature, such as hospice

_____ **2.** a type of insurance that covers injuries caused by the insured or injuries that occurred on the insured's property

_____ **3.** a rule that states that the insurance policy of a policyholder whose birthday comes first in the year is the primary payer for all dependents

_____ **4.** information that explains the medical claim in detail, including the amount filled, amount allowed, amount of subscriber liability, amount paid, and notations of any noncovered services with explanations; also known as remittance advice (RA) EOB

_____ **5.** insurance that provides a monthly, prearranged payment to an individual who cannot work as a result of an injury, illness, or disability

_____ **6.** a national health insurance program for Americans aged 65 and older, as well as some patients under age 65 who meet specific criteria

_____ **7.** the process of clarifying and reviewing past-due accounts by age from the first date of billing

**a.** accounts payable [LO17.7]

**b.** accounts receivable [LO17.7]

**c.** age analysis [LO17.9]

**d.** allowed charge [LO17.1]

**e.** balance billing [LO17.1]

**f.** benefits [LO17.1]

**g.** birthday rule [LO17.1]

**h.** capitation [LO17.1]

**i.** Centers for Medicare and Medicaid Services (CMS) [LO17.1]

**j.** CHAMPVA (Civilian Health and Medical Program for Veterans Administration) [LO17.1]

**k.** charge slip [LO17.1]

**l.** class action lawsuit [LO17.1]

**m.** clearinghouse [LO17.5]

**n.** coinsurance [LO17.1]

_____ 8. an insurance plan's list of approved prescription medications

_____ 9. a type of insurance that covers the expenses of dependents of veterans with total, permanent, service-connected disabilities; covers the surviving dependents of veterans who die in the line of duty or as a result of service-connected disabilities

_____ 10. a legal principle that limits payments by insurance companies to 100% of the covered expenses

_____ 11. the Medicare fee-for-service plan that allows the beneficiary to choose any licensed physician certified by Medicare

_____ 12. money owed by a business; the practice's expenses

_____ 13. money paid as punishment for intentionally breaking the law

_____ 14. private insurance that Medicare beneficiaries can purchase to reduce the gaps in Medicare coverage; the amount they would have to pay from their own pockets after receiving Medicare benefits

_____ 15. a medical procedure that is not required to sustain life, but for which the patient or physician requests payment from a third-party payer; some such procedures are paid for by third-party payers, whereas others are not

_____ 16. formerly a major type of health plan, which repays policyholders for the costs of health care due to illness and injuries

_____ 17. a negative balance on an account that occurs when more money than is owed is paid to the practice

_____ 18. an account that has only one charge, usually for a small amount, for a patient who does not come in regularly

_____ 19. the billing of a patient for the difference between a higher, usual fee and the lower, allowed charge

_____ 20. a group that takes nonstandard medical billing software formats and translates them into the standard EDI format

**o.** coordination of benefits [LO17.1]

**p.** credit [LO17.1]

**q.** credit balance [LO17.1]

**r.** credit bureau [LO17.10]

**s.** cycle billing [LO17.8]

**t.** damages [LO17.1]

**u.** deductible [LO17.1]

**v.** disability insurance [LO17.1]

**w.** disclosure statement [LO17.11]

**x.** elective procedure [LO17.1]

**y.** electronic data interchange (EDI) [LO17.5]

**z.** exclusion [LO17.1]

**aa.** explanation of benefits (EOB) [LO17.1]

**bb.** fee-for-service [LO17.2]

**cc.** fee schedule [LO17.2]

**dd.** formulary [LO17.1]

**ee.** health maintenance organization (HMO) [LO17.1]

**ff.** liability insurance [LO17.1]

**gg.** lifetime maximum benefit [LO17.1]

**hh.** Medicaid [LO17.3]

**ii.** Medicare [LO17.3]

**jj.** Medicare Advantage plans [LO17.3]

**kk.** Medigap [LO17.3]

**ll.** open-book account [LO17.9]

**mm.** Original Medicare Plan [LO17.3]

**nn.** overpayment [LO17.7]

**oo.** palliative care [LO17.1]

_____ **21.** a managed care plan that establishes a network of providers to perform services for plan members

_____ **22.** the process of the provider contacting the insurance plan to see if the proposed procedure is a covered service under the patient's insurance plan

_____ **23.** an expense that is not covered by a particular insurance policy, such as an eye exam or dental care

_____ **24.** a form similar to an invoice; often contains a courteous reminder to the patient that payment is due

_____ **25.** a system that sends statements to groups of patients every few days, spreading the work of billing all patients over the period of a month, while billing each patient only once

_____ **26.** a program that provides health-care benefits for dependents of military personnel and military retirees

_____ **27.** physicians who enroll in managed care plans; contracts with MCOs stipulates their fees

_____ **28.** the total sum that a health plan will pay out over the patient's lifetime

_____ **29.** a payment structure in which a health maintenance organization prepays an annual set fee per patient to a physician

_____ **30.** the payment system used by Medicare; establishes the relative value units for services, replacing the provider consensus on usual fees

_____ **31.** a written description of agreed terms of payment; also called a federal Truth in Lending statement

_____ **32.** PPOs, HMOs, private fee-for-service plans, and Medicare medical savings accounts that provide Medicare beneficiaries with plan coverage choices in addition to the traditional Medicare plan

_____ **33.** the amount that is the most the payer will pay any provider for each procedure or service; the payer's payment is based on this allowed charge

**pp.** participating physicians [LO17.1]

**qq.** preauthorization [LO17.1]

**rr.** precertification [LO17.1]

**ss.** preferred provider organization (PPO) [LO17.1]

**tt.** premium [LO17.1]

**uu.** punitive damages [LO17.1]

**vv.** referral [LO17.1]

**ww.** remittance advice (RA) [LO17.5]

**xx.** resource-based relative value scale (RBRVS) [LO17.4]

**yy.** single-entry account [LO17.7]

**zz.** skips [LO17.10]

**aaa.** statement [LO17.8]

**bbb.** statute of limitations [LO17.12]

**ccc.** TRICARE [LO17.1]

**ddd.** X12837 Health Care Claim [LO17.5]

_____ **34.** a health-care organization that provides specific services to individuals and their dependents who are enrolled in the plan; physicians enrolled in the organization agree to provide certain services in exchange for a prepaid fee or capitation payment

_____ **35.** the original record of services performed for a patient and the charges for those services

_____ **36.** an extension of time to pay for services, which are provided on trust

_____ **37.** payment made that is more than the amount billed; results in a credit balance

_____ **38.** income or money owed to a business; the practice's income

_____ **39.** an authorization from a medical practice for a patient to have specialized services performed by another practice; often required for insurance purposes

_____ **40.** an account that is open to charges made occasionally as needed

_____ **41.** transmission of electronic medical insurance claims from providers to payers, using the necessary information systems

_____ **42.** a list of common services and procedures (performed by a physician) and the charges of each

_____ **43.** a company that provides information about the credit worthiness of a person seeking credit

_____ **44.** people who move leaving no forwarding information in the hopes that they will not be found

_____ **45.** payment for medical services

_____ **46.** a fixed percentage of covered charges paid by the insured person after a deductible has been met

_____ **47.** the basic annual cost of health-care insurance

_____ **48.** the process of the provider contacting the insurance plan to see if the proposed procedure is a covered service under the patient's insurance plan

_____ **49.** information that explains the medical claim in detail, including the amount filled, amount allowed, amount of subscriber liability, amount paid, and notations of any noncovered services with explanations; also known as remittance advice (RA)

_____ **50.** a state law that sets a time limit on when a collection suit on a past-due account can legally be filed

_____ **51.** money paid as compensation for violating legal rights

_____ **52.** an electronic claim transaction that is the HIPAA Health Care Claim or Equivalent Encounter Information

_____ **53.** a fixed dollar amount that must be paid (yearly) by the insured before additional expenses are covered by the insurer

_____ **54.** a federally funded health cost assistance program for low-income, blind, and disabled patients and for families receiving aid for dependent children; foster children; and children with birth defects

_____ **55.** a congressional agency designed to handle Medicare and Medicaid insurance claims; formerly known as the Health Care Financing Administration

_____ **56.** a lawsuit in which one or more people sue a company or other legal entity that allegedly wronged all of them in the same way

## Multiple-Choice Certification Questions

There may be more than one answer; circle the letter of the choice that best completes each statement or answers each question.

**1.** [LO17.5] The physician or provider of health care who submits insurance claims must obtain a National Provider Identifier number issued by
   a. the AMA.
   b. CMS.
   c. an MCO.
   d. the CDC.
   e. the ICD.

**2.** [LO17.2] TRICARE has three choices of health-care benefits including
   a. Prime, Extra, Basic.
   b. Extra, Basic, Civilian.
   c. Prime, Extra, Standard.
   d. Standard, Basic, Prime.
   e. Basic, Standard, Civilian.

**3.** [LO17.1] A patient who has emphysema might have which of the following abbreviations written on his medical record, signifying his chronic condition?
   a. CHF
   b. CABG
   c. PTCA
   d. COPD
   e. AHF

**4.** [LO17.5] Workers' compensation insurance requires employers to report any workplace accident or incident to the state labor department within
   a. 12 hours.
   b. 24 hours.
   c. 36 hours.
   d. 48 hours.
   e. 64 hours.

**5.** [LO17.1] Which of the following abbreviations would relate to reports from a radiologist or x-ray department?
   a. IVP, MRI
   b. PFT, FAS
   c. CXR, CT
   d. SOM, HPV
   e. Answers (a) and (c)

**6.** [LO17.5] The primary purpose of the coordination of benefits is to
   a. ensure that the insured person's medical bills are paid in full.
   b. allow physicians to charge differently based on the patient's insurance.
   c. determine the patient's eligibility for medical services.
   d. prevent duplication of payment.
   e. require insurance companies to pay the bill in full.

**7.** [LO17.1] Which of the following statements accurately describes the "birthday rule"?
   a. All states are required by federal law to adopt the birthday rule.
   b. The birthday rule only applies when determining coverage for dependents.
   c. When a husband and wife both carry insurance, the policy that has been in effect the shortest amount of time is the primary insurance.
   d. The husband's insurance always becomes the primary insurance.
   e. None of the above.

**8.** [LO17.1] The explanation of benefits received from the insurance company is now referred to or called the
   a. disclosure statement.
   b. remittance advice.
   c. formulary.
   d. coordination of benefits.
   e. receivable statement.

**9.** [LO17.1] Billing a patient for the difference between a higher, usual fee and a lower, allowed charge is called _____ and is not allowed by participating physicians.
   a. capitation
   b. assignment of benefits
   c. coordination of benefits

d. third-party billing
e. balance billing

10. **[LO17.3]** Under Medicare Part B, patients are required to annually pay
   a. a premium.
   b. a fee for service.
   c. coinsurance.
   d. a processing fee.
   e. none of the above.

11. **[LO17.3]** Medicare Part A does not pay for
   a. inpatient expenses up to 90 days for each benefit period.
   b. medical care at home.
   c. outpatient hospital services.
   d. psychiatric hospitalization.
   e. respite care.

12. **[LO17.3]** Patients enrolled in the Original Medicare Plan may purchase additional coverage under a
   a. Medicare Part A plan.
   b. coinsurance plan.
   c. Medigap plan.
   d. Medicare Advantage plan.
   e. fee-for-service plan.

13. **[LO17.3]** Which of the following is a Medicare plan that charges a monthly premium and a small copayment for each office visit, but no deductible?
   a. Medicare managed care plan
   b. Medicare preferred provider organization plan
   c. Medicare private fee-for-service plan
   d. Original Medicare Plan
   e. Medigap plan

14. **[LO17.1]** At the time of service, if required by the managed care plan, the administrative medical assistant collects
   a. the deductible.
   b. the copayment.
   c. the premium.
   d. the coinsurance.
   e. nothing.

15. **[LO17.4]** The nationally uniform relative value of a procedure is based on which of the following three things?
   a. The physician's specialty, the cost of living, and insurance rates
   b. The age of the patient, the diagnosis of the patient, and the geographic area of the practice
   c. The amount billed by the physician, the cost of the procedure, and the copayment of the patient
   d. The physician's work, the practice's overhead, and the cost of malpractice insurance
   e. The fee schedule of the physician, the geographic area of the practice, and the diagnosis of the patient

16. **[LO17.4]** Under the concept of the resource-based relative value scale (RBRVS) used by Medicare, the fee for a procedure is based on
   a. a formula based on using the relative value, the geographic adjustment factor, and a conversion factor.
   b. the generally accepted fee that a physician charges for difficult or complicated services.
   c. the average fee that a physician charges for a service or procedure.
   d. the 90th percentile of fees charges for a procedure by similar physicians in the same area.
   e. a formula based on the physician's fee schedule and the geographic area's cost of living.

**17.** [LO17.2] The major types of health plans are
   a. fee-for-service and workers' compensation.
   b. workers' compensation and managed care.
   c. managed care and fee-for-service.
   d. disability and private plan.
   e. answers (a) and (c).

**18.** [LO17.3] Which of the following statements accurately relates to Medicare benefits?
   a. The Medicare Part A hospital plan begins after the patient has been in the hospital 3 days.
   b. To be eligible for Medicare Part A the beneficiary is required to be at least 65 years old and no longer employed.
   c. Once a person is enrolled in Medicare Part A, she is automatically enrolled in Part B.
   d. Medicare Part A covers only 190 days of psychiatric care.
   e. The Original Medicare Plan requires the beneficiary to pay 50% of disallowed charges.

**19.** [LO17.5] Which of the following is true of workers' compensation insurance?
   a. Medical costs arising from an auto accident while on the way to work are covered under worker's compensation.
   b. Death benefits are allowed if the death occurred in a work-related setting.
   c. Rehabilitation costs are covered if required because of a work-related injury.
   d. Payment is made to a patient for a temporary disability due to a work-related illness.
   e. Answers (b) and (d).

**20.** [LO17.11] If a patient and a physician enter into a unilateral agreement about the patient's outstanding bill, the patient will
   a. pay the debt over a period of months.
   b. immediately pay the bill in full.
   c. need to seek a different physician for future medical care.
   d. not be allowed to be seen by the physician until the bill is paid in full.
   e. do none of the above.

**21.** [LO17.11] The Truth in Lending Act covers or regulates
   a. the fees a physician can charge patients.
   b. insurance companies' reimbursement policies.
   c. credit agreements that involve more than four payments.
   d. the amount of money the patient can be responsible for paying after the insurance company has paid its portion.
   e. the method of releasing credit reports.

**22.** [LO17.5] Which of the following is *true* concerning disability insurance?
   a. Disability insurance may be offered by the employer at the employee's expense.
   b. Disability insurance is not health insurance.
   c. Disability insurance does not cover medical expenses.
   d. Disability insurance can be either short-term or long-term.
   e. All of the above.

**23.** [LO17.10] When initially contacting a patient with the intent to collect a bill, you should
   a. demand immediate payment in full.
   b. be friendly, cordial, and sympathetic.
   c. require a partial payment by the next day.
   d. threaten the patient with legal action if the bill is not paid.
   e. inform the patient that medical services are no longer available from your physician.

**24.** [LO17.3] If a patient covered by the Original Medicare Plan sees a participating physician and has a bill for medical services in the amount of $200 and the Medicare-allowed charge is $100, what are the amounts that each party will pay?
   a. Medicare $80; patient $20
   b. Medicare $50; patient $50
   c. Medicare $100; patient $0

d. Medicare $90; patient $10

e. None of the above

**25.** [LO17.5] A reason that a medical practice might use a clearinghouse for electronic claims processing is

a. the clearinghouse can take a standard formatted claim and translate it into a nonstandard format.

b. the medical practice does not have the translation software necessary to process the claims.

c. a clearinghouse may process all the medical practice claims or just those for specific insurance companies.

d. answers (a) and (b).

e. answers (b) and (c).

# True or False

Decide whether each statement is true or false. In the space at the left, write "T" for true or "F" for false. On the lines provided, rewrite the false statements to make them true.

_____ **1.** [LO17.2] CHAMPVA covers the expenses of the dependents of veterans with total, permanent, service-connected disabilities.

_____

_____ **2.** [LO17.2] TRICARE is a Medicaid program.

_____

_____ **3.** [LO17.2] A managed care organization (MCO) sets up agreements with physicians as well as with enrolled policyholders.

_____

_____ **4.** [LO17.1] Copayments are made to insurance companies.

_____

_____ **5.** [LO17.4] The RBRVS system is the basis for the Medicare payment system.

_____

_____ **6.** [LO17.2] Preferred provider organizations (PPOs) never allow members to receive care from physicians outside the network.

_____

_____ **7.** [LO17.1] Exclusions are expenses covered by an insurance company.

_____

_____ **8.** [LO17.1] An overpayment occurs when payment on an account is more than the amount billed and results in a credit balance.

_____

_____ **9.** [LO17.1] A deductible is a fixed-dollar amount that must be met in full on the first visit each year to a physician.

_____

_____ **10.** [LO17.5] The X12 837 Health Care Claim is also known as the "universal claim."

_____

## Sentence Completion

In the space provided, write the word or phrase that best completes each sentence.

**1.** [LO17.2] Managed care plans pay their participating physicians in one of two ways, either by _____ fees or a _____ called capitation.

**2.** [LO17.3] Medicare managed care plans charge a monthly _____ and a small _____ for each office visit, but not a _____.

**3.** [LO17.3] In 2008, CMS announced aggressive new steps to find and prevent _____, _____, and _____ in Medicare.

**4.** [LO17.3] Do not submit a claim to Medicaid without _____ of Medicaid membership and benefit _____.

**5.** [LO17.5] Using the direct transmission of electronic claims, providers need the necessary information systems, including a _____ and _____ technology.

**6.** [LO17.1] HIPAA rules set standards for protecting individually identifiable health information when transmitted electronically. Medical offices must protect the _____, _____, and _____ of this information.

**7.** [LO17.1] A doctor may treat some patients free of charge or for just the amount covered by the patient's insurance. This practice is known as _____ _____.

**8.** [LO17.9] Age analysis is the process of _____ and _____ past-due accounts by _____ from the _____ date of billing.

**9.** [LO17.11] The Truth in Lending Act requires creditors to provide applicants with _____ and _____ credit costs and terms, clearly and obviously.

**1.** _____
_____

**2.** _____
_____

**3.** _____
_____

**4.** _____
_____

**5.** _____
_____

**6.** _____

**7.** _____
_____

**8.** _____

**9.** _____
_____

**10.** [LO17.10] According to the AMA, it is appropriate to assess _____ _____ or late charges on past-due accounts if the patient is notified in _____.

10. _____

_____

# Apply Your Knowledge

## Short Answer

Write the answer to each question on the lines provided.

**1.** [LO17.5] List the three major methods used to transmit claims electronically.

_____

_____

_____

**2.** [LO17.5] Explain why the X12 837 Health Care Claim must be used for Medicare claims.

_____

_____

_____

**3.** [LO17.1] What is the purpose of the coordination of benefits in insurance policies?

_____

_____

_____

**4.** [LO17.3] What does an eligible individual have to do to receive Medicare Part B benefits?

_____

_____

_____

**5.** [LO17.5] List at least five tasks the administrative medical assistant will perform to support the insurance claims process.

_____

_____

_____

# Problem-Solving Activities

Follow the directions for each activity.

**1.** [LO17.5] Extracting Information from the Remittance Advice Form

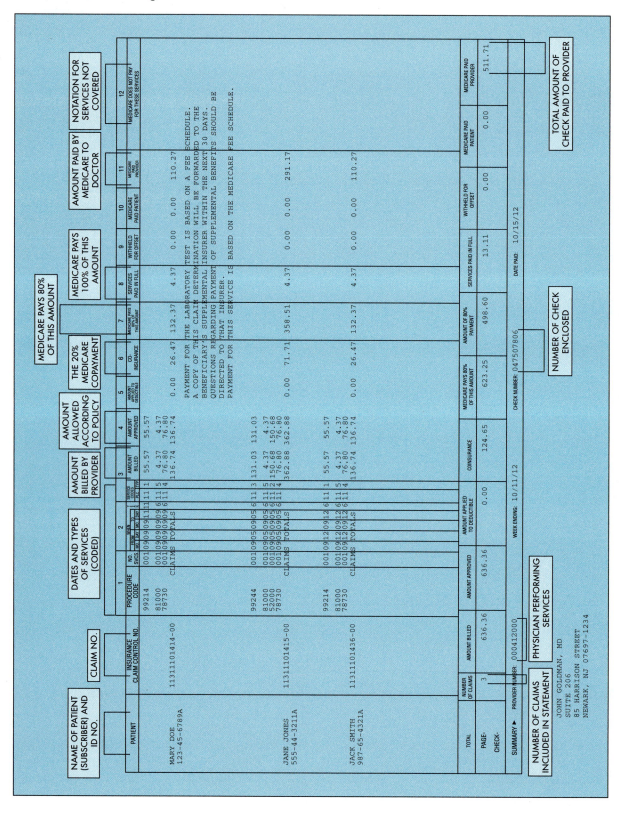

a. Refer to the remittance advice form.

b. Locate the following information on the form and fill in the blank with the appropriate information.

- Jane Jones' identification number:

_____

- Total amount billed for Mary Doe:

_____

- Physician's provider number:

_____

- The reimbursement check number:

_____

- Jack Smith's copayment amount:

_____

- Total amount of check the physician received:

_____

- Jane Jones' procedure code for billed amount $150.68:

_____

- Amount paid to physician on Jack Smith's account:

_____

- Payment amount approved for Mary Doe's procedure 81000:

_____

- Amount Medicare paid to Jane Jones:

_____

**2.** [LO17.9] Accounts Receivable—Age Analysis

a. Using the Accounts Receivable—Age Analysis Table on the next page, enter the following patients' account information in the table. At the end of the entries, complete the Total Age Analysis amounts for the practice.

1. Mary Simmons charged services on August 12 and has a balance of $300 with the entire amount over 120 days. She has been sent three notices by the office and was just sent a certified letter requesting payment on her account. She has made no payments to the account.

2. Frank Brown has a balance of $140, which was charged on September 30. He made a payment on October 5; $40 is 60 days past due and the remainder 90 days past due. An initial notice was sent to him requesting a payment on this account.

3. Harvey Jenson has a balance of $600 for services charged on November 8. He made four payments on the account, the last of which was received on November 30. He has not been sent a notice of payment due.

4. Theodore Thomas has a balance of $720 charged on September 18. He made a payment on October 15. His insurance company, Blue Cross Blue Shield, has been billed for the charges.

5. Adam Cooper has a balance of $1400 charged on June 1. He has made no payment on this account and has no insurance. This account was turned over to a collections agency on December 15.

6. Sally Carson has a balance of $75 charged on November 1. She has made no payment to the account, and a Medicare claim was filed.

# ACCOUNTS RECEIVABLE–AGE ANALYSIS

Date: _____

| Patient | Balance | Date of Charges | Most Recent Payment | 30 days | 60 days | 90 days | 120 days | Remarks |
|---------|---------|-----------------|---------------------|---------|---------|---------|----------|---------|
|         |         |                 |                     |         |         |         |          |         |
|         |         |                 |                     |         |         |         |          |         |
|         |         |                 |                     |         |         |         |          |         |
|         |         |                 |                     |         |         |         |          |         |
|         |         |                 |                     |         |         |         |          |         |
|         |         |                 |                     |         |         |         |          |         |
| TOTAL   |         |                 |                     |         |         |         |          |         |

# Thinking Critically

Write your response to each case study question on the lines provided.

## Case 1 [LO17.10]

Brenda is the office manager for the medical clinic where you are employed as an administrative medical assistant. There are several patient accounts with large unpaid balances, and payments have not been made for weeks or in some cases several months. The physician has asked you to assist Brenda in contacting these patients about their delinquent accounts to try and collect some or all the money owed on these accounts. Brenda asks you to observe her first call to a patient who owes $250 on a bill that is over 3 months old. She threatens the patient that, if some payment is not made by the end of the week, the account will be turned over to a collection agency. She also tells the patient that the physician may not be able to treat her until this bill is settled. You know that this is an inappropriate way to talk to a patient about this type of issue. Even though you know Brenda is your supervisor, you know that you should talk with her about this approach to collecting bills.

1. What should you tell Brenda about the way she handled this call?

_____

_____

_____

2. What did Brenda say that was inappropriate as a method to collect the debt?

_____

_____

_____

## Case 2 [LO17.3]

Herlinda and Cindy are co-workers in a family practice medical office. In the employee break room, Herlinda mentions that some of the patients in the practice receive Medicaid benefits and she doesn't understand why she has to pay for health-care benefits when these patients get their health care paid for. She believes that anyone on Medicaid is a burden to taxpayers. Cindy disagrees with Herlinda about this topic.

1. What information should Cindy discuss with Herlinda about the patients that are receiving Medicaid assistance?

_____

_____

_____

2. What would be the alternative for these patients if Medicaid were not available to them?

_____

_____

_____

## Case 3 [LO17.2]

Mr. Lewis, a new patient, arrives at your office for his first visit. His neighbor is a patient of your office and speaks highly about the physician. As you are checking him in, you discover that he is enrolled in a PPO insurance plan; however, your physician is not in the network for Mr. Lewis's plan. You explain to Mr. Lewis that he can still see your physician but that he will be responsible for paying a higher percentage of the charges for the visit and that he may also be subject to a deductible. Mr. Lewis is upset and angry that he was not informed of this when he made the appointment.

1. How could this incident have been avoided?

_____

_____

_____

2. Is there anything you can do to assist Mr. Lewis?

_____

_____

_____

# Demonstrate Your Knowledge

**Student Name:** _____

## Procedure 17–1: Verifying Workers' Compensation Coverage

**GOAL:** To verify workers' compensation coverage before accepting a patient

**MATERIALS:** Telephone, paper, pencil

**METHOD:** To pass this procedure the minimum required score is _____% or all elements must meet "satisfactory" ability on the final demonstration. The first box may be used as a practice or final demonstration, with the evaluator placing **S for Satisfactory** or **U for Unsatisfactory** if that is the grading criteria. The second box may be used as a final demonstration with a **grade point** written in the box.

| STEPS | POSSIBLE POINTS | S/U | POINTS EARNED |
|---|---|---|---|
| 1. Call the patient's employer and verify that the accident or illness occurred on the employer's premises or at an employment-related work site. | 15 | | |
| 2. Obtain the employer's approval to provide treatment. Be sure to write down the name and title of the person giving approval, as well as his phone number. | 20 | | |
| 3. Ask the employer for the name of its workers' compensation insurance company. (Employers are required by law to carry such insurance. It is a good policy to notify your state labor department about any employer you encounter that does not have workers' compensation insurance, although you are not required to do so.) You may wish to remind the employer to report any workplace accidents or injuries that result in a workers' compensation claim to the state labor department within 24 hours of the incident. | 15 | | |
| 4. Contact the insurance company and verify that the employer does indeed have a policy with the company and that the policy is in good standing. | 15 | | |
| 5. Obtain a claim number for the case from the insurance company. This claim number is used on all bills and paperwork. | 15 | | |
| 6. At the time the patient starts treatment, create a patient record. If the patient is already one of the practice's regular patients, create separate medical and financial records for the workers' compensation case. | 20 | | |
| **Total Points (if applicable)** | 100 | | |

**Comments:** _____

_____

_____

**Final Evaluator's Signature:** _____

**Date:** _____

## CAAHEP Competencies Achieved

VII. C (3) Discuss workers' compensation as it applies to patients

VII. P (4) Obtain precertification, including documentation

VII. P (5) Obtain preauthorization, including documentation

VII. P (6) Verify eligibility for managed care services

VII. A (1) Demonstrate assertive communication with managed care and/or insurance providers

## ABHES Competencies Achieved

8. r. Apply third-party guidelines

8. s. Obtain managed care referrals and precertification

## Procedure 17–2: Submitting a Request for Prior Authorization

**GOAL:** To submit a request for prior authorization

**MATERIALS:** Patient medical chart with planned procedure and CPT code, diagnosis and ICD-9 code for proof of medical necessity, patient financial record or the following information: patient name, address, DOB, subscriber name and relationship to patient if not the same, insurance policy group and ID numbers

**METHOD:** To pass this procedure the minimum required score is _____ % or all elements must meet "satisfactory" ability on the final demonstration. The first box may be used as a practice or final demonstration, with the evaluator placing **S for Satisfactory** or **U for Unsatisfactory** if that is the grading criteria. The second box may be used as a final demonstration with a **grade point** written in the box.

| STEPS | POSSIBLE POINTS | S/U | POINTS EARNED |
|---|---|---|---|
| 1. Place call to insurance carrier or access Web site if available. | 10 | | |
| 2. When you reach the nurse manager for the patient's policy, explain that you would like to obtain prior authorization for the requested procedure. She will ask a series of questions regarding the patient, procedure, and diagnosis. Answer these questions utilizing the assembled materials from the patient's medical and financial records. | 50 points for step 2 *or* 3 | | |
| 3. If obtaining authorization via the insurance carrier Web site, access the website utilizing your user ID and password. Enter the prior authorization area of the Web site and enter the required information using the assembled materials from the patient's medical and financial records. | 50 points for step 2 *or* 3 | | |
| 4. When prior authorization is obtained, carefully record the authorization number and the name and extension number of the person issuing the authorization (if obtained over the phone). If the authorization is obtained via a Web site, print out the authorization documentation. | 20 | | |
| 5. Place the authorization number and/or documentation in the patient medical and financial record for future reference as it will be required when submitting the patient's health insurance claim. | 20 | | |
| **Total Points (if applicable)** | 100 | | |

**Comments:** _____

_____

_____

**Final Evaluator's Signature:** _____

**Date:** _____

## CAAHEP Competencies Achieved

VII. C (4) Describe procedures for implementing both managed care and insurance plans

VII. P (4) Obtain precertification, including documentation

VII. P (5) Obtain preauthorization, including documentation

VII. P (6) Verify eligibility for managed care services

VII. A (1) Demonstrate assertive communications with managed care and/or insurance providers

## ABHES Competencies Achieved

8. r. Apply third-party guidelines

8. s. Obtain managed care referrals and precertification

## Procedure 17–3: Tracking Insurance Claims Submissions

**GOAL:** To create a spreadsheet to track insurance claims submission

**MATERIALS:** CMS-1500 claims prepared for submission or record of CMS-1500 claims submitted electronically; spreadsheet or grid for handwritten record with pen; or computer with software program such as MS Excel, allowing for creation of a spreadsheet
(*Note:* An insurance claim register can be found at the end of this study guide.)

**METHOD:** To pass this procedure the minimum required score is _____ % or all elements must meet "satisfactory" ability on the final demonstration. The first box may be used as a practice or final demonstration, with the evaluator placing **S for Satisfactory** or **U for Unsatisfactory** if that is the grading criteria. The second box may be used as a final demonstration with a **grade point** written in the box.

| STEPS | POSSIBLE POINTS | S/U | POINTS EARNED |
|---|---|---|---|
| 1. Using Figure 17–8 as a guide, create columns with the following (or similar) headings: Patient Name (and/or account number); Insurance Company; Claim Filing Date and Amount; Insurance Response and Date of Response; Date Resubmitted; Payment Date; Payment Amount; Patient Balance; Date of Patient Billing. | 20 | | |
| 2. Using the list of claims being submitted, complete the blanks for patient name, insurance company, date of submission, and amount of the claim. | 20 | | |
| 3. When the RA (EOB) is received, complete the date and response columns, including whether the claim is paid, rejected, or denied, or a request was made for more information. | 15 | | |
| 4. If resubmission is required, enter the date of resubmission. | 15 | | |
| 5. If payment is received, enter the date of receipt and the amount of the payment. | 15 | | |
| 6. Record patient balance (if any) and the date the patient is billed. | 15 | | |
| **Total Points (if applicable)** | 100 | | |

Comments: _____

_____

_____

Final Evaluator's Signature: _____

Date: _____

## CAAHEP Competencies Achieved

None

## ABHES Competencies Achieved

8. d. Apply concepts for office procedures

8. i. Perform billing and collection procedures

## Procedure 17–4: Completing the CMS-1500 Claim Form

**GOAL:** To complete the CMS-1500 claim form correctly

**MATERIALS:** Patient record, CMS-1500 form, typewriter or computer, patient ledger card or charge slip
*(Note: A blank CMS-1500 form can be found at the end of this study guide.)*

**METHOD:** To pass this procedure the minimum required score is _____% or all elements must meet "satisfactory" ability on the final demonstration. The first box may be used as a practice or final demonstration, with the evaluator placing **S for Satisfactory** or **U for Unsatisfactory** if that is the grading criteria. The second box may be used as a final demonstration with a **grade point** written in the box.

| STEPS | POSSIBLE POINTS | S/U | POINTS EARNED |
|---|:---:|:---:|:---:|
| *(Note: The numbers below correspond to the numbered fields on the CMS-1500 form.)*<br>1. Place an X in the appropriate insurance box. | 1 | | |
| 1a. Enter the insured's insurance identification number as it appears on the insurance card. | 2 | | |
| 2. Enter the patient's name in this order: last name, first name, middle initial (if any). | 2 | | |
| 3. Enter the patient's birth date using an 8-digit format. Indicate the sex of the patient—male or female. | 1 | | |
| 4. If the insured and the patient are the same person, enter "SAME." If not, enter the policy-holder's name. | 2 | | |
| 5. Enter the patient's mailing address, city, state, zip code, and telephone number. | 2 | | |
| 6. Enter the patient's relationship to the insured. If they are the same, mark SELF. | 1 | | |
| 7. Enter the insured's mailing address, city, state, zip code, and telephone number. If this address is the same as the patient's, enter "SAME." For Medicare, leave blank. | 2 | | |
| 8. Indicate the patient's marital, employment, and student status by placing an X in the boxes. | 0 | | |
| 9. Enter the last name, first name, and middle initial of any other insured person whose policy might cover the patient. If the claim is for Medicare and the patient has a Medigap policy, enter the patient's name again. | 2 | | |
| 9a. Enter the policy or group number for the other insured person. | 1 | | |
| 9b. Enter the date of birth and sex of the other insured person (field 9). | 1 | | |

*(Continued)*

| STEPS | POSSIBLE POINTS | S/U | POINTS EARNED |
|---|---|---|---|
| 9c. Enter the other insured's employer or school name. | 2 | | |
| 9d. Enter the other insured's insurance plan or program name. If the plan is Medigap and CMS has assigned it a nine-digit number called PAYERID, enter that number here. | 2 | | |
| 10. Place Xs in the appropriate "YES" or "NO" boxes to indicate whether the patient's place of employment, an auto accident, or other type of accident precipitated the patient's condition. If an auto accident is responsible, for "PLACE," enter the two-letter state postal abbreviation for the location of the accident. | 1 | | |
| 11. Enter the insured's policy group number. For Medicare claims, fill out this section only if there is other insurance primary to Medicare; otherwise, enter "NONE" and leave fields 11a—d blank. | 2 | | |
| 11a. Enter the insured's date of birth and sex as in field 3, if the insured is not the patient. | 1 | | |
| 11b. Enter the employer's name or school name here. This information will determine if Medicare is the primary payer. | 1 | | |
| 11c. Enter the insurance plan or program name. | 1 | | |
| 11d. Place an X to indicate "YES" or "NO" related to another health benefit plan. | 1 | | |
| 12. The patient or an authorized representative signs and dates the form here. If a representative signs, have the representative indicate the relationship to the patient. If signatures are on file, this may be noted by inserting "Signature on File," or for some payers, the abbreviation "SOF" is also acceptable. | 2 | | |
| 13. Have the insured (the patient or another individual) sign here. If signatures are on file, this may be noted by inserting "Signature on File," or for some payers, the abbreviation "SOF" is also acceptable. | 2 | | |
| 14. Enter the date of the current illness, injury, or pregnancy, using eight digits. | 2 | | |
| 15. Enter date patient was first seen for illness or injury. Leave it blank for Medicare. | 0 | | |
| 16. Enter the dates the patient is or was unable to work. This information could signal a workers' compensation claim. | 1 | | |

*(Continued)*

| STEPS | POSSIBLE POINTS | S/U | POINTS EARNED |
|---|---|---|---|
| 17. Enter the name of the referring physician, clinical laboratory, or other referring source. | 2 | | |
| 17a. Depending on insurance carrier instructions, enter an approved 2-digit qualifier (refer to Table 17–1) in the small space and the appropriate referring provider identifier next to it. If the carrier requires only the NPI, leave this box blank. | 2 | | |
| 17b. Enter the referring provider NPI number. | 2 | | |
| 18. If the patient was hospitalized during this encounter, enter dates here. | 1 | | |
| 19. Use your payer's current instructions for this field. In many cases it may be left blank. | 2 | | |
| 20. Place an X in the "YES" box if a laboratory test was performed outside the physician's office, and enter the test price if you are billing for these tests. Place an X in the "NO" box if the test was done in the office of the physician who is billing the insurance company. | 1 | | |
| 21. Enter the code number for each diagnosis or nature of injury (see Chapter 18). Enter up to four codes in order of importance. | 5 | | |
| 22. Enter the Medicaid resubmission code and original reference number if applicable. | 2 | | |
| 23. Enter the prior authorization number if required by the payer. | 2 | | |
| 24. The six service lines in block 24 are divided horizontally to accommodate NPI and other proprietary identifiers per insurance carrier instructions. Otherwise, use the nonshaded areas. | 2 | | |
| 24A. Enter the date of each service, procedure, or supply provided. Add the number of days for each, and enter them, in chronological order, in field 24G. | 2 | | |
| 24B. Enter the two-digit place-of-service code. | 1 | | |
| 24C. "EMG" stands for emergency care. Check with insurer to see if this information is needed. If it is required and emergency care was provided, enter "Y"; if it is not required or care was not on an emergency basis, leave this field blank. | 1 | | |

*(Continued)*

| STEPS | POSSIBLE POINTS | S/U | POINTS EARNED |
|---|---|---|---|
| 24D. Enter the CPT/HCPCS codes with modifiers for the procedures, services, or supplies provided (see Chapter 20). | 5 | | |
| 24E. Enter the diagnosis code (or its reference number—1, 2, 3, or 4—depending on carrier regulations) that applies to that procedure, as listed, in field 21. | 0 | | |
| 24F. Enter the dollar amount of the fee charged. | 2 | | |
| 24G. Enter the days or units on which the service was performed. | 2 | | |
| 24H. This field is Medicaid-specific for early periodic screening diagnosis and treatment programs. | 2 | | |
| 24I. If required by the insurance carrier, enter the appropriate non-NPI identifier here. If not required, leave this area blank. | 2 | | |
| 24J. If a non-NPI number is required by the carrier, enter the PIN identified in 24I in the shaded area. Use the nonshaded area below this to enter the provider's NPI in 24I. | 2 | | |
| 25. Enter the physician's or care provider's federal tax identification number or Social Security number. | 2 | | |
| 26. Enter the patient's account number assigned by your office, if applicable. | 2 | | |
| 27. Place an X in the "YES" box to indicate that the physician will accept Medicare or TRICARE assignment of benefits. | 1 | | |
| 28. Enter the total charge for the service. | 2 | | |
| 29. Enter the amount already paid by any primary insurance company or the patient, if it pertains to his deductible. | 2 | | |
| 30. Enter the balance due your office. For primary Medicare claims, leave blank. | 2 | | |
| 31. Have the physician or service supplier sign and date the form here. In most cases, because claims are filed electronically, the signature is on file and the typed name of the provider is acceptable in this block. | 2 | | |
| 32. Enter the name and address of the organization or individual who performed the services. If the services were performed in the patient's home, leave this field blank. | 2 | | |
| 32a. In field 32a, enter the NPI for the service facility. | 2 | | |

*(Continued)*

| STEPS | POSSIBLE POINTS | S/U | POINTS EARNED |
|---|---|---|---|
| 32b. If required by the insurance carrier, enter the appropriate two-digit qualifier immediately followed by the identification number being used. Do not place any spaces or punctuation between the qualifier and the identification number. | 2 | | |
| 33. List the billing physician's or supplier's name, address, zip code, and phone number. | 2 | | |
| 33a. Enter the NPI of the billing provider. | 2 | | |
| 33b. If required by the insurance carrier, enter the non-NPI qualifier, immediately followed by the identification number being used. Do not place any spaces or punctuation between the qualifier and the identification number. | 2 | | |
| **Total Points (if applicable)** | 100 | | |

Comments: _____

_____

_____

Final Evaluator's Signature: _____

Date: _____

## CAAHEP Competencies Achieved

VII. C (8) Describe processes for filing insurance claims both manually and electronically

VII. C (9) Describe guidelines for third-party claims

VII. P (3) Complete insurance claim forms

## ABHES Competencies Achieved

8. u. Prepare and submit insurance claims

## Procedure 17–5: Completing the Encounter Form (Superbill)

**GOAL:** To complete an encounter form or superbill accurately (make sure the doctor's name and address appear on the form)

**MATERIALS:** Superbill, patient ledger card, patient information sheet, fee schedule, insurance code list, pen *(Note: A superbill can be found at the end of this study guide.)*

**METHOD:** To pass this procedure the minimum required score is _____% or all elements must meet "satisfactory" ability on the final demonstration. The first box may be used as a practice or final demonstration, with the evaluator placing **S for Satisfactory** or **U for Unsatisfactory** if that is the grading criteria. The second box may be used as a final demonstration with a **grade point** written in the box.

| STEPS | POSSIBLE POINTS | S/U | POINTS EARNED |
|---|---|---|---|
| 1. From the patient ledger card and information sheet, fill in the patient data, such as name, sex, date of birth, and insurance information. | 10 | | |
| 2. Fill in the place and date of service. | 5 | | |
| 3. Attach the superbill to the patient's medical record, and give them both to the doctor. | 5 | | |
| 4. Accept the completed superbill from the patient after the patient sees the doctor. Make sure that the doctor has indicated the diagnosis and the procedures performed. Also make sure that an appropriate diagnosis is listed for each procedure. | 10 | | |
| 5. If the doctor has not already recorded the charges, refer to the fee schedule for procedures that are marked. Then fill in the charges next to those procedures. | 10 | | |
| 6. List the total charges for the visit and the previous balance (if any). | 10 | | |
| 7. Calculate the subtotal. | 10 | | |
| 8. Fill in the amount and type of payment (cash, check, money order, or credit card) made by the patient during this visit. | 10 | | |
| 9. Calculate and enter the new balance. | 10 | | |
| 10. Have the patient sign the authorization-and-release section of the superbill. | 10 | | |
| 11. Keep a copy of the superbill for the practice records. Give the original to the patient along with one copy to file with the insurer. | 10 | | |
| **Total Points (if applicable)** | 100 | | |

**Comments:** _____

_____

_____

**Final Evaluator's Signature:** _____

**Date:** _____

## CAAHEP Competencies Achieved

VI. P (2) Perform accounts receivable procedures, including:

      b. Perform billing procedures

VI. A (1) Demonstrate sensitivity and professionalism in handling accounts receivable activities with clients

## ABHES Competencies Achieved

8. i. Perform billing and collection procedures

8. k. Perform accounts receivable procedures

## Procedure 17–6: Preparing an Age Analysis

**GOAL:** To create and examine an age analysis

**MATERIALS:** Computer, patient accounts, ledger cards (if being done by hand), accounts receivable aging record analysis form (optional), policy and procedure manual, pen
*(Note:* An age analysis can be found at the end of this study guide.)

**METHOD:** To pass this procedure the minimum required score is _____% or all elements must meet "satisfactory" ability on the final demonstration. The first box may be used as a practice or final demonstration, with the evaluator placing **S for Satisfactory** or **U for Unsatisfactory** if that is the grading criteria. The second box may be used as a final demonstration with a **grade point** written in the box.

| STEPS | POSSIBLE POINTS | S/U | POINTS EARNED |
|---|---|---|---|
| 1. Using the reporting section of your billing computer program, create an age analysis report for patients and insurance companies. This also can be done manually by pulling patient ledger cards, noting balances due and dates of last payments. Use Figure 17–16 as a guide to create a spreadsheet for your findings. | 15 | | |
| 2. Review the accounting report. Check the report—highlight for proposed actions for each account, according to your office policy. | 10 | | |
| 3. Mark the accounts that are under 31 days as "No action to be taken at this time." | 5 | | |
| 4. Bills that are unpaid at more than 31 days should be marked as "Contact or follow up with insurance company." | 10 | | |
| 5. Accounts that are 31—60 days old should be marked according to your office policy. An initial phone call may be made inquiring as to payment arrangements. | 10 | | |
| 6. Accounts that are 61—90 days old should be marked according to your office policy. Make notations such as "Account Past Due." A follow-up phone call and/or more insistent statement message letter for payment may be in order. | 10 | | |
| 7. Accounts that are 91—120 days old should be marked according to your office policy. A last phone call to attempt discussing the account and more insistent collection statement/letter should be sent. | 10 | | |

*(Continued)*

| | | | |
|---|---|---|---|
| 8. For accounts older than 120 days, make sure you review previous collection attempts. At this point, after it is discussed with the physician, a letter stating the account will be turned over to the collection agency will be sent, with a specific date listed in the letter. This letter should be mailed by certified, return-receipt mail. | 10 | | |
| 9. Record all actions that have been taken beside each account. | 10 | | |
| 10. Finally, write follow-up letters to patients and document any agreements that you and the patient have discussed via telephone. Be sure to keep a copy in the financial record of any correspondence mailed to the patient. | 10 | | |
| **Total Points (if applicable)** | 100 | | |

**Comments:** _____

_____

_____

**Final Evaluator's Signature:** _____

**Date:** _____

## CAAHEP Competencies Achieved

VI. C (8) Describe common periodic financial reports

VI. C (10) Identify procedures for preparing patient accounts

VI. P (3) Utilize computerized office billing systems

## ABHES Competencies Achieved

8. i. Perform billing and collection procedures

8. k. Perform accounts receivable procedure

8. w. Use manual or computerized bookkeeping systems

# 18 ICD-9-CM Coding

## Test Your Knowledge

### Vocabulary Review

Match the key terms in the right column with the definitions in the left column by placing the letter of each correct answer in the space provided.

_____ **1.** the notation within the ICD-9 using the directions *See or See also* after the main term in the index; notes that another term may be appropriate when coding the referenced diagnosis

_____ **2.** a code set based on a system maintained by the World Health Organization; use is mandated by HIPAA for reporting patient diseases, conditions, and signs and symptoms

_____ **3.** the patient's primary reason for seeking care

_____ **4.** the alphanumeric designation used to communicate the diagnosis to the third-party payer on the health-care claim form

_____ **5.** a process of finding, correcting, and preventing illegal medical office practices

_____ **6.** one of two ways diagnoses are listed in the ICD-9-CM; diagnoses appear in alphabetic order with their corresponding diagnosis code(s)

_____ **7.** a type of ICD-9 code that identifies external causes of injuries and illnesses such as accidents and poisonings

**a.** Alphabetic Index [LO18.3]

**b.** chief complaint [LO18.3]

**c.** compliance plan [LO18.3]

**d.** conventions [LO18.2]

**e.** cross-reference [LO18.3]

**f.** diagnosis [LO18.3]

**g.** diagnosis code [LO18.3]

**h.** E code [LO18.4]

**i.** *International Classification of Diseases, Ninth Revision, Clinical Modification (ICD-9-CM)* [LO18.1]

**j.** primary diagnosis [LO18.3]

**k.** principal diagnosis [LO18.3]

**l.** Tabular List [LO18.3]

**m.** V code [LO18.4]

_____ **8.** one of two ways that diagnoses are listed in the ICD-9-CM; diagnosis codes are listed in numeric order with additional instructions regarding the use of the code for each diagnosis

_____ **9.** the first diagnosis listed for outpatient claims as the *primary* reason for the patient's visit

_____ **10.** the condition for which the patient is seeking care

_____ **11.** the first diagnosis listed for inpatient claims as the *principal* reason found, after study, for the patient's hospitalization

_____ **12.** an ICD-9 code used to identify health-care encounters for reasons other than illness or injury, such as annual physical exams, immunizations, and normal childbirth

_____ **13.** a list of abbreviations, punctuation, symbols, typefaces, and instructional notes appearing in the beginning of ICD-9; provides guidelines for using the code set

## Multiple-Choice Certification Questions

There may be more than one answer; circle the letter of the choice that best completes each statement or answers each question.

**1.** **[LO18.1]** The use of ICD-9 codes is mandated by _____ for reporting patients' diseases and conditions.
 a. AAPC
 b. DHS
 c. HIPAA
 d. CPT
 e. AHIMA

**2.** **[LO18.4]** An example of a condition that requires the use of a V code is
 a. chronic bronchitis.
 b. a fractured tibia.
 c. influenza.
 d. an annual checkup.
 e. an acute back sprain.

**3.** **[LO18.5]** The ICD-10 diagnoses coding program is scheduled to be introduced in
 a. 2012.
 b. 2013.
 c. 2014.
 d. 2015.
 e. 2016.

**4.** [LO18.1] One of the reasons the ICD-9-CM was originally created was to classify statistics of patient "morbidity," which means
   a. death.
   b. surgeries.
   c. wellness.
   d. sickness.
   e. None of the above.

**5.** [LO18.2] The WHO developed "O" codes, which are used to track
   a. obstetrical conditions.
   b. oncology diseases.
   c. otology-related illnesses.
   d. obstructive diseases.
   e. All of the above.

**6.** [LO18.2] When a condition or disease cannot be described more specifically, the abbreviation that may be used is
   a. NOS.
   b. SPN.
   c. NOT.
   d. SNO.
   e. NOP.

**7.** [LO18.3] Which of the following descriptions accurately reflects the difference between acute and chronic?
   a. A chronic condition is more serious than an acute condition.
   b. Chronic conditions may worsen from time to time and become acute.
   c. The onset of an acute illness is slow and lasts a long time.
   d. If a patient has an acute and chronic illness, the acute code is listed first, followed by the chronic code.
   e. Answers (b) and (d).

**8.** [LO18.4] An E code is used to
   a. describe chronic illness.
   b. explain how an injury happened.
   c. describe the treatment the patient received.
   d. assign the benefits the patient will receive.
   e. Answers (c) and (d).

**9.** [LO18.3] Appendix D of the ICD-9-CM lists categories related to
   a. auto accidents.
   b. chronic conditions.
   c. pediatric injuries.
   d. accidents that happen in a personal home or dwelling.
   e. industrial injuries.

**10.** [LO18.2] Codes are updated and new ICD-9 manuals are available
   a. every 6 months.
   b. every year.
   c. as needed when new codes are developed.
   d. every 2 years.
   e. every 10 years.

**11.** [LO18.2] ICD-9-CM codes are made up of
   a. 1–3 digits.
   b. 2–4 digits.
   c. 3–5 digits.
   d. 2–6 digits.
   e. 5–8 digits.

**12.** **[LO18.3]** When choosing an ICD-9 code, you would need to have
   a. a ledger card.
   b. an encounter form.
   c. a remittance advice.
   d. a superbill.
   e. Answer (b) or (d).

**13.** **[LO18.2]** NOS, NEC, brackets, and parentheses are examples of
   a. abbreviations.
   b. exclusions.
   c. conventions.
   d. encounter terms.
   e. None of the above.

**14.** **[LO18.3]** To find an ICD-9 code for a patient with the diagnosis gastroesophageal reflux disease, you would look in Chapter _____ of the ICD-9-CM.
   a. 2
   b. 3
   c. 9
   d. 10
   e. 12

**15.** **[LO18.3]** Which of the following statements is true concerning M codes?
   a. M codes are found in the Tabular List.
   b. Parentheses are used around M codes.
   c. Neoplasms are coded using M codes.
   d. M codes are found in the CPT manual.
   e. Answers (b) and (c).

**16.** **[LO18.3]** When you code malignant neoplasms, the primary site is
   a. the location where the cancer originated.
   b. the area where the cancer has spread.
   c. the place where chemotherapy drugs are injected.
   d. the metastatic location of the cancer.
   e. None of the above.

**17.** **[LO18.3]** Appendix B of the ICD-9-CM was officially deleted in 2004. It contained the glossary of
   a. spinal disorders.
   b. mental disorders.
   c. obstetrical conditions.
   d. pediatric congenital disorders.
   e. work-related injuries.

**18.** **[LO18.2]** The abbreviation NEC is used when
   a. there is more than one diagnosis.
   b. the physician does not have a final diagnosis.
   c. a patient has a serious illness.
   d. there is not a code that is specific enough to use.
   e. the physician is a specialist.

**19.** **[LO18.2]** When two codes will be required to completely code a diagnosis, the code will appear with
   a. slanted brackets.
   b. parentheses.
   c. a colon.
   d. no punctuation.
   e. a semicolon.

**20.** **[LO18.2]** When the word "excludes" is found in the ICD-9-CM, it means that
   a. it is a supplementary code.
   b. it is the primary code.

c. the entry is not classified as part of the preceding code.

d. it is a nonessential code.

e. the code is incomplete without another digit.

**21.** **[LO18.2]** When the phrase "code first underlying disease" appears beneath a coded condition, you will

a. not use this code as the first code.

b. use the primary diagnosis code first.

c. use this code as the first code.

d. place the primary code after this code.

e. Answers (a) and (b).

**22.** **[LO18.2]** Which of the following statements accurately describes the use of conventions found in the tabular index?

a. Italicization is used for all exclusion notes.

b. Boldface is used for all codes and titles in the tabular index.

c. "Use additional code" means you will list the primary code as the second code.

d. A colon is used to separate primary and secondary codes.

e. Answers (a) and (b).

**23.** **[LO18.4]** A patient who is seen at your clinic to receive a flu shot will have the insurance claim coded using a(n) _____ code.

a. E

b. M

c. O

d. V

e. B

**24.** **[LO18.4]** Which of the following would *not* be coded using a V code?

a. Blood pressure exam

b. Poisoning

c. Colonoscopy

d. Immunization

e. Pap smear

**25.** **[LO18.2]** Chapter 17 of the Tabular List classifies

a. injuries and poisoning.

b. female disorders.

c. metastatic conditions.

d. pregnancy complications.

e. mental disorders.

## True or False

Decide whether each statement is true or false. In the space at the left, write "T" for true or "F" for false. On the lines provided, rewrite the false statements to make them true.

_____ **1.** **[LO18.2]** The ICD-9-CM has two parts, Volume 1, the Alphabetic Index, and Volume 2, the Tabular List.

_____

_____ **2.** **[LO18.2]** The Alphabetic Index is organized by the condition, not by the body part in which the condition occurs.

_____

_____ **3.** [LO18.2] The Tabular List includes 17 chapters and supplementary V and E codes.

_____

_____ **4.** [LO18.4] V codes are used to identify encounters such as illness or injury.

_____

_____ **5.** [LO18.5] Transitioning to ICD-10-CM will be easier because the codes will be simpler to understand.

_____

_____ **6.** [LO18.1] One of the purposes of the ICD-9-CM is to study health-care costs.

_____

_____ **7.** [LO18.3] When you code neoplasms, the secondary site is the area where the cancer originated.

_____

_____ **8.** [LO18.3] Appendix D lists the Classification of Industrial Accidents According to Agency, and the codes are listed on all insurance forms.

_____

_____ **9.** [LO18.2] Most of the NOS codes end with the number 9.

_____

_____ **10.** [LO18.2] The brace symbol, }, is used to enclose a series of terms.

_____

## Sentence Completion

In the space provided, write the word or phrase that best completes each sentence.

**1.** [LO18.3] The physician establishes a _____ that describes the primary condition for which a patient is receiving care.

**2.** [LO18.3] The Alphabetic Index is _____ used alone because it does not contain all the information.

**3.** [LO18.2] If the diagnostic statement is "The patient presents with blindness," the main term _____ is located in the Alphabetic Index.

**4.** [LO18.3] The diseases, conditions, and injuries in the Tabular List are organized into chapters according to the _____ or _____ _____.

**1.** _____

_____

**2.** _____

_____

**3.** _____

_____

**4.** _____

_____

5. **[LO18.4]** Insurance carriers, such as _____, do not cover V codes.

6. **[LO18.5]** PCS is used only in the _____ _____ setting by those reporting ICD-9-CM procedure codes.

7. **[LO18.5]** Because of the flexibility and _____ of the ICD-10-CM coding system, it is possible to provide more _____ in the coding of many conditions.

8. **[LO18.1]** The ICD-9-CM was originally created for the classification of patient _____, which means sickness and _____ or death statistics.

9. **[LO18.3]** Appendix E of the ICD-9-CM consists of a listing of the _____ _____ Categories used.

10. **[LO18.2]** Parentheses are used around descriptions in the Alphabetic Index that do not affect the code, that is, _____ or supplementary terms.

5. _____
_____

6. _____
_____

7. _____
_____

8. _____
_____

9. _____
_____

10. _____
_____

# Apply Your Knowledge

## Short Answer

Write the answer to each question on the lines provided.

1. **[LO18.3]** Explain the three- to five-digit code structure used in determining an ICD-9-CM coding system.

_____

_____

_____

2. **[LO18.5]** Why is there a mandate to transition from the ICD-9-CM manual to the ICD-10-CM?

_____

_____

_____

3. **[LO18.1]** List six reasons for the use of the ICD-9 codes.

_____

_____

_____

**4.** [LO18.1] Explain the difference between the use of the abbreviations NOS and NEC.

_____

_____

_____

**5.** [LO18.3] What is the difference between an acute and a chronic condition or illness?

_____

_____

_____

## Problem-Solving Activities

Follow the directions for each activity.

**1.** [LO18.3] ICD-9-CM Coding Exercise
 a. Using an ICD-9 coding manual, locate the appropriate diagnosis codes for the following diseases or conditions.

| DIAGNOSIS/CONDITION | ICD-9 DIAGNOSIS CODE |
|---|---|
| Diabetes with unspecified complication | |
| Stress fracture of the tibia | |
| Burn, first degree, forearm | |
| Corneal abrasion not due to contact lenses | |
| Cellulitis of the right knee | |
| Neuralgia of sciatic nerve | |
| Uncomplicated senile dementia | |
| Acute vein thrombosis of the calf | |
| Mild dysplasia of the cervix | |
| Genital herpes, unspecified | |
| Frostbite of the foot | |
| Sprain of elbow at the radiohumeral joint | |
| First-degree sunburn | |
| Acute cholecystitis with gallstones in ducts | |
| Acute, benign pericarditis, idiopathic | |
| Bell's palsy | |
| Poisoning (hypersensitivity) by penicillin | |
| Breech delivery, buttocks presentation | |
| Group B Streptococcus Pneumonia | |

# Thinking Critically

Write your response to each case study question on the lines provided.

## Case 1 [LO18.3]

Henry Warner is an established patient at Dr. Frazier's office. He has a longtime history of COPD. The physician has been treating Henry with bronchodilator therapy, oxygen, and steroids when weather changes cause Henry's breathing to worsen. Today Henry has an appointment to see the doctor because of weakness, a nonproductive cough, and an elevated temperature. Upon examination, the physician determines that Henry has an upper respiratory infection. He orders a CBC (complete blood count), chest x-ray and pulse oximetry. These examinations and laboratory tests are performed in the clinic.

**1.** What conditions should be coded for this patient? What are the codes and where do you locate them?

_____

_____

_____

**2.** What procedures should be coded for this office visit? What are the codes and where do you locate them?

_____

_____

_____

## Case 2 [LO18.3]

Annette is a new employee at the Frazier Medical Clinic. During her first week of her employment she is asked to do the insurance processing for claims submission. Although she was trained in her schooling how to do coding, Annette is not sure of her coding skills but accepts the task without saying anything to her supervisor. Later in the day she is noticeably struggling, trying to find the proper codes to complete some of the insurance forms. You approach Annette to offer help, and she says, "It's all right, I'm doing fine." Hearing that, you walk away and continue with your tasks.

**1.** Knowing that she was not confident with her skills, how could Annette have handled the situation when her supervisor asked her to do the insurance processing tasks?

_____

_____

_____

**2.** When Annette refused any assistance from you with the coding, is there anything else you could have done to assist with the problem?

_____

_____

_____

## Case 3 [LO18.3]

Sally Schmidt arrived at your office seeking urgent care for a laceration on her hand. While she was washing dishes, a drinking glass broke and she cut her hand in the fleshy area between the thumb and index finger. When she returns to the reception desk to check out, the encounter form states that she received sutures for a 3 cm laceration. Later that day you are coding the insurance form for Sally and retrieve her medical record. The physician entry for today's visit indicates that she received sutures for a 1.5 cm laceration.

1. What action should you take to properly code this claim?

_____

_____

_____

2. Why is it critical to verify medical information prior to coding an insurance claim?

_____

_____

_____

# Demonstrate Your Knowledge

**Student Name:** _____

## Procedure 18–1: Locating an ICD-9-CM Code

**GOAL:** To analyze diagnoses and locate the correct ICD-9 code

**MATERIALS:** Patient record, charge slip or superbill, ICD-9-CM

**METHOD:** To pass this procedure the minimum required score is _____ % or all elements must meet "satisfactory" ability on the final demonstration. The first box may be used as a practice or final demonstration, with the evaluator placing **S for Satisfactory** or **U for Unsatisfactory** if that is the grading criteria. The second box may be used as a final demonstration with a **grade point** written in the box.

| STEPS | POSSIBLE POINTS | S/U | POINTS EARNED |
|---|---|---|---|
| 1. Locate the patient's diagnosis.<br>  a. This information may be located on the superbill (encounter form) or elsewhere in the patient's chart. If it is on the superbill, verify documentation in the medical chart. | 20 | | |
| 2. Find the diagnosis in the ICD-9 Alphabetic Index. Look for the condition first, then locate the indented subterms that make the condition more specific. Read all cross-references to check all the possibilities for a term, including its synonyms and any eponyms. | 20 | | |
| 3. Locate the code from the Alphabetic Index in the ICD-9 Tabular List. | 20 | | |
| 4. Read all information to find the code that corresponds to the patient's specific disease or condition.<br>  a. Study the list of codes and descriptions. Be sure to pick the most specific code available. Check for the symbol that shows that 4th (and) 5th digits may be required. | 20 | | |
| 5. Carefully record the diagnosis code(s) on the insurance claim and proofread the numbers.<br>  a. Be sure that all necessary codes are given to completely describe each diagnosis. Check for instructions stating an additional code is needed. If more than one code is needed, be sure instructions are followed and the codes are listed in the correct order. | 20 | | |
| **Total Points (if applicable)** | 100 | | |

**Comments:** _____

_____

_____

**Final Evaluator's Signature:** _____

**Date:** _____

## CAAHEP Competencies Achieved

VIII. C (3) Describe how to use the most current diagnostic coding classification system

VIII. P (2) Perform diagnostic coding

VIII. A (1) Work with the physician to achieve the maximum reimbursement

## ABHES Competencies Achieved

8. t. Perform diagnostic and procedural coding

## Procedure 18–2: Locating a V Code

**GOAL:** To analyze the patient record (or encounter form) and decide whether a V code is an appropriate diagnosis code

**MATERIALS:** Patient record, superbill or encounter form, ICD-9-CM

**METHOD:** To pass this procedure the minimum required score is _____% or all elements must meet "satisfactory" ability on the final demonstration. The first box may be used as a practice or final demonstration, with the evaluator placing **S for Satisfactory** or **U for Unsatisfactory** if that is the grading criteria. The second box may be used as a final demonstration with a **grade point** written in the box.

| STEPS | POSSIBLE POINTS | S/U | POINTS EARNED |
|---|---|---|---|
| 1. Locate the patient's diagnosis. This information may be located on the superbill (encounter form) or elsewhere in the patient's chart. If it is on the superbill, verify documentation in the medical chart. | 20 | | |
| 2. If the reason for the patient encounter relates to a physician exam, immunization, well child visit, or other visit where there is no diagnosis or condition of illness found, a V code will be used to code the reason for the visit (diagnosis). | 0 | | |
| 3. Find the diagnosis in the ICD-9 Alphabetic Index. Look for the condition first, and then locate any indented subterms that make the condition more specific. Read all cross-references. | 20 | | |
| 4. Locate the code from the Alphabetic Index in the V code area of the ICD-9 Tabular List. | 20 | | |
| 5. Read all descriptive information to find the code that corresponds to the patient's specific reason for today's visit. Be sure to pick the most specific code available. Check for the symbol that shows that a fourth and possibly a fifth digit is required. | 20 | | |
| 6. Carefully record the diagnosis code(s) on the insurance claim and proofread the numbers. Be sure that no other codes are required to describe the patient's reason for the visit. Check for instructions stating an additional code is needed. If more than one code is needed, be sure instructions are followed and the codes are listed in the correct order. | 20 | | |
| **Total Points (if applicable)** | 100 | | |

**Comments:** _____

_____

_____

**Final Evaluator's Signature:** _____

**Date:** _____

### CAAHEP Competencies Achieved

VIII. C (3) Describe how to use the most current diagnostic coding classification system

VIII. P (2) Perform diagnostic coding

VIII. A (1) Work with the physician to achieve the maximum reimbursement

### ABHES Competencies Achieved

8. t. Perform diagnostic and procedural coding

**Student Name:** _____

## Procedure 18–3: Locating an E Code

**GOAL:** To analyze the patient record (or encounter form) and decide whether an E code is necessary to completely code the encounter

**MATERIALS:** Patient record, superbill or encounter form, ICD-9-CM

**METHOD:** To pass this procedure the minimum required score is _____% or all elements must meet "satisfactory" ability on the final demonstration. The first box may be used as a practice or final demonstration, with the evaluator placing **S for Satisfactory** or **U for Unsatisfactory** if that is the grading criteria. The second box may be used as a final demonstration with a **grade point** written in the box.

| STEPS | POSSIBLE POINTS | S/U | POINTS EARNED |
|---|---|---|---|
| 1. Locate the patient's diagnosis. This information may be located on the superbill (encounter form) or elsewhere in the patient's chart. If it is on the superbill, verify documentation in the medical chart. | 20 | | |
| 2. If the patient's diagnosis begs the question, "How did that happen?", an E code is required to give the insurance carrier as much information as possible. | 0 | | |
| 3. After coding the diagnosis of the condition requiring treatment, open the ICD-9 to the external cause Alphabetic Index or, if necessary, use the Table of Drugs and Chemicals. Find the appropriate description in the ICD-9 Alphabetic Index, looking for the condition first, and then locate any indented subterms that make the condition more specific. Read all cross-references. | 20 | | |
| 4. Locate the code from the Alphabetic Index in the E code area of the ICD-9 Tabular List. | 20 | | |
| 5. Read all descriptive information to find the code that corresponds to how the patient's current condition came about. Be sure to pick the most specific code available. Check for the symbol that shows that a fourth and possibly a fifth digit is required; many E codes require these. | 20 | | |
| 6. Carefully record the diagnosis code(s) on the insurance claim and proofread the numbers. E codes are always secondary, so be sure that the primary diagnosis code is listed first. Check for instructions stating an additional code is needed. If more than one code is needed, be sure instructions are followed and the codes are listed in the correct order. | 20 | | |
| **Total Points (if applicable)** | 100 | | |

**Comments:** _____

_____

_____

**Final Evaluator's Signature:** _____

**Date:** _____

## CAAHEP Competencies Achieved

VIII. C (3) Describe how to use the most current diagnostic coding classification system

VIII. P (2) Perform diagnostic coding

VIII. A (1) Work with the physician to achieve the maximum reimbursement

## ABHES Competencies Achieved

8. t. Perform diagnostic and procedural coding

## Test Your Knowledge

### Vocabulary Review

Match the key terms in the right column with the definitions in the left column by placing the letter of each correct answer in the space provided.

_____ **1.** causes and severity of illnesses

_____ **2.** within the Alphabetic Index, subdivisions of the ICD-10 chapters containing a clinical description of the code range and the guidelines for coding; within the tabular index, codes consisting of four or five characters specifying the level of complexity of the diagnosis

_____ **3.** the cause of disease or condition

_____ **4.** the 3-digit code subdivisions of ICD-10

_____ **5.** a specialized agency of the United Nations (UN) that acts as a coordinating authority on international public health

_____ **6.** *International Classification of Diseases, Tenth Revision, Clinical Modification*

_____ **7.** divisions of ICD-10 named either for a body system or specific disease type

_____ **8.** causes of death

**a.** categories [LO19.2]

**b.** chapters [LO19.2]

**c.** etiology [LO19.2]

**d.** ICD-10-CM [LO19.1]

**e.** morbidity [LO19.2]

**f.** mortality [LO19.2]

**g.** subcategories [LO19.2]

**h.** World Health Organization (WHO) [LO19.1]

# Multiple-Choice Certification Questions

There may be more than one answer; circle the letter of the choice that best completes each statement or answers each question.

1. **[LO19.1]** The ICD-10-CM is published via the Internet by separate agencies, which are the
   a. NCHS and CDC.
   b. CDC and CMS.
   c. FDC and CMS.
   d. NCHS and CMS.
   e. FDC and NCHS.

2. **[LO19.2]** The first step in the procedure to locate the appropriate code in the ICD-10 is to
   a. identify the expanded diagnosis phrase.
   b. identify the main term in the Alphabetic Index.
   c. locate the main term in the Tabular List.
   d. determine if there is a secondary diagnosis.
   e. None of the above.

3. **[LO19.2]** Which of the following statements is *true* concerning the "x" character used in the ICD-10 coding?
   a. The "x" means that a shorter code must be used.
   b. The "x" is used as a placeholder for future expansion of the subcategory.
   c. The "x" is used for a nonexistent digit when a sixth or seventh digit is required for code specificity.
   d. The "x" is always used in the fifth digit place.
   e. Answers (b) and (c).

4. **[LO19.1, 19.2]** In the Alphabetic Index, brackets within a code are used
   a. to indicate manifestation (secondary) codes.
   b. to enclose supplementary words.
   c. to enclose modifiers.
   d. if an exclusion exists.
   e. None of the above.

5. **[LO19.2]** "Excludes1" is a note that indicates
   a. codes that are always attached together.
   b. codes that cannot appear together.
   c. the patient's condition must be congenital.
   d. the patient's condition is an acquired one.
   e. the patient's condition is neither acquired nor congenital.

6. **[LO19.1]** Which of the following statements represents a feature of the ICD-10?
   a. V codes are still included in the ICD-10.
   b. There are less than 45,000 codes in the ICD-10.
   c. The format of the ICD-10 codes includes 3–7 characters.
   d. E codes will be used in the ICD-10 version the same as in the ICD-9.
   e. None of the above.

7. **[LO19.2]** When you apply the guidelines for laterality codes, right and left would be coded using
   a. R = right and L = left.
   b. 0 = right and 1 = left.
   c. 1 = right and 2 = left.
   d. D = right (*dextro*-) and S = left (*sinistro*-).
   e. Answers (b) or (d).

8. **[LO19.3]** Which of the following code ranges would be used when a person may or may not be sick but has an encounter for medical services?
   a. A00–B99
   b. F00–F99

c. P00–P96
d. R00–R99
e. Z00–Z99

9. **[LO19.3]** A patient who is being treated for diabetes mellitus would typically have codes related to Chapter
   a. 2.
   b. 3.
   c. 4.
   d. 5.
   e. 6.

10. **[LO19.2]** When coding a pregnancy with multiple gestations, which coding digit is used to specify the number of fetuses in utero?
    a. Fourth
    b. Fifth
    c. Seventh
    d. Eighth
    e. None of the above.

11. **[LO19.2]** In Chapter 19 of the ICD-10, the letters A, D, and S are referred to as
    a. extensions.
    b. subcategories.
    c. categories.
    d. etiologies.
    e. diagnoses.

12. **[LO19.2]** A patient who sustained an injury from being burned with battery acid would have codes from code range
    a. V01–Y98.
    b. S00–T98.
    c. M00–M99.
    d. H60–H95.
    e. E00–E90.

13. **[LO19.1]** The Z codes found in the ICD-10 are similar to the _____ codes that are in the ICD-9-CM.
    a. C
    b. D
    c. E
    d. M
    e. V

14. **[LO19.2]** An infant born with spina bifida would have diagnostic codes from Chapter
    a. 17.
    b. 16.
    c. 15.
    d. 14.
    e. 13.

15. **[LO19.2]** A patient who is diagnosed with an adenoma would require diagnostic codes from Chapter
    a. 5.
    b. 4.
    c. 3.
    d. 2.
    e. 1.

16. **[LO19.5]** Which of the following would not be a consideration when planning for the implementation of the ICD-10?
    a. Updating the encounter forms
    b. Recoding the billing system
    c. Accommodating the needs of the practice
    d. Writing new procedures
    e. Ensuring compliance by October 1, 2018

17. **[LO19.2]** Hypertension is a disease that is coded using codes found in Chapter
    a. 9.
    b. 8.
    c. 7.
    d. 6.
    e. 5.

18. **[LO19.2]** The code T36 is used to code
    a. diabetes mellitus due to an underlying condition with hyperosmolarity.
    b. influenza due to H1N1 influenza virus.
    c. age-related osteoporosis with current pathological fracture.
    d. influenza due to identified avian influenza virus with other manifestations.
    e. poisoning by, adverse effect of and underdosing of systemic antibiotics.

19. **[LO19.2]** When a provider has not given enough information to choose a more specific code, the convention used is
    a. CMRS.
    b. ADQ.
    c. Z00–Z99.
    d. NEC.
    e. NOS.

20. **[LO19.2]** The note "Excludes2" indicates that
    a. the condition is excluded as not part of the condition represented by the code.
    b. one code is used for more than one condition.
    c. a separate code is used for all related conditions.
    d. codes cannot appear together.
    e. if the patient has more than two conditions, additional codes are not necessary.

21. **[LO19.3]** Which of the following codes relates to a patient with diabetes mellitus and an underlying condition?
    a. M80–M90
    b. J09–J10
    c. S00–S10
    d. E08–E13
    e. R65–R68

22. **[LO19.2]** When a patient has an abnormal clinical or laboratory finding involving the kidneys and it is unassociated with the patient's diagnosis, codes would be found in Chapter
    a. 16.
    b. 17.
    c. 18.
    d. 19.
    e. 20.

23. **[LO19.2]** A patient with a psychological disorder such as bipolar or manic depression would have codes found in Chapter
    a. 1.
    b. 2.
    c. 3.
    d. 4.
    e. 5.

**24.** [LO19.2] Burns are classified by the extent of the burn based on the
   a. agent that caused the burn.
   b. treatment required.
   c. location of the burn on the body.
   d. rule of nines.
   e. code of burns.

**25.** [LO19.2] A patient diagnosed with a malignant tumor would have codes associated with code range
   a. C00–D48.
   b. E00–E90.
   c. O00–O99.
   d. R00–R99.
   e. U00–U99.

## True or False

Decide whether each statement is true or false. In the space at the left, write "T" for true or "F" for false. On the lines provided, rewrite the false statements to make them true.

_____ **1.** [LO19.2] The statement "Excludes1" means that you should always use the code listed above the Exclude1 note.

_____

_____ **2.** [LO19.1] One purpose for the ICD-10 is to provide decreased specificity of diagnostic codes.

_____

_____ **3.** [LO19.2] Primary codes must relate to the systemic disorder or underlying condition causing the secondary problem.

_____

_____ **4.** [LO19.1] Many other countries in the world have adopted at least some version of the ICD-10-CM.

_____

_____ **5.** [LO19.2] To accurately code a diagnosis, the coder must first obtain a copy of the patient's billing information.

_____

_____ **6.** [LO19.1] The abbreviations NEC and NOS are no longer used in the ICD-10-CM.

_____

_____ **7.** [LO19.2] Parentheses are used to enclose supplemental or nonessential information that will not affect the code selection.

_____

_____ **8.** [LO19.2] When you code for HIV positivity, it is adequate for the provider to only state "known HIV" or "positive HIV."

_____

_____ **9.** [LO19.2] A patient who has an elevated blood pressure should always have a diagnosis code for hypertension.

_____

_____**10.** [LO19.2] The neoplasm table includes neoplasms listed by anatomical location.

_____

## Sentence Completion

In the space provided, write the word or phrase that best completes each sentence.

**1.** [LO19.2] To accurately code a diagnosis, the coder must first obtain a(n) _____ _____ description from the medical record.

**2.** [LO19.2] _____ are used in the Alphabetic Index and indicate manifestation (secondary) codes.

**3.** [LO19.2] Burns are classified by depth of the burn and are classified as _____ degree, _____ degree, or _____ degree.

**4.** [LO19.3] Codes in Chapter 20 identify _____, _____, _____, and _____ an accident or injury occurred.

**5.** [LO19.3] Chapter 19 includes three extensions, which are the _____ encounter, extension A; the _____ encounter, extension D; and the _____ encounter, extension S.

**6.** [LO19.2] A category has _____ characters and a subcategory has _____-_____ characters.

**7.** [LO19.3] The codes within Chapter 20 are used for data in determining _____ and _____ strategies for injuries.

**8.** [LO19.5] The first step toward implementing the new coding system is identifying the _____ _____ within your practice.

**9.** [LO19.2] In the ICD-10, instead of a separate section, external causes are included as _____-_____ codes.

**10.** [LO19.1] The ICD-10 uses a(n) _____ to hold a place for future expansion of the code's specificity.

1. _____
   _____

2. _____
   _____

3. _____
   _____

4. _____
   _____

5. _____
   _____

6. _____
   _____

7. _____
   _____

8. _____
   _____

9. _____
   _____

10. _____
    _____

# Apply Your Knowledge

## Short Answer

Write the answer to each question on the lines provided.

1. **[LO19.1, 19.2]** What is the difference between the Alphabetic Index and the Tabular List?

_____

_____

_____

2. **[LO19.1]** Explain the difference between a category and a subcategory. Be specific.

_____

_____

_____

3. **[LO19.3]** What is a combination code and when is it used?

_____

_____

_____

4. **[LO19.3]** Explain what laterality codes are and when they are used.

_____

_____

_____

5. **[LO19.5]** List six items a medical practice should consider when planning for the transition from the ICD-9-CM to the ICD-10-CM.

_____

_____

_____

## Problem-Solving Activities

Follow the directions for each activity.

1. **[LO19.5]** Transitioning from ICD-9-CM to ICD-10-CM
   a. You have been asked by your physician to make a presentation to the office staff about the office's transition from using the ICD-9-CM to the ICD-10-CM. You are asked to make this presentation in a training session that will last not more than 1 hour.
   b. Using PowerPoint software, develop a presentation that will introduce the employees to the basic differences between the two versions of the ICD coding process. You should plan to use between 15–20 slides.
   c. Access information for this project on the Internet utilizing information from Web sites including www.ahima.org or www.aapc.com.

2. **[LO19.1]** What is the World Health Organization (WHO)?
   a. Write a two-page document that describes what the World Health Organization (WHO) is and how it is involved with the ICD-10-CM coding system. Access information about the WHO at the Web site www.who.int.
   b. Within your document, provide information about how the WHO uses the information from the data it receives from ICD coding.

## Thinking Critically

Write your response to each case study question on the lines provided.

### Case 1 [LO19.5]

Mary Stevens, the practice manager, just attended a seminar on the new ICD-10-CM. She arrives back to the clinic and seems very anxious to start the transition process for the employees. She talks nonstop about the seminar and how great it was to learn about the new ICD-10 and how it will be used. Two of your co-workers don't seem to be as eager about the change that will need to take place. In the employee break room, you overhear them talking about how much work it will be to change and how they don't want to be a part of it.

1. Why is it important for the entire office staff to embrace the change from the ICD-9-CM to the ICD-10-CM?

   _____

   _____

   _____

2. What kind of interaction or encouragement can you provide to the co-workers?

   _____

   _____

   _____

### Case 2 [LO19.5]

The office where you are employed has decided to convert to electronic health records and prepare for the transition from the ICD-9 to the ICD-10. The staff seems overwhelmed with all the change, and they question whether they will be able to do this. As patients come into the office, some staff members are sharing their concerns with the patients in a complaining manner. There are comments being made to some patients as they check in, like "They are asking us to do too much change at one time" and "We will probably make so many mistakes." All these comments are quite concerning to you.

**1.** Why is it important not to involve patients in the operations or the affairs of an office?

_____

_____

_____

**2.** What actions will make an easier transition for both of these major projects?

_____

_____

_____

## Case 3 [LO19.5]

There are six administrative medical assistants employed at your medical office. All but two of them are nationally certified. The certified assistants also participate frequently in seminars and continuing education sessions. The seminars include topics such as new office technology, electronic health records management, and updates on HIPAA guidelines and mandates. The two uncertified assistants don't understand why anyone would want to volunteer their personal time to go to these meetings and think they are a waste of time.

**1.** Why is it important to become certified in a profession?

_____

_____

_____

**2.** What are the benefits of attending seminars?

_____

_____

_____

# Demonstrate Your Knowledge

**Student Name:** _____

## Procedure 19–1: Coding from the ICD-10

**GOAL:** To analyze diagnoses and locate the correct ICD-10 code

**MATERIALS:** Patient record; charge slip or superbill; access to ICD-10-CM codes on the CMS Web site, www.cms.hhs.gov/ICD10/01_Overview.asp, or access to a draft copy of 2010 ICD-10-CM manual (*Note:* A superbill is available at the end of this study guide.)

**METHOD:** To pass this procedure the minimum required score is _____ % or all elements must meet "satisfactory" ability on the final demonstration. The first box may be used as a practice or final demonstration, with the evaluator placing **S for Satisfactory** or **U for Unsatisfactory** if that is the grading criteria. The second box may be used as a final demonstration with a **grade point** written in the box.

| STEPS | POSSIBLE POINTS | S/U | POINTS EARNED |
|---|---|---|---|
| 1. Locate the patient's diagnosis. This information may be located on the superbill (encounter form) or elsewhere in the patient's chart. If it is on the superbill, verify documentation in the medical chart. | 20 | | |
| 2. Find the diagnosis in the ICD-10 Alphabetic Index. Look for the condition first, then locate the indented subterms that make the condition more specific. Read all cross-references to check all the possibilities for a term, including its synonyms and any eponyms. | 20 | | |
| 3. Following the directions in the alpha index, locate the code or code range from the Alphabetic Index in the ICD's Tabular List. | 20 | | |
| 4. Read all information and instructions carefully to find the code that exactly corresponds to the patient's specific disease or condition. a. Study the list of codes and descriptions. Be sure to pick the most specific code available. b. Watch for instructions advising of the need for additional codes as well as instructions regarding coding sequence and need for sixth and seventh digits or placeholders. | 20 | | |
| 5. Document the chosen codes carefully, remembering sequencing instructions. | 20 | | |
| **Total Points (if applicable)** | 100 | | |

**Comments:** _____

_____

_____

**Final Evaluator's Signature:** _____

**Date:** _____

## CAAHEP Competencies Achieved

VIII. C (3) Describe how to use the most current diagnostic coding classification system

VIII. P (2) Perform diagnostic coding

VIII. A (1) Work with the physician to achieve the maximum reimbursement

## ABHES Competencies Achieved

8. t. Perform diagnostic and procedural coding

## Test Your Knowledge

### Vocabulary Review

Match the key terms in the right column with the definitions in the left column by placing the letter of each correct answer in the space provided.

_____ **1.** similar care being provided by more than one physician

_____ **2.** A reference with the most commonly used system of procedure codes; the HIPAA required code set for physician procedures

_____ **3.** the period of time after many procedures for follow-up care that is considered included in the payment for that procedure

_____ **4.** One or more two-digit alphanumeric codes assigned in addition to the five-digit CPT code to show that some special circumstance applies to the service or procedure performed by the physician

_____ **5.** any CPT code that includes more than one procedure in its description

_____ **6.** codes that represent medical procedures, such as surgery and diagnostic tests, and medical services, such as an examination to evaluate a patient's condition

_____ **7.** codes used when discussing with the patient and family questions or concerns regarding one or more of the following: diagnostic results and

**a.** add-on code **[LO20.5]**

**b.** bundled code **[LO20.2]**

**c.** code linkage **[LO20.7]**

**d.** concurrent care **[LO20.5]**

**e.** consultation **[LO20.5]**

**f.** counseling **[LO20.5]**

**g.** critical care **[LO20.5]**

**h.** Current Procedural Terminology (CPT) **[LO20.1]**

**i.** downcoding **[LO20.2]**

**j.** E/M (evaluation/management) code **[LO20.3]**

**k.** established patient **[LO20.5]**

**l.** global period **[LO20.2]**

**m.** HCPCS (Healthcare Common Procedural Coding System) Level II codes **[LO20.6]**

**n.** modifier **[LO20.5]**

**o.** new patient **[LO20.5]**

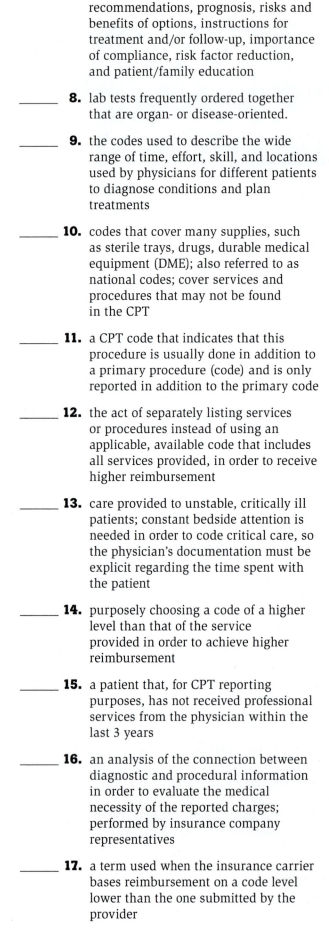

recommendations, prognosis, risks and benefits of options, instructions for treatment and/or follow-up, importance of compliance, risk factor reduction, and patient/family education

_____ **8.** lab tests frequently ordered together that are organ- or disease-oriented.

_____ **9.** the codes used to describe the wide range of time, effort, skill, and locations used by physicians for different patients to diagnose conditions and plan treatments

_____ **10.** codes that cover many supplies, such as sterile trays, drugs, durable medical equipment (DME); also referred to as national codes; cover services and procedures that may not be found in the CPT

_____ **11.** a CPT code that indicates that this procedure is usually done in addition to a primary procedure (code) and is only reported in addition to the primary code

_____ **12.** the act of separately listing services or procedures instead of using an applicable, available code that includes all services provided, in order to receive higher reimbursement

_____ **13.** care provided to unstable, critically ill patients; constant bedside attention is needed in order to code critical care, so the physician's documentation must be explicit regarding the time spent with the patient

_____ **14.** purposely choosing a code of a higher level than that of the service provided in order to achieve higher reimbursement

_____ **15.** a patient that, for CPT reporting purposes, has not received professional services from the physician within the last 3 years

_____ **16.** an analysis of the connection between diagnostic and procedural information in order to evaluate the medical necessity of the reported charges; performed by insurance company representatives

_____ **17.** a term used when the insurance carrier bases reimbursement on a code level lower than the one submitted by the provider

**p.** panel [LO20.5]

**q.** procedure code [LO20.5]

**r.** unbundling [LO20.2]

**s.** upcoding [LO20.7]

_____ **18.** care provided at the request of other
health-care providers

_____ **19.** a patient who has been seen by the
physician within the last 3 years;
important determination when using
E/M codes

## Multiple-Choice Certification Questions

There may be more than one answer; circle the letter of the choice that best completes each statement or answers each question.

**1.** **[LO20.1]** The organization that publishes the *Current Procedural Terminology* reference manual is
a. HIPAA.
b. AMA.
c. AAMA.
d. WHO.
e. CMS.

**2.** **[LO20.2]** The maximum composition of a CPT code is five CPT code numbers plus
a. 1 two-digit modifier.
b. 2 two-digit modifiers.
c. 3 two-digit modifiers.
d. 2 three-digit modifiers.
e. 3 three-digit modifiers.

**3.** **[LO20.2]** When a medical facility uses published superbills or encounter forms with the CPT codes already on them for procedures, it is important to update the forms with the new codes when they are available in
a. January.
b. March.
c. June.
d. September.
e. December.

**4.** **[LO20.6]** HCPCS Level II codes are also called
a. modifiers.
b. national codes.
c. professional codes.
d. AMA codes.
e. DME codes.

**5.** **[LO20.6]** HCPCS Level I codes are also known as
a. E/M codes.
b. national codes.
c. AMA codes.
d. modifiers.
e. CPT codes.

**6.** **[LO20.2]** Health-care claims must comply with rules imposed by
a. federal law.
b. state law.
c. payer requirements.
d. insurance carrier requirements.
e. All of the above.

7. **[LO20.5]** Which of the following would *not* be a possible result of an inaccurately coded claim?
   a. Denied claim
   b. Reduced payment
   c. Loss of hospital privileges
   d. Fines and other sanctions
   e. None of the above.

8. **[LO20.7]** To avoid the risk of fraud, medical offices should have
   a. an encounter form.
   b. a software program for electronic billing.
   c. a certified administrative medical assistant.
   d. a compliance plan.
   e. Answers (a) and (b).

9. **[LO20.4]** When a surgeon provides and administers general anesthesia, the modifier used with the surgical procedure is
   a. 22.
   b. 23.
   c. 32.
   d. 47.
   e. 50.

10. **[LO20.2]** A red dot next to a CPT code in the manual denotes that this code is
    a. a new code for this edition.
    b. revised from a previous edition.
    c. used when coding vaccines pending approval.
    d. used when moderate sedation was used with the procedure.
    e. being removed this year.

11. **[LO20.7]** Which of the following statements describes the function or result of unbundling?
    a. Codes are broken down into more than one code.
    b. It is used to create higher reimbursement.
    c. It is not allowed as an acceptable practice.
    d. It is used to consolidate more than one coded procedure.
    e. Answers (a), (b), and (c).

12. **[LO20.1]** The range of codes used to code radiology procedures is
    a. 00100–01999.
    b. 10021–69990.
    c. 80048–89356.
    d. 70010–79999.
    e. 99500–99602.

13. **[LO20.7]** A patient recovering from a surgical procedure is now seen by the physician for an unrelated problem. The unrelated problem is billed
    a. bundled with the code for the surgical procedure if it is still within the global period.
    b. separately using a modifier.
    c. at the end of the global period for the surgical procedure.
    d. Applying answers (a) and (c).
    e. Applying answers (b) and (c).

14. **[LO20.2]** When you submit a claim for immunizations
    a. two codes are required, one for the injection and one for the vaccine or toxoid given.
    b. one code is used for both the injection and the vaccine or toxoid given.
    c. an E/M code is required for all submissions.
    d. the vaccine is the only item coded and submitted.
    e. Answers (b) and (c) apply.

15. [LO20.7] Insurance fraud includes practices such as billing
    a. only once for a service.
    b. for procedures that are related to the patient's condition.
    c. separately for services that are bundled in a single procedure code.
    d. for medically necessary procedures.
    e. for a service that was performed.

16. [LO20.5] When a service such as a consult is required by the insurance carrier or a governmental or regulatory agency, the CPT modifier used is called
    a. Unrelated Services.
    b. Mandated Services.
    c. Technical Component.
    d. Professional Component.
    e. Increased Procedural Services.

17. [LO20.5] The subheading area of the CPT coding manual provides the
    a. general section name, such as Surgery.
    b. general body system.
    c. procedures performed.
    d. body area for the body system.
    e. detailed body system.

18. [LO20.2] The # sign is used to
    a. note that codes are out of numeric sequence.
    b. denote that the code is new for the new edition of the CPT manual.
    c. tell the user that the code has been revised.
    d. separate codes in a section.
    e. designate codes that are pending approval.

19. [LO20.5] When a physician meets with a patient and the family to discuss questions or concerns regarding the patient's prognosis, it is coded as
    a. concurrent care.
    b. critical care.
    c. a consultation.
    d. an evaluation.
    e. counseling.

20. [LO20.7] The term "code creep" is also known as
    a. unbundling.
    b. downcoding.
    c. underbilling.
    d. upcoding.
    e. bundling.

21. [LO20.1] The range of codes for the evaluation and management section of the CPT manual is
    a. 99201–99499.
    b. 90281–99199.
    c. 99100–99140.
    d. 99500–99602.
    e. 99602–99800.

22. [LO20.2] Which of the following is used to determine the level of E/M code that is used?
    a. The age of the patient
    b. The specific insurance carrier the patient uses
    c. The extent of the examination that the physician conducted
    d. The level of medication the physician prescribes for the patient
    e. The geographic location of the medical practice

**23.** [LO20.6] Which of the following would *not* be coded using the HCPCS Level II codes?
   a. Durable medical equipment
   b. Procedures performed by the physician
   c. Emergency transport services
   d. Drugs and injections
   e. Routine venipuncture and Pap smear

**24.** [LO20.3] Which of the following is *not* a subcategory title used as a type of E/M code?
   a. Hospital Inpatient Services
   b. Consultations
   c. Office/Other Outpatient Services
   d. OB/GYN Services
   e. Critical Care Services

**25.** [LO20.3] Which of the following elements are included when coding using the problem-focused level of service?
   a. CC and HPI
   b. CC and ROS
   c. HPI and PFSH
   d. ROS and HPI
   e. CC and PFSH

## True or False

Decide whether each statement is true or false. In the space at the left, write "T" for true or "F" for false. On the lines provided, rewrite the false statements to make them true.

_____ **1.** [LO20.2] The CPT manual is updated every 6 months in January and June.

_____

_____ **2.** [LO20.3] E/M codes are often considered the most important of all CPT codes because they can be used by all physicians in any medical specialty.

_____

_____ **3.** [LO20.2] The period of time that is covered for follow-up care is called the entire period of service.

_____

_____ **4.** [LO20.2] To code a laboratory testing panel correctly, the physician must order each test listed within the panel and there must be a need for each of them.

_____

_____ **5.** [LO20.7] Claims fraud occurs when physicians or others falsely represent their services or charges to payers.

_____

_____ **6.** [LO20.4] The modifier 54, surgical care only, means that the surgeon did not provide the pre- or post-op care.

_____

_____ **7.** **[LO20.2]** The blue triangle symbol tells the user that this is a new symbol not used in previous editions of the CPT manual.

_____

_____ **8.** **[LO20.2]** Concurrent care is a term used to describe a situation where a patient is being cared for by one physician who is a specialist.

_____

_____ **9.** **[LO20.3]** The expanded problem-focused level of service includes a review of the past family and/or social history of the patient.

_____

_____ **10.** **[LO20.3]** The most difficult level of E/M code to document is the MDM or medical decision making level.

_____

## Sentence Completion

In the space provided, write the word or phrase that best completes each sentence.

**1.** **[LO20.2]** To make coding processes more efficient, medical offices often list frequently used procedures and their applicable CPT codes on _____.

**2.** **[LO20.2]** HCPCS was developed by the CMS, which stands for _____ for _____ and _____ Services.

**3.** **[LO20.2]** Claims processing must comply with the rules imposed by _____ and _____ law and with _____ requirements.

**4.** **[LO20.7]** When performing a code review or coding audit, the processor needs to ensure that there is a clear and correct link between each _____ and _____.

**5.** **[LO20.7]** Claims fraud occurs when physicians or others falsely represent their _____ or _____ to payers.

**6.** **[LO20.2]** A compliance plan is a process for _____, _____, and _____ illegal medical office practices.

**7.** **[LO20.2]** CPT symbols include triangles pointing toward each other, which indicate _____ or _____ text information.

**1.** _____
_____

**2.** _____
_____

**3.** _____
_____

**4.** _____
_____

**5.** _____
_____

**6.** _____
_____

**7.** _____
_____

**8.** **[LO20.3]** The levels for coding a patient history include _____ focused, _____ _____ focused, _____, and _____.

**9.** **[LO20.7]** When unbundling is done intentionally or repeatedly to receive more payment than is correct, you and the practice can come under investigation for _____.

**10.** **[LO20.3]** The complexity levels of medical decision making (MDM) include, _____-_____ MDM, _____-_____ MDM, and _____-_____ MDM.

**8.** _____
_____

**9.** _____
_____

**10.** _____
_____

# Apply Your Knowledge

## Short Answer

Write the answer to each question on the lines provided.

**1.** **[LO20.7]** Cite seven possible consequences of inaccurate coding and incorrect billing.

_____

_____

_____

**2.** **[LO20.1]** List the six main sections found in the CPT coding manual, in the sequence they are found from the beginning of the manual to the end.

_____

_____

_____

**3.** **[LO20.2]** What are the items needed to properly perform CPT coding?

_____

_____

_____

**4.** **[LO20.7]** When you perform a coding audit, what are the key points to remember to check?

_____

_____

_____

**5.** **[LO20.7]** When a medical office develops a compliance plan, the compliance officer and committee should write the plan with four main objectives. List the four main intended goals of a compliance plan.

_____

_____

_____

## Problem-Solving Activities

Follow the directions for this activity.

**1.** **[LO20.5]** Solving the CPT/ICD Puzzle
   a. For each of the following scenarios, provide the CPT and ICD codes that appropriately apply to the services provided:
   - A new patient is seen for a high school sports physical examination. The physician discovers a heart murmur and orders an electrocardiogram with interpretation, a complete blood count, and a urinalysis.
   - An established patient is seen for a follow-up blood pressure check and to receive a flu shot.
   - An established patient is seen to have an incision and drainage of a Bartholin's gland abscess. A bacterial culture is performed. The patient receives an injection of Penicillin G Procaine, 600,000 units.
   - An established patient is seen in the emergency room following an accidental fall. She has a fractured tibia that requires the application of a short leg cast.
   - An established patient with diabetes is seen by the physician for a 15-minute visit to evaluate her diabetes. The physician orders a glucose test using a monitoring device. The patient also receives a pneumococcal vaccine.

## Thinking Critically

Write your response to each case study question on the lines provided.

### Case 1 [LO20.7]

Mary Ann and Sarah work as administrative medical assistants in an internal medicine practice. Mary Ann has been doing the insurance processing for the clinic for over 2 years. Sarah is newly hired from the externship she completed at this practice. As Mary Ann orients Sarah to the practice coding procedures, Sarah asks many questions about the level of E/M codes used for some of the patient visits that don't appear to be appropriate. Mary Ann tells Sarah to just continue coding the way the office has always done it in the past.

**1.** How should Sarah respond to Mary Ann's request to just do things the way they've always done it?

_____

_____

_____

**2.** Since Sarah is a newly graduated and employed administrative medical assistant, how can she maintain a professional and confident approach in this situation?

_____

_____

_____

## Case 2 [LO20.7]

John is employed as an administrative medical assistant in a general surgical practice clinic. A patient is seen in the office for a postoperative visit following a routine appendectomy 5 days ago. As the patient and his mother approach the reception area, the patient's mother asks why there is a charge of $25.00 to see the surgeon that day.

**1.** How should John respond to the patient's mother?

_____

_____

_____

**2.** What is the potential coding or billing problem surrounding this situation?

_____

_____

_____

## Case 3 [LO20.3]

Karen is the coding specialist for a family practice. The encounter forms are preprinted with the E/M codes for the different levels of care provided. She notices that most of the patients that are seen for basic problems have the encounter form box checked by the physician for detailed level of care. This occurs for many patients who only see the physician for 10–15 minutes.

**1.** Why should Karen be concerned about the physician's choice for the level of care provided to these patients?

_____

_____

_____

**2.** Why is it critical for Karen to discuss this matter with the physician?

_____

_____

_____

# Demonstrate Your Knowledge

**Student Name:** _____

## Procedure 20–1: Locating a CPT Code

**GOAL:** To locate correct CPT codes

**MATERIALS:** Patient record, superbill or charge slip, CPT manual

**METHOD:** To pass this procedure the minimum required score is _____% or all elements must meet "satisfactory" ability on the final demonstration. The first box may be used as a practice or final demonstration, with the evaluator placing **S for Satisfactory** or **U for Unsatisfactory** if that is the grading criteria. The second box may be used as a final demonstration with a **grade point** written in the box.

| STEPS | POSSIBLE POINTS | S/U | POINTS EARNED |
|---|---|---|---|
| 1. Find the services listed on the superbill (if used) and in the patient's record. Check the patient's record to see which services were documented. For E/M procedures, note whether the patient is a new or established patient and then look for clues as to the location of the service, extent of history, examination, and medical decision making that were involved. | 20 | | |
| 2. Look up the procedure code(s) in the alphabetic index of the CPT manual.<br> a. Verify the code number in the numeric index, reading all notes and guidelines for that section. | 10 | | |
| b. If a code range is noted, look up the range and choose the correct code from the range given. If the correct description is not found, start the process again. Use the same process if multiple codes are given, looking each one up in the numeric index until the correct code description is found. | 10 | | |
| 3. Determine appropriate modifiers. Check section guidelines and Appendix A to choose a modifier if needed to explain a situation involving the procedure being coded, such as bilateral procedure, surgical team, or a discontinued procedure. | 20 | | |
| 4. Carefully record the procedure code(s) on the health-care claim, or, if the office is computerized, enter the codes into the office billing system for placement on an electronic health claim form. Usually the primary procedure, the one that is the primary reason for the encounter or visit, is listed first. | 20 | | |

*(Continued)*

| STEPS | POSSIBLE POINTS | S/U | POINTS EARNED |
|---|---|---|---|
| 5. Match each procedure with its corresponding diagnosis. The primary procedure is often (but not always) matched with the primary diagnosis. | 20 | | |
| Total Points (if applicable) | 100 | | |

**Comments:** _____

_____

_____

**Final Evaluator's Signature:** _____

**Date:** _____

## CAAHEP Competencies Achieved

VIII. C (1) Describe how to use the most current procedural coding system

VIII. C (2) Define upcoding and why it should be avoided

VIII. P (1) Perform procedural coding

VIII. A (1) Work with the physician to achieve the maximum reimbursement

## ABHES Competencies Achieved

8. t. Perform diagnostic and procedural coding

Student Name: _____

## Procedure 20–2: Locating a HCPCS Code

**GOAL:** To locate the proper HCPCS code for a service or piece of equipment

**MATERIALS:** HCPCS manual, patient record, charge slip or superbill

**METHOD:** To pass this procedure the minimum required score is _____% or all elements must meet "satisfactory" ability on the final demonstration. The first box may be used as a practice or final demonstration, with the evaluator placing **S for Satisfactory** or **U for Unsatisfactory** if that is the grading criteria. The second box may be used as a final demonstration with a **grade point** written in the box.

| STEPS | POSSIBLE POINTS | S/U | POINTS EARNED |
|---|---|---|---|
| 1. Locate the service, supplies, and equipment requiring a HCPCS code from the encounter form or from the patient's record. If an encounter form is used, verify procedure completions in the medical record. | 20 | | |
| 2. Use the index at the back of the manual to locate the section in which the category of codes is found. | 20 | | |
| 3. Find the code or code range by seeking first the initial letter and then the four-digit number. They are arranged alphabetically and numerically. Make sure you read the description thoroughly and determine the correct code. Do not code from the index. | 20 | | |
| 4. Make sure the code is valid for the type of insurance the patient carries. | 20 | | |
| 5. Enter the correct code(s) on the superbill or encounter form (if necessary) and, if the office uses a computerized billing program, in the patient's computerized record so that it can be used for billing purposes. Otherwise, place the HCPCS code in block 24d of the 1500 claim form for submission to the insurance carrier. Match each HCPCS code with the appropriate diagnosis code to demonstrate medical necessity. | 20 | | |
| **Total Points (if applicable)** | 100 | | |

**Comments:** _____

_____

_____

**Final Evaluator's Signature:** _____

**Date:** _____

## CAAHEP Competencies Achieved

VIII. C (1) Describe how to use the most current procedural coding system

VIII. C (4) Describe how to use the most current HCPCS coding

VIII. P (1) Perform procedural coding

VIII. A (1) Work with the physician to achieve the maximum reimbursement

## ABHES Competencies Achieved

8. t. Perform diagnostic and procedural coding

## Test Your Knowledge

### Vocabulary Review

Match the key terms in the right column with the definitions in the left column by placing the letter of each correct answer in the space provided.

_____ **1.** a statement that shows the cash on hand at the beginning of a period, the income and disbursements made during the period, and the new amount of cash on hand at the end of the period

_____ **2.** this act requires employers to pay a percentage of each employee's income up to a certain dollar amount

_____ **3.** a certificate of guaranteed payment, which may be purchased from a bank, a post office, or some convenience stores

_____ **4.** a person who receives a payment

_____ **5.** a debit to an account

_____ **6.** the legal right to act as the attorney or agent of another person, including handling that person's financial matters

_____ **7.** Social Security and Medicare taxes that are withheld from what is earned by the employee, with the employer matching contributions

_____ **8.** the process of logging charges and receipts in a chronological list each day; used in the single-entry system of bookkeeping

**a.** ABA number [LO21.3]

**b.** bookkeeping [LO21.1]

**c.** cash flow statement [LO21.5]

**d.** cashier's check [LO21.3]

**e.** certified check [LO21.3]

**f.** charge [LO21.2]

**g.** check [LO21.3]

**h.** counter check [LO21.3]

**i.** dependent [LO21.6]

**j.** endorse [LO21.3]

**k.** Federal Insurance Contributions Act (FICA) [LO21.6]

**l.** Federal Unemployment Tax Act (FUTA) [LO21.6]

**m.** gross earnings [LO21.6]

**n.** journalizing [LO21.5]

_____ **9.** a fraction appearing in the upper-right corner of all printed checks that identifies the geographic area and specific bank on which the check is drawn

_____ **10.** take-home pay, calculated by subtracting total deductions from gross earnings

_____ **11.** A comparison of the office's financial records with bank records to ensure that they are consistent and accurate; usually done when the monthly checking account statement is received from the bank

_____ **12.** cash kept on hand in the office for small purchases

_____ **13.** a payer's check written and signed by the payer, which is stamped by the bank, indicating the bank has already drawn money from the payer's account to guarantee that the check will be paid

_____ **14.** an act that governs some states; the resulting taxes are filed along with FUTA taxes

_____ **15.** legally transferable from one person to another

_____ **16.** a person who depends on another person for financial support

_____ **17.** a check made out to one recipient and given in payment to another, as with one made out to a patient rather than the medical practice

_____ **18.** the systematic recording of business transactions

_____ **19.** a person who pays a bill or writes a check

_____ **20.** money withheld from employees' paychecks and held in a separate account that must be used to pay taxes to appropriate government agencies

_____ **21.** a list showing how often an employee is paid, such as weekly, biweekly, or monthly

_____ **22.** a business check with an attached stub, which is kept as a receipt

**o.** limited check **[LO21.3]**

**p.** money order **[LO21.3]**

**q.** negotiable **[LO21.3]**

**r.** net earnings **[LO21.6]**

**s.** patient ledger card **[LO21.1]**

**t.** pay schedule **[LO21.6]**

**u.** payee **[LO21.3]**

**v.** payer **[LO21.3]**

**w.** pegboard system **[LO21.2]**

**x.** petty cash fund **[LO21.8]**

**y.** power of attorney **[LO21.3]**

**z.** Form 941: Employer's Quarterly Federal Tax Return **[LO21.7]**

**aa.** reconciliation **[LO21.3]**

**bb.** State Unemployment Tax Act (SUTA) **[LO21.6]**

**cc.** tax liability **[LO21.7]**

**dd.** third-party check **[LO21.3]**

**ee.** traveler's check **[LO21.3]**

**ff.** voucher check **[LO21.3]**

_____ **23.** a special bank check that allows a depositor to draw funds from his own account only, as when he has forgotten his checkbook

_____ **24.** a form submitted to the IRS every 3 months that summarizes the federal income and employment taxes withheld from employees' paychecks

_____ **25.** to sign or stamp the back of a check with the proper identification of the person or organization to whom the check is made out, to prevent the check from being cashed if it is stolen or lost

_____ **26.** a check purchased and signed at a bank and later signed over to a payee

_____ **27.** the total amount an employee earns before deductions

_____ **28.** a bank check issued by a bank on bank paper and signed by a bank representative; usually purchased by individuals who do not have checking accounts

_____ **29.** a card containing information needed for insurance purposes, including the patient's name, address, telephone number, Social Security number, insurance information, employer's name, and any special billing instructions; also includes the name of the person who is responsible for charges if this is anyone other than the patient

_____ **30.** a bookkeeping system that uses a lightweight board with pegs on which forms can be stacked, allowing each transaction to be entered and recorded on four different bookkeeping forms at once; also called the one-write system

_____ **31.** a check that is void after a certain time limit; commonly used for payroll

_____ **32.** a bank draft or order written by a payer that directs the bank to pay a sum of money on demand to the payee

# Multiple-Choice Certification Questions

There may be more than one answer; circle the letter of the choice that best completes each statement or answers each question.

1. **[LO21.1]** An example of an accounts receivable item is
   a. the monthly lease due on the office space.
   b. the outstanding balance on a patient's ledger card.
   c. the employees' biweekly salary.
   d. the insurance premium for professional liability.
   e. Answers (a), (c), and (d).

2. **[LO21.3]** If a patient's check does not clear, due to nonsufficient funds, the practice should
   a. not allow the patient to be seen by the physician.
   b. abandon the patient by not providing future care.
   c. adjust the account accordingly, adding the amount back to the account.
   d. send a collections letter to the patient.
   e. write off the amount of the check.

3. **[LO21.3]** When a check for payment from a patient is received some time after the patient's visit, the administrative medical assistant should
   a. hold it until the end of the week and do a batch entry of all checks received that week.
   b. deposit it in the bank and wait for it to clear, then post it to the patient's ledger card.
   c. place it with all the other checks received that day and post them the following day after the checks have been deposited.
   d. staple the envelope to the check and hold it until the end of the week.
   e. record it on the patient's ledger card and day sheet on the day received.

4. **[LO21.3]** The ABA number on a check appears
   a. as a fraction in the top-right side of the check.
   b. next to the routing number on the bottom of the check.
   c. below the signature line on the front of the check.
   d. on the back of the check above the endorsement line.
   e. adjacent to the account number on the check.

5. **[LO21.3]** A third-party check
   a. should never be accepted under any circumstances.
   b. is always written to the practice.
   c. can be accepted if it is from the patient's health insurance company.
   d. may be accepted as payment in full on the patient's account.
   e. should be deposited and credited to the patient's account when it clears the bank.

6. **[LO21.3]** Medical practices prefer electronic banking because
   a. it improves productivity.
   b. cash flow is usually increased.
   c. there is improved accuracy in banking records.
   d. Answers (a) and (c) only.
   e. Answers (a), (b), and (c).

7. **[LO21.3]** What is the reconciled ending balance for a checking account with a balance of $1,800.00 on the month-end statement from the bank, $3,200.00 deposited during that month and $600.00 in outstanding checks that have not yet posted to the account?
   a. $600.00
   b. $800.00
   c. $1,000.00
   d. $1,200.00
   e. $1,800.00

**8.** [LO21.3] A patient's beginning account balance is $30.00. The charge for medical services today is $40.00. A payment is made on the account today in the amount of $50.00. What is the current balance due on this account?
a. $0.00
b. $10.00
c. $20.00
d. $30.00
e. $40.00

**9.** [LO21.1] When an insurance company makes a payment to a medical practice for services rendered to a patient and the patient also makes a payment on the account, causing it to exceed the allowed charges, it is called
a. account imbalance.
b. excessive billing.
c. payment reconciliation.
d. overpayment.
e. incorrect billing.

**10.** [LO21.3] Sequentially, the first step in reconciling a bank account is to
a. check the closing balance on the previous bank statement against the opening statement balance on the new bank statement.
b. place all the redeemed checks in numerical order.
c. ensure that all deposits have posted.
d. place a check mark on all checks if they are listed on the bank statement.
e. subtract any service charges from the ending balance on the bank statement.

**11.** [LO21.4] An example of an accounts payable item is
a. unemployment taxes for employees.
b. the unpaid balance on a patient's account.
c. posted charges for a hospitalized patient.
d. the current charge for a surgical procedure performed in the medical office.
e. the cost of oxygen therapy for a patient who is homebound.

**12.** [LO21.4] Which of the following is *not* a recommended practice to properly manage office and medical supplies?
a. Order only the necessary supplies.
b. Buy only generic products when available because they are much cheaper.
c. Get the best quality supplies for the best price.
d. Order only in proper amounts.
e. Buy from reputable suppliers.

**13.** [LO21.6] Which of the following is a payroll duty that is performed on or before January 31 of each year?
a. Have each employee complete a new Form I-9.
b. Deposit employer Social Security taxes into the proper bank account.
c. Provide each employee with a Form W-2.
d. Calculate the annual Medicare taxes.
e. Withhold annual FICA taxes from each employee.

**14.** [LO21.3] A best practice for depositing checks is to
a. send all checks collected in one envelope through the mail to the bank.
b. collect all checks for a 1-week period of time and deposit them all at one time.
c. deposit checks on a daily basis in person at the bank.
d. endorse all the checks at the end of the week and make a single deposit.
e. mail the checks individually to the bank so if lost, only one check is missing.

**15.** [LO21.3] Which of the following features is not available with all medical office electronic banking software programs?
a. Record deposits
b. Manage payroll
c. Pay bills
d. Display a checkbook
e. Balance a checkbook

**16.** [LO21.7] The employer identification number (EIN)
a. is required by law for federal tax accounting purposes.
b. is obtained by completing Form I-9.
c. allows an employer to be exempt from paying payroll taxes.
d. is not required for employers with less than 50 employees.
e. is obtained by filing an application with the state unemployment office.

**17.** [LO21.7] Federal income tax is withheld from an employee's payroll
a. every week.
b. once a year.
c. monthly.
d. every payday.
e. quarterly.

**18.** [LO21.6] Gross earnings refers to
a. the amount of money earned yearly after all deductions have been taken out.
b. the annual salary an employee makes after FICA is deducted.
c. the total amount of income earned before deductions.
d. the amount of money an employee earns each month after the employee's medical insurance premium is deducted.
e. the hourly wage earned after taxes.

**19.** [LO21.6] Which of the following is acceptable for documentation on Form I-9?
a. U.S. passport
b. Driver's license and Social Security account number card
c. Permanent resident card
d. Birth certificate and federal ID card
e. All of the above.

**20.** [LO21.6] The Employee's Withholding Allowance Certificate is also referred to as the
a. Form W-2.
b. Form W-4.
c. Form I-9.
d. Form SS-4.
e. Form 940.

**21.** [LO21.6] What is the gross income per pay period for an employee who is paid biweekly, works 40 hours a week, and earns $15.00 per hour?
a. $400.00
b. $600.00
c. $800.00
d. $1,000.00
e. $1,200.00

**22.** [LO21.3] Which of the following is *not* a type of checking account that a physician would have?
a. Personal account and business account
b. Business account and interest-earning account
c. Indirect account and direct-interest account
d. Payroll account and insurance account
e. Answers (c) and (d).

**23.** [LO21.1] A patient's ledger card would *not* include the
   a. patient's insurance policy number.
   b. physician's DEA number.
   c. physician's practice name and address.
   d. patient's full name.
   e. patient's work phone number.

**24.** [LO21.3] Which of the following conditions should be met in order for a check to be negotiable?
   a. The check must be written and signed by the payer.
   b. The check must be payable to the payee.
   c. The check must include the amount of money to be paid.
   d. The check must have the name of the bank on the check.
   e. All of the above.

**25.** [LO21.2] Which formula would be used to balance a day sheet or a patient's ledger?
   a. Previous balance + Today's charges − (Payments + Adjustments) = Current balance
   b. Current balance + Today's charges − (Payments + Adjustments) = Previous balance
   c. Previous balance − Today's charges + (Payments − Adjustments) = Current balance
   d. Current balance − Today's charges + (Payments − Adjustments) = Current balance
   e. Previous balance − Today's charges − (Payments − Adjustments) = Current balance

## True or False

Decide whether each statement is true or false. In the space at the left, write "T" for true or "F" for false. On the lines provided, rewrite the false statements to make them true.

_____ **1.** [LO21.6] Form I-9 is a document that is required for employment eligibility verification.

_____

_____ **2.** [LO21.2] Patient accounting methods within a medical practice may be computerized or manual, with the manual method being the most commonly used type of system.

_____

_____ **3.** [LO21.5] The summary of charges, receipts, and disbursements is not summarized until the end of each fiscal year.

_____

_____ **4.** [LO21.1] The total charges and total receipts in any summary should be almost the same. They may not be identical because some bills may not have been fully collected.

_____

_____ **5.** [LO21.3] The face or front of every check contains two important items: the ABA number and the endorsement area.

_____

_____ **6.** [LO21.3] Electronic banking can improve productivity, cash flow, and accuracy.

_____

_____ **7.** [LO21.1] Of the many elements used in a practice's accounting system, the daily log and patient ledger cards are used primarily for accounts payable.

_____

_____ **8.** [LO21.5] The statement of income and expense, also known as a cash flow statement, highlights the practice's profitability.

_____

_____ **9.** [LO21.6] The Fair Labor Standards Act requires that employees are paid double time, plus normal holiday pay, for all hours worked on a company-approved holiday.

_____

_____ **10.** [LO21.7] Each quarter, employers are required to file a Form 941: Employer's Quarterly Federal Tax Return with the IRS, summarizing the federal income and FICA taxes withheld from employees' paychecks.

_____

## Sentence Completion

In the space provided, write the word or phrase that best completes each sentence.

**1.** [LO21.2] The choice of an accounting system is based on the _____ and _____ of the practice.

**2.** [LO21.1] In the daily log you enter the name of each patient seen that day. Across from the name, you record the _____ provided, the fee _____, and the _____ received.

**3.** [LO21.1] The charge slips/receipts are _____. This numbering promotes good cash control and theoretically prevents _____.

**4.** [LO21.3] NSF payments are first deducted from the office _____ account. The patient's account is then updated with a _____ _____ for the amount of the check, adding that amount back to the patient _____.

**5.** [LO21.3] To prevent theft of checks, always put the checkbook in a _____ _____ place when it is not in use and file deposit receipts promptly. If they are lost, you have no _____.

**6.** [LO21.6] For hourly employees, the Fair Labor Standards Act mandates payment of _____ times the normal hourly wage for all hours worked beyond the normal _____ hours in a regular workday.

1. _____
   _____

2. _____
   _____

3. _____
   _____

4. _____
   _____

5. _____
   _____

6. _____
   _____

7. [LO21.6] For the latest FICA tax percentages and level of taxable earnings, check the IRS _____ _____.

8. [LO21.1] Every day, you must update the accounts receivable record, which shows the total _____ to the practice.

9. [LO21.3] A check that is _____ is legally transferable from one person to another.

10. [LO21.3] A physician is likely to have three different types of checking accounts: a _____ account, a _____ account for office expenses, and a(n) _____ earning account.

7. _____
   _____

8. _____
   _____

9. _____
   _____

10. _____
    _____

# Apply Your Knowledge

## Short Answer

Write the answer to each question on the lines provided.

1. [LO21.1] Describe the importance of accuracy in bookkeeping and banking.

_____

_____

_____

2. [LO21.2] Cite one advantage and one disadvantage to using a double-entry accounting system.

_____

_____

_____

3. [LO21.4] List the three main types or groups of accounts payable and give one example of an accounts payable item for each group.

_____

_____

_____

4. [LO21.3] Why is it advantageous to make frequent bank deposits?

_____

_____

_____

**5.** [LO21.6] What is the purpose of the Fair Labor Standards Act?

_____

_____

_____

## Problem-Solving Activities

Follow the directions for each activity.

**1.** [LO21.5] Creating a Record of Office Disbursements
   a. Using the form provided on the facing page, complete a monthly Record of Office Disbursements using the following transactions for the month of July 2013. Ensure that the entries are in order of occurrence.
   - PSS Medical Supply, 7/3, check 3970, $414.32, medical supplies
   - Clean Quick Janitorial Service, 7/15, check 3980, $175.00, cleaning service
   - My Florist, 7/3, check 3969, $45.00, flowers Mary Garcia birthday
   - Medlab Service Center, 7/20, check 3986, $200, repair ECG machine
   - U.S. Postal Service, 7/5, check 3971, $47.00, stamps
   - National Geographic Society, 7/30, check 3991, $58.00, magazine subscription
   - LLC Rental Co., 7/5, check 3972, $1850.00, office rent
   - Office Max, 7/16, check 3981, $88.47, general office supplies
   - American Insurance Co., check 3990, 7/30, $800.00, general liability insurance premium
   - U. S. Postal Service, 7/21, check 3987, $68.00, postage
   - Central Laundry, 7/10, check 3975, $130.00, lab coats/linens
   - Cheesecake Factory, 7/16, check 3982, $126.75, employee luncheon
   - Western Gas Company, 7/29, check 3989, $684.79, gas and electric
   - Staples Office Supply, 7/6, check 3973, $45.64, case copy paper
   - Cox Cable, 7/28, check 3988, $97.59, telephone, Internet
   - ABC Plumbing, 7/11, check 3976, $385.00, replace sink
   - Monument Insurance, 7/19, check 3985, $525.00, professional liability insurance premium
   - Waste Management, 7/10, check 3974, $75.00, medical waste disposal
   - JW Marriott Hotel, 7/14, check 3979, $379.00, lodging conference
   - AMT, 7/17, check 3983, $95.00, certification Cheryl Adams
   - FedEx, 7/17, check 3984, $18.87, shipping
   - Safeguard, 7/12, check 3977, $48.00, medical records off-site storage
   - Aquariums Plus, 7/12, check 3978, $129.00, fish tank service
   - Shelby Pharmacy Wholesalers, 7/31, check 3992, $325.57, pharmacy supplies
   - Costco, 7/14, check 3968, $148, employee lounge supplies

# Record of Office Disbursements
## 2013

### TYPES OF EXPENSES

| DATE | PAYEE | CK. NO. | TOTAL AMOUNT | RENT | UTILITIES | POSTAGE | LAB/ X-RAY | MEDICAL SUPPLIES | OFFICE SUPPLIES | WAGES | INSURANCE | TAXES | TRAVEL | MISC. |
|------|-------|---------|--------------|------|-----------|---------|------------|------------------|-----------------|-------|-----------|-------|--------|-------|
| | | | | | | | | | | | | | | |
| | | | | | | | | | | | | | | |
| | | | | | | | | | | | | | | |
| | | | | | | | | | | | | | | |
| | | | | | | | | | | | | | | |
| | | | | | | | | | | | | | | |
| | | | | | | | | | | | | | | |
| | | | | | | | | | | | | | | |
| | | | | | | | | | | | | | | |
| | | | | | | | | | | | | | | |
| | | Total | | | | | | | | | | | | |

# Thinking Critically

Write your response to each case study question on the lines provided.

## Case 1 [LO21.3]

After seeing the doctor, Fred McMann, a patient, is checking out at the reception area. He hands you a check for $20.00 to cover the copay amount. When you access his ledger card to record the payment, it states that he is a "cash pay" patient due to prior problems he had with several nonsufficient funds checks.

**1.** What is the appropriate response to Mr. McMann when he hands you his check?

_____

_____

_____

**2.** What course of action will prevent this from happening in the future?

_____

_____

_____

## Case 2 [LO21.5]

You are assigned the task of completing the office monthly disbursement journal, and this is the first time you have been asked to do this. As you enter the numerous monthly expenditures on the log sheet, you realize there are some items that are ordered frequently and in greater quantity than expected. These expenses include office and administrative supplies such as printed letterhead, business envelopes, copy and fax paper, pens, notebooks, file folders, etc. It was not apparent until now that the office consumed so many administrative supplies each month.

**1.** Why is it important to be concerned about the expenditures for the practice?

_____

_____

_____

**2.** What are some recommendations you might make to the practice manager to better control the use of administrative supplies?

_____

_____

_____

# Demonstrate Your Knowledge

**Student Name:** _____

## Procedure 21–1: Posting Charges, Payments, and Adjustments

**GOAL:** To maintain a system that promotes accurate record keeping for the practice

**MATERIALS:** Daily log sheets, patient ledger cards, and check register, or computerized bookkeeping system; summaries of charges, receipts, and disbursements
(*Note:* A daily log and patient ledger card are available at the end of this study guide.)

**METHOD:** To pass this procedure the minimum required score is _____% or all elements must meet "satisfactory" ability on the final demonstration. The first box may be used as a practice or final demonstration, with the evaluator placing **S for Satisfactory** or **U for Unsatisfactory** if that is the grading criteria. The second box may be used as a final demonstration with a **grade point** written in the box.

| STEPS | POSSIBLE POINTS | S/U | POINTS EARNED |
|---|---|---|---|
| 1. Use a new log (day) sheet each day. For each patient seen that day, record the patient name, the relevant charges, and any payments received, calculating any necessary adjustments and new balances. If you're using a computerized system, enter the patient's name or account number, the relevant charge, and any payments received and adjustments made in the appropriate areas. The computer will calculate the new balances. The day sheets will also be used to do month-end reports and MUST be balanced before the next business day's transactions can be added to the system. | 20 | | |
| 2. Create a ledger card for each new patient, and maintain a ledger card for all existing patients. The ledger card should include the patient's name, address, home and work telephone numbers, and insurance company. It should also contain the name of the guarantor (if different from the patient). Update the ledger card every time the patient incurs a charge or makes a payment. Be sure to adjust the account balance after every transaction. In a computerized system, a patient record is the same as a ledger card. This record must also be maintained and updated as this is the most up-to-date financial record for each patient's account. | 20 | | |

*(Continued)*

| STEPS | POSSIBLE POINTS | S/U | POINTS EARNED |
|---|---|---|---|
| 3. Record all deposits accurately in the check register. File the deposit receipt—with a detailed listing of checks, cash, and money orders deposited—for later use in reconciling the bank statement. The deposit amount should match the amount of money collected by the practice for that day. | 20 | | |
| 4. When paying bills for the practice, enter each check in the check register accurately, including the check number, date, payee, and amount before writing the check. | 20 | | |
| 5. Prepare and/or print a summary of charges, receipts, and disbursements every month, quarter, or year, as directed. Be sure to double-check all entries and calculations from the monthly summary before posting them to the quarterly summary. Also, double-check the entries and calculations from the quarterly summary before posting them to the yearly summary. | 20 | | |
| **Total Points (if applicable)** | 100 | | |

Comments: _____

_____

_____


Final Evaluator's Signature: _____


Date: _____

### CAAHEP Competencies Achieved

VI. C (1) Explain basic bookkeeping computations

VI. C (13) Discuss types of adjustments that may be made to a patient's account

VI. P (2) Perform accounts receivable procedures including:

      a. Post entries on a day sheet

      d. Post adjustments

VI. P (3) Utilize computerized office billing systems

### ABHES Competencies Achieved

8. h. Post entries on a day sheet

8. m. Post adjustments

## Procedure 21-2: Posting a Nonsufficient Funds (NSF) Check

**GOAL:** To post a nonsufficient funds (NSF) check to a patient's account

**MATERIALS:** Computer, returned check, patient ledger sheet, calculator (optional), daily log sheet (optional) (*Note:* A daily log and patient ledger card are available at the end of this study guide.)

**METHOD:** To pass this procedure the minimum required score is _____% or all elements must meet "satisfactory" ability on the final demonstration. The first box may be used as a practice or final demonstration, with the evaluator placing **S for Satisfactory** or **U for Unsatisfactory** if that is the grading criteria. The second box may be used as a final demonstration with a **grade point** written in the box.

| STEPS | POSSIBLE POINTS | S/U | POINTS EARNED |
|---|---|---|---|
| 1. Locate the patient's account on the computer or pull the patient's ledger card for manual processes. | 20 | | |
| 2. Use your medical facility code for an NSF check or charge (if used) and using today's date, create a new charge log for the patient. Use the code and the description *Check returned by bank* in the description column. | 20 | | |
| 3. In the Payment/Adjustment column, insert the amount of the NSF check in parentheses as it was never actually received and the parentheses informs you to "do the opposite of usual"; in this case add the payment to the balance instead of subtracting it. | 20 | | |
| 4. Add the amount of the NSF check to the previous balance and insert that figure in the Current Balance column. | 20 | | |
| 5. On the next line, also using today's date, add the description of "NSF Office Fee" with the office charge for NSF checks returned by the bank. Add this charge to the previous balance to obtain the new current balance. | 20 | | |
| **Total Points (if applicable)** | 100 | | |

| DAILY LOG—Total Care Clinic, PC | | | | | | | |
|---|---|---|---|---|---|---|---|
| DATE | PATIENT | CODE | TODAY'S CHARGE | PAYMENTS/ ADJUSTMENT | CURRENT BALANCE | PREVIOUS BALANCE | PROVIDER |
| 3/22 | Ashley Wilkens | Payment-Ck #102 | | 15.00 | 0.00 | 15.00 | WC |
| 3/30 | Ashley Wilkens | (NSF) Ck returned by bank | | (15.00) | 15.00 | 0.00 | WC |
| 3/30 | Ashley Wilkens | NSF Office fee | 35.00 | | 50.00 | 15.00 | WC |
| | | | | | | | |

**Comments:** _____

_____

_____

**Final Evaluator's Signature:** _____

**Date:** _____

## CAAHEP Competencies Achieved

VI. C (13) Discuss types of adjustments that may be made to a patient's account

VI. P (2) Perform accounts receivable procedures including:

      a.  Post entries on a day sheet

      g.  Post nonsufficient fund (NSF) checks

VI. P (3) Utilize computerized office billing systems

## ABHES Competencies Achieved

8. h. Post entries on a day sheet

8. p. Post nonsufficient funds (NSF)

8. w. Use manual or computerized bookkeeping systems

Student Name: _____

## Procedure 21–3: Processing a Credit Balance

**GOAL:** To process a credit balance

**MATERIALS:** Daily log sheet or day sheet, checks, ledger card, computer, calculator, RA (Remittance Advice) or Explanation of Benefits (EOB)
(*Note:* A daily log and patient ledger card are available at the end of this study guide.)

**METHOD:** To pass this procedure the minimum required score is _____% or all elements must meet "satisfactory" ability on the final demonstration. The first box may be used as a practice or final demonstration, with the evaluator placing **S for Satisfactory** or **U for Unsatisfactory** if that is the grading criteria. The second box may be used as a final demonstration with a **grade point** written in the box.

| STEPS | POSSIBLE POINTS | S/U | POINTS EARNED |
|---|---|---|---|
| 1. Locate the patient's account in the computer or pull the patient's ledger card for paper-based systems. | 10 | | |
| 2. Review the policy manual to make sure you are following the guidelines for posting credit balances. | 10 | | |
| 3. Review the EOB and check to be sure that the payment is being credited to the correct patient account. | 15 | | |
| 4. Post the payment to the patient's account by writing (or keying) the remittance amount in the paid column. | 15 | | |
| 5. Subtract the payment amount from the previous balance and insert the new balance in the balance column. Check calculations carefully, particularly if it appears that an overpayment has been made. | 15 | | |
| 6. Review the account thoroughly in case more insurance payments are expected on the patient's account. | 15 | | |
| 7. Adjust the credit balance off the patient's account by issuing a refund (see Procedure 21–4). | 20 | | |
| **Total Points (if applicable)** | 100 | | |

Comments: _____

_____

_____

**Final Evaluator's Signature:** _____

**Date:** _____

## CAAHEP Competencies Achieved

VI. C (13) Discuss types of adjustments that may be made to a patient's account

VI. P (2) Perform accounts receivable procedures including:

      a. Post entries on a day sheet

      e. Process a credit balance

VI. P (3) Utilize computerized office billing systems

## ABHES Competencies Achieved

8. h. Post entries on a day sheet

8. n. Process credit balances

**Student Name:** _____

## Procedure 21–4: Processing Refunds to Patients

**GOAL:** To process refunds to patients

**MATERIALS:** Payment (check), ledger card, computer, calculator, Remittance Advice (RA) or Explanation of Benefits (EOB)
(*Note:* A patient ledger card is available at the end of this study guide.)

**METHOD:** To pass this procedure the minimum required score is _____% or all elements must meet "satisfactory" ability on the final demonstration. The first box may be used as a practice or final demonstration, with the evaluator placing **S for Satisfactory** or **U for Unsatisfactory** if that is the grading criteria. The second box may be used as a final demonstration with a **grade point** written in the box.

| STEPS | POSSIBLE POINTS | S/U | POINTS EARNED |
|---|---|---|---|
| 1. Calculate and determine the amount to be refunded (from Procedure 21–3). | 20 | | |
| 2. Write a check to the patient for the amount to be refunded. | 20 | | |
| 3. Ask the physician or business manager to sign the check so that it can be given or mailed to the patient. | 20 | | |
| 4. Post the refund as a negative payment (credit) to the patient's ledger card, or to the patient's account if a computerized system is being used. Using parentheses around the figure is a common way to record credits. | 20 | | |
| 5. Make a copy of the check, retaining a copy in the patient's financial record. Give or mail the check to the patient. If the check is being mailed, be sure to verify the patient's address prior to mailing and utilize certified return receipt mail to be sure the patient receives the check. | 20 | | |
| **Total Points (if applicable)** | 100 | | |

**Comments:** _____

_____

_____

**Final Evaluator's Signature:** _____

**Date:** _____

## CAAHEP Competencies Achieved

VI. C (13) Discuss types of adjustments that may be made to a patient's account

VI. P (2) Perform accounts receivable procedures including:

      a. Post entries on a day sheet

      f. Process refunds

 VI. P (3) Utilize computerized office billing systems

## ABHES Competencies Achieved

8. h. Post entries on a day sheet

8. o. Process refunds

8. w. Use manual or computerized bookkeeping systems

## Procedure 21–5: Making a Bank Deposit

**GOAL:** To prepare cash and checks for deposit and to deposit them properly into a bank account

**MATERIALS:** Bank deposit slip and items to be deposited, such as checks, cash, and money orders (*Note:* A bank deposit slip is available at the end of this study guide.)

**METHOD:** To pass this procedure the minimum required score is _____ % or all elements must meet "satisfactory" ability on the final demonstration. The first box may be used as a practice or final demonstration, with the evaluator placing **S for Satisfactory** or **U for Unsatisfactory** if that is the grading criteria. The second box may be used as a final demonstration with a **grade point** written in the box.

| STEPS | POSSIBLE POINTS | S/U | POINTS EARNED |
|---|:---:|:---:|:---:|
| 1. Divide the bills, coins, checks, and money orders into separate piles. | 10 | | |
| 2. Sort the bills by denomination, from largest to smallest. Then stack them, portrait side up, in the same direction. Total the amount of the bills, and write this amount on the deposit slip on the line marked currency or cash. | 10 | | |
| 3. If you have enough coins to fill coin wrappers, put them in wrappers of the proper denomination. If not, count the coins, and put them in the deposit bag. Total the amount of coins, and write this amount on the deposit slip on the line marked "Coin." | 10 | | |
| 4. Review all checks and money orders to be sure they are properly endorsed with a restrictive endorsement. List each check on the deposit slip, including the check number and amount. | 10 | | |
| 5. List each money order on the deposit slip. Include the notation "money order" or "MO" and the name of the writer. | 10 | | |
| 6. Calculate the total deposit (total of amounts or currency, coin, checks, and money orders). Write this amount on the deposit slip on the line marked "Total." If you do not use deposit slips that record a copy for the office, photocopy the deposit slip for your office records. | 10 | | |
| 7. Record the total amount of the deposit in the office checkbook register. | 10 | | |
| 8. If you plan to make the deposit in person, place the currency, coins, checks, and money orders in a deposit bag. If you cannot make the deposit in person, put the checks and money orders in a special bank-by-mail envelope, or put all deposit items in an envelope and send it by registered mail. | 10 | | |

*(Continued)*

| STEPS | POSSIBLE POINTS | S/U | POINTS EARNED |
|---|---|---|---|
| 9. Make the deposit in person or by mail. | 10 | | |
| 10. Obtain a deposit receipt from the bank. File it with the copy of the deposit slip in the office for later use when reconciling the bank statement. | 10 | | |
| **Total Points (if applicable)** | 100 | | |

**Comments:** _____

_____

_____


**Final Evaluator's Signature:** _____

**Date:** _____

## CAAHEP Competencies Achieved

VI. C (3) Describe banking procedures

VI. C (4) Discuss precautions for accepting checks

VI. C (5) Compare types of endorsement

VI. P (1) Prepare bank deposits

## ABHES Competencies Achieved

8. g. Prepare and reconcile a bank statement and deposit record

## Procedure 21–6: Reconciling a Bank Statement

**GOAL:** To ensure that the bank record of deposits, payments, and withdrawals agrees with the practice's record of deposits, payments, and withdrawals

**MATERIALS:** Previous bank statement, current bank statement, reconciliation worksheet (if not part of current bank statement), deposit receipts, red pencil, check stubs or checkbook register, returned checks (*Note:* A bank reconciliation form is available at the end of this study guide.)

**METHOD:** To pass this procedure the minimum required score is _____% or all elements must meet "satisfactory" ability on the final demonstration. The first box may be used as a practice or final demonstration, with the evaluator placing **S for Satisfactory** or **U for Unsatisfactory** if that is the grading criteria. The second box may be used as a final demonstration with a **grade point** written in the box.

| STEPS | POSSIBLE POINTS | S/U | POINTS EARNED |
|---|---|---|---|
| 1. Check the closing balance on the previous statement against the opening balance on the new statement. The balances should match. If they do not, call the bank. | 5 | | |
| 2. Record the closing balance from the new statement on the reconciliation worksheet (Figure 21–9). This worksheet usually appears on the back of the bank statement. | 5 | | |
| 3. Check each deposit receipt against the bank statement. Place a red check mark in the upper right corner of each receipt that is recorded on the statement. Total the amount of deposits that do not appear on the statement. Add this amount to the closing balance on the reconciliation worksheet. | 15 | | |
| 4. Put the redeemed checks in numerical order. (Your bank may send you several sheets consisting of photocopies or scans of the checks instead of the actual checks.) | 10 | | |
| 5. Compare each redeemed check with the bank statement, making sure that the amount on the check agrees with the amount on the statement. Place a red check mark in the upper-right corner of each redeemed check that is recorded on the statement. Also, place a check mark on the check stub or check register entry. Any checks that were written but that do not appear on the statement and were not returned as redeemed are considered "outstanding" checks. You can find these easily on the check stubs or checkbook register because they have no red check mark. | 15 | | |

*(Continued)*

| STEPS | POSSIBLE POINTS | S/U | POINTS EARNED |
|---|---|---|---|
| 6. List each outstanding check separately on the worksheet, including its check number and amount. Total the outstanding checks, and subtract this total from the bank statement balance. | 15 | | |
| 7. If the statement shows that the checking account earned interest, add this amount to the checkbook balance. | 10 | | |
| 8. If the statement lists such items as a service charge, check printing charge, or automatic payment, subtract them from the checkbook balance. | 15 | | |
| 9. Compare the new checkbook balance with the new bank statement balance. They should match. If they do not, repeat the process, rechecking all calculations. Double-check the addition and subtraction in the checkbook register. Review the checkbook register to make sure you did not omit any items. Ensure that you carried the correct balance forward from one register page to the next. Double-check that you made the correct additions or subtractions for all interest earned and charges. | 10 | | |
| 10. If your work is correct, and the balances still do not agree, call the bank to determine if a bank error has been made. Contact the bank promptly because the bank may have a time limit for corrections. The bank may consider the bank statement correct if you do not point out an error within a specified time. Check with your individual bank for their policy. | 0 | | |
| **Total Points (if applicable)** | 100 | | |

**Comments:** _____

_____

_____


**Final Evaluator's Signature:** _____

**Date:** _____

## CAAHEP Competencies Achieved

VI. C (3) Describe banking procedures

VI. C (4) Discuss precautions for accepting checks

VI. C (5) Compare types of endorsement

VI. P (1) Prepare bank deposits

## ABHES Competencies Achieved

8. g. Prepare and reconcile a bank statement and deposit record

**Student Name:** _____

## Procedure 21-7: Setting Up the Accounts Payable System

**GOAL:** To set up an accounts payable system

**MATERIALS:** Disbursements journal, petty cash record, payroll register, pen
(*Note:* A record of office disbursements is available at the end of this study guide.)

**METHOD:** To pass this procedure the minimum required score is _____ % or all elements must meet "satisfactory" ability on the final demonstration. The first box may be used as a practice or final demonstration, with the evaluator placing **S for Satisfactory** or **U for Unsatisfactory** if that is the grading criteria. The second box may be used as a final demonstration with a **grade point** written in the box.

| STEPS | POSSIBLE POINTS | S/U | POINTS EARNED |
|---|---|---|---|
| **Setting Up the Disbursements Journal** | | | |
| 1. Write in column headings for the basic information about each check: date, payee's name, check number, and check amount. | 9 | | |
| 2. Write in column headings for each type of business expense, such as rent and utilities. | 10 | | |
| 3. Write in column headings (if space is available) for deposits and the account balance. | 10 | | |
| 4. Record the data from completed checks under the appropriate column headings. | 10 | | |
| 5. Be sure to subtract payments from the balance and add deposits to it. | 11 | | |
| **Setting Up the Payroll Register** | | | |
| 1. Write in column headings for check number, employee name, earnings to date, hourly rate, hours worked, regular earnings, overtime hours worked, and overtime earnings. | 9 | | |
| 2. Write in column headings for total gross earnings for the pay period and gross taxable earnings. | 10 | | |
| 3. Write in column headings for each deduction. These may include federal income tax, Federal Insurance Contributions Act (FICA) tax, state income tax, local income tax, and various voluntary deductions. | 10 | | |
| 4. Write in a column heading for net earnings. | 10 | | |
| 5. Each time you write payroll checks, record earnings and deduction data under the appropriate column headings on the payroll register. | 11 | | |
| **Total Points (if applicable)** | 100 | | |

**Comments:** _____

_____

_____

**Final Evaluator's Signature:** _____

**Date:** _____

## CAAHEP Competencies Achieved

VI. C (6) Differentiate between accounts payable and accounts receivable

VI. C (7) Compare manual and computerized bookkeeping systems used in ambulatory health care

VI. C (10) Identify procedures for preparing patient accounts

## ABHES Competencies Achieved

8. j. Perform accounts payable procedures

## Procedure 21–8: Generating Payroll

**GOAL:** To handle the practice's payroll as efficiently and accurately as possible for each pay period

**MATERIALS:** Employees' time cards, employees' earnings records, payroll register, IRS tax tables, check register
(*Note:* An employee earnings record and a payroll register are available at the end of this study guide.)

**METHOD:** To pass this procedure the minimum required score is _____% or all elements must meet "satisfactory" ability on the final demonstration. The first box may be used as a practice or final demonstration, with the evaluator placing **S for Satisfactory** or **U for Unsatisfactory** if that is the grading criteria. The second box may be used as a final demonstration with a **grade point** written in the box.

| STEPS | POSSIBLE POINTS | S/U | POINTS EARNED |
|---|---|---|---|
| 1. Calculate the total regular and overtime hours worked, based on the employee's time card. Enter those totals under the appropriate headings on the payroll register. | 9 | | |
| 2. Check the pay rate on the employee earnings record. Then multiply the hours worked (including any paid vacation or paid holidays, if applicable) by the rates for regular time and overtime (time and a half or double time). This yields gross earnings. | 9 | | |
| 3. Enter the gross earnings under the appropriate heading on the payroll register. Subtract any nontaxable benefits, such as health-care or retirement programs. | 9 | | |
| 4. Using IRS tax tables and data on the employee earnings record, determine the amount of federal income tax to withhold based on the employee's marital status and number of exemptions. Also compute the amount of FICA tax to withhold for Social Security (6.2%) and Medicare (1.45%). | 10 | | |
| 5. Following state and local procedures, determine the amount of state and local income taxes (if any) to withhold based on the employee's marital status and number of exemptions. | 9 | | |
| 6. Calculate the employer's contributions to FUTA and to the state unemployment fund, if any. Post these amounts to the employer's account. | 9 | | |
| 7. Enter any other required or voluntary deductions, such as health insurance or contributions to a 401(k) fund. | 9 | | |
| 8. Subtract all deductions from the gross earnings to get the employee's net earnings. | 9 | | |

*(Continued)*

| STEPS | POSSIBLE POINTS | S/U | POINTS EARNED |
|---|---|---|---|
| 9. Enter the total amount withheld from all employees for FICA under the headings for Social Security and Medicare. Remember that the employer must match these amounts. Enter other employer contributions, such as for federal and state unemployment taxes, under the appropriate headings. | 9 | | |
| 10. Fill out the check stub, including the employee's name, date, pay period, gross earnings, all deductions, and net earnings. Make out the paycheck for the net earnings. | 9 | | |
| 11. Deposit each deduction in a tax liability account. | 9 | | |
| **Total Points (if applicable)** | 100 | | |

**Comments:** _____

_____

_____

**Final Evaluator's Signature:** _____

**Date:** _____

**CAAHEP Competencies Achieved**

None

**ABHES Competencies Achieved**

None

# 22 Practice Management

## Test Your Knowledge

### Vocabulary Review

Match the key terms in the right column to the definitions in the left column by placing the letter of each correct answer in the space provided.

_____ **1.** a special form required by a facility when an adverse outcome or event with risk of liability occurs; also called an occurrence report

_____ **2.** forms that address the potentially hazardous substances used and that provide workers and emergency personnel with the procedures for handling these substances if a spill or accident occurs

_____ **3.** a list of meeting topics and the order in which they will be addressed

_____ **4.** a model showing the supervisory structure and reporting relationships between different functions and positions in an organization

_____ **5.** Description of personnel protective equipment and other safety engineering devices and processes; instructions of what an employee should do if an exposure occurs

_____ **6.** a nurse practitioner or physician assistant

_____ **7.** a plan and processes ensuring that the practice's services meet or exceed the requirements and standards

**a.** agenda [LO22.2]

**b.** budget [LO22.2]

**c.** chain of command [LO22.1]

**d.** exposure control plan [LO22.3]

**e.** I-9 form [LO22.5]

**f.** organizational chart [LO22.1]

**g.** quality assurance [LO22.4]

**h.** midlevel provider [LO22.1]

**i.** probationary period [LO22.6]

**j.** Material Safety Data Sheets (MSDS) [LO22.3]

**k.** sexual harassment [LO22.6]

**l.** W-2 tax form [LO22.5]

**m.** incident report [LO22.4]

**n.** risk management [LO22.4]

**o.** W-4 tax form [LO22.6]

_____ **8.** term first used in the military to demonstrate how each rank is accountable to those directly superior and how the authority passes from one link in the chain to the next, or top to bottom

_____ **9.** an allotted period of time when a new employee may be terminated without cause; a trial period

_____ **10.** unwelcome verbal, visual, or physical conduct of a sexual nature that is severe or pervasive and affects working conditions or creates a hostile work environment

_____ **11.** employment eligibility verification certifying the employee's U.S. citizenship, legal alien status, or legal authorization to work in this country

_____ **12.** the employer's statement of how much gross income the organization paid the employee for the year and the taxes withheld on this form

_____ **13.** a process to continually asses, identify, correct, and monitor functions of the medical office to prevent negative outcomes and minimize exposure to risk

_____ **14.** the predicted expenses and revenues to operate a practice over a given period of time

_____ **15.** a form stating the number of deductions an employee wishes to claim on income tax

_____ **16.** statements of intent, commitments, or goals of the practice that also prescribe the correct method for performing or carrying out individual parts of these goals

_____ **17.** facilitation of communication between parties experiencing unresolved issues

_____ **18.** the formal manner in which employees may express disagreement with management

_____ **19.** issues between employees and employers

_____ **20.** a synopsis of human relations policies

**p.** policies and procedures (P&P) [LO22.2]

**q.** grievance process [LO22.6]

**r.** employee handbook [LO22.5]

**s.** labor relations [LO22.6]

**t.** mediation [LO22.6]

# Multiple-Choice Certification Questions

There may be more than one answer; circle the letter of the choice that best completes each statement or answers each question.

1. [LO22.2] Which of the following duties is not usually performed by the practice manager?
   a. Evaluating employees
   b. Taking vital signs
   c. Hiring an administrative medical assistant
   d. Ensuring that employees are trained
   e. Terminating a medical assistant

2. [LO22.1] In a typical organizational structure of a physician-owned practice, the
   a. administrative medical assistant directly reports to the physician at all times.
   b. office manager reports to the administrative medical assistants.
   c. physician is solely responsible for all office activities.
   d. practice manager reports to the corporate board of directors.
   e. administrative medical assistant reports to the practice manager.

3. [LO22.1] If you are following the chain of command for your organization, when a problem arises you should initially report to your
   a. receptionist.
   b. supervisor.
   c. physician.
   d. co-worker.
   e. practice manager.

4. [LO22.2] A medical practice budget could be negatively affected by
   a. increased patient payments.
   b. decreased use of office supplies.
   c. increased patient load.
   d. decreased revenue.
   e. new contractual agreements for annual sports physicals.

5. [LO22.3] To ensure that the medical practice EHR system has secure communication between the provider and outside entities, the practice should use a system that is certified by
   a. AHIMA.
   b. CCHIT.
   c. OSHA.
   d. Medicare.
   e. the CDC.

6. [LO22.3] If an accidental chemical spill occurs in the workplace, the employee needs to access a/an _____ for instructions on dealing with the cleanup of the spill.
   a. MSDS sheet
   b. OSHA manual
   c. CDC advisor
   d. local poison control center advisor
   e. administrative manual

7. [LO22.2] At least 1 week prior to a staff meeting, the office manager should
   a. decide where to hold the meeting.
   b. put out a call for agenda items.
   c. send around a sign-in sheet.
   d. determine when the subsequent meetings will be held.
   e. notify the physician of the meeting.

8. **[LO22.6]** Mediating appropriate issues between staff members is the responsibility of the
   a. human resources department.
   b. risk management department.
   c. staff and employees.
   d. recruiting staff.
   e. quality assurance team.

9. **[LO22.5]** The qualifications and requirements for the administrative medical assistant position would be found
   a. in a procedure manual.
   b. in the job description.
   c. in the MSDS binder.
   d. in a QA manual.
   e. on the organizational chart.

10. **[LO22.1]** In a company-owned medical practice, the person who has ultimate responsibility is the
    a. administrative medical assistant.
    b. office manager.
    c. chief executive officer.
    d. physician.
    e. physician's designee.

11. **[LO22.3]** Maintaining an entryway free of ice and other hazards is considered what area of management?
    a. Human resources
    b. Quality assurance
    c. Health and safety
    d. Legal and business
    e. Organizational

12. **[LO22.4]** If a patient slips and falls on a slippery floor in the medical office, this accident falls under
    a. human resources.
    b. quality assurance.
    c. health and safety.
    d. legal and business.
    e. risk management.

13. **[LO22.4]** If a patient falls on a slippery floor, the type of form that must be initiated is a/n
    a. I-9.
    b. W-2.
    c. grievance.
    d. incident report.
    e. W-4.

14. **[LO22.2]** An effective practice manager should possess all the following attributes *except*
    a. fairness.
    b. firmness.
    c. judgmental attitude.
    d. tact.
    e. open-mindedness.

15. **[LO22.5]** The Equal Pay Act prohibits pay discrimination based on
    a. ability.
    b. age.
    c. ethnicity.
    d. gender.
    e. disability.

**16.** [LO22.5] Which of the following topics would be covered in the benefits section of an employee handbook?
a. A leave of absence from work
b. Payroll amounts
c. 401(k) plan
d. Safety and security
e. ADA policy

**17.** [LO22.5] A newly hired employee is required to complete a Form I-9, which is used to
a. state the number of deductions the employee wishes to claim for income tax.
b. certify citizenship or other legal status to work in the United States.
c. arrange for direct deposit of payroll checks into a bank account.
d. assign a beneficiary for the life insurance policy provided by the employer.
e. identify the person to contact in case of emergency.

**18.** [LO22.5] Which of the following is an accurate statement regarding the human relations department of a medical practice?
a. It is the only department that does not involve the patient.
b. The human relations department deals with people services.
c. This department assists the employer with the hiring process.
d. HR also is known as the personnel department.
e. All of the above are accurate.

**19.** [LO22.5] According to the FMLA requirements, how many weeks is an employee allowed to take leave from work without pay?
a. 6 weeks
b. 8 weeks
c. 10 weeks
d. 12 weeks
e. 15 weeks

**20.** [LO22.5] Components of a typical job description include
a. requirements and qualifications.
b. the number of holidays that are included as paid time off.
c. the criteria for enrolling in the 401(k) plan.
d. instructions for handling emergencies and incidents.
e. a copy of the organizational chart for the practice.

**21.** [LO22.5] Which of the following is *not* protected from discrimination under the EEOC?
a. Race
b. Color
c. Child care
d. Religion
e. Sex or gender

**22.** [LO22.6] When a medical practice has a probationary period to evaluate a new employee, the customary time period is
a. 120 days.
b. 90 days.
c. 60 days.
d. 30 days.
e. 2 weeks.

**23.** [LO22.6] An employee who feels unjustly treated should
a. contact an attorney.
b. write a letter to the board of directors.
c. bring up the topic at the next staff meeting.
d. follow the steps of the grievance process.
e. file a complaint with the EEOC.

**24.** [LO22.3] Which information would you expect to find in the office safety manual?
   a. Location of the MSDS manuals
   b. OSHA compliance requirements
   c. Disaster plan
   d. Aseptic practices
   e. All of the above.

**25.** [LO22.4] An incident report should never include
   a. the identification of the injured party.
   b. assumptions.
   c. the medical treatment provided.
   d. statements.
   e. names of witnesses.

## True or False

Decide whether each statement is true or false. In the space at the left, write "T" for true or "F" for false. On the lines provided, rewrite the false statements to make them true.

_____ **1.** [LO22.1] The medical director is in charge of the physician assistants and nurse practitioners.

_____

_____ **2.** [LO22.1] Since the administrative medical assistants work closely with the physicians, it is appropriate to ask the physician for time off from work.

_____

_____ **3.** [LO22.2] It is not anticipated that the practice manager will have communication or interaction with bankers and lawyers.

_____

_____ **4.** [LO22.3] If the medical practice is renting office space, the practice manager has no responsibility for the facility safety.

_____

_____ **5.** [LO22.5] The human resources department is probably the only department in the medical clinic that does not involve the patient.

_____

_____ **6.** [LO22.6] Under FMLA regulations, an employer is required to pay the employee's salary up to 12 weeks when he or she is on leave from work.

_____

_____ **7.** [LO22.5] In order for sexual harassment to have taken place, the victim must prove there was a physical encounter with the accused person.

_____

_____ **8.** [LO22.5] The company's policy on protective personal equipment would be found in the safety manual.

_____

_____ **9.** [LO22.2] The practice manager is usually responsible for ensuring that the budgeted expenses and revenues are met.

_____

_____ **10.** [LO22.4] When using the problem-solving model to resolve a quality assurance issue, it is important to "close the loop."

_____

## Sentence Completion

In the space provided, write the word or phrase that best completes each sentence.

**1.** [LO22.1] The organizational design and chart show the _____ structure and _____ relationship between different functions and positions within the medical practice.

**2.** [LO22.1] When the administrative medical assistant has a complaint, it is not appropriate to go outside the _____ _____ _____ with a complaint, even if the complaint if about your supervisor.

**3.** [LO22.2] The role of the practice manager is to ensure that all communication is _____, _____, _____, and HIPAA compliant.

**4.** [LO22.5] Other names for the human relations department are personnel _____, personnel _____, or people _____.

**5.** [LO22.6] The EEOC prohibits job discrimination for _____, _____, _____, _____ or _____ _____.

**6.** [LO22.4] When an adverse event occurs in the medical practice, a/an _____ _____ is completed.

**7.** [LO22.3] The medical practice must comply with the health and safety regulations established by _____.

**8.** [LO22.1] Most states require that, when a medical assistant is involved in a clinical aspect of patient care, he or she must be supervised by a _____.

**9.** [LO22.4] A frayed electrical wire would be a concern for facility management and _____ _____.

**10.** [LO22.2, LO22.3, LO22.4] It is recommended that all medical practice manuals are reviewed at least _____.

**1.** _____
_____

**2.** _____
_____

**3.** _____
_____

**4.** _____
_____

**5.** _____
_____

**6.** _____
_____

**7.** _____
_____

**8.** _____
_____

**9.** _____
_____

**10.** _____
_____

# Apply Your Knowledge

## Short Answer

Write the answer to each question on the lines provided.

1. **[LO22.2]** Provide at least six items that are the responsibility of the health-care administrator or practice manager.

_____

_____

_____

_____

2. **[LO22.1]** Explain the difference between the role of the physician and the physician assistant.

_____

_____

_____

3. **[LO22.4]** Explain the difference between risk management and quality assurance.

_____

_____

_____

_____

4. **[LO22.5]** Why is it recommended that an employee keep a copy of the documents that are provided for his or her personnel file? Documents include items such as immunizations, performance reviews, training and in-service.

_____

_____

_____

5. **[LO22.6]** Explain the purpose of a probationary period for a new employee.

_____

_____

_____

_____

**6.** [LO22.5] List at least five items that are included in a job description.

_____

_____

_____

_____

## Problem-Solving Activities

Follow the directions for each activity.

**1.** [LO22.2, LO22.5] Building a Training Checklist
   a. You have been asked to design a training checklist that will be used to ensure that all new employees of the medical clinic are trained and oriented in all necessary areas of the office practice.
   b. You will complete the following training checklist, filling in at least 20 items that should be included in a new employee orientation.

| TRAINING ITEM | TRAINER SIGNATURE/DATE COMPLETED | EMPLOYEE SIGNATURE/DATE COMPLETED |
|---|---|---|
| 1. | | |
| 2. | | |
| 3. | | |
| 4. | | |
| 5. | | |
| 6. | | |
| 7. | | |
| 8. | | |
| 9. | | |
| 10. | | |
| 11. | | |
| 12. | | |
| 13. | | |
| 14. | | |
| 15. | | |
| 16. | | |
| 17. | | |
| 18. | | |
| 19. | | |
| 20. | | |

**2.** [LO22.2] Staff Meeting Agenda
  a. Develop an agenda that will be used at the next staff meeting of the Total Care Clinic on Wednesday, November 14, 2012, at 2:00 P.M.
  b. Information to be presented at the meeting includes the following items. Organize the topics appropriately to develop the agenda.
   • Announce new physician starting at the clinic, Dr. James Thomas.
   • Approve prior minutes and agenda.
   • Update the status of the building renovation.
   • Announce that CPR class will be held next month for new employees.
   • Discuss the office hours during holiday as well as the holiday party.
   • Provide an update on EHR software implementation.

## Thinking Critically

Write your response to each case study question on the lines provided.

### Case 1 [LO22.5]

Anna and Stephanie, administrative medical assistants, have worked at the same medical clinic for over 5 years. A new employee, Greg, has been hired to work in the back office as a phlebotomist. During a lunch break in the employee lounge, Greg, Anna, and Stephanie engage in a conversation about dating since all three are single. Greg begins to make inappropriate comments about couples dating. These comments make Anna and Stephanie uncomfortable. They try to change the subject, but Greg continues to make inappropriate sexual comments about couples dating. Anna and Stephanie leave the employee lounge, and as they leave, Greg says, "What's the matter, girls? Can't you lighten up and have fun?"

**1.** What is the main problem with Greg's behavior?

_____

_____

_____

_____

**2.** How could situations like this be avoided in the workplace?

_____

_____

_____

_____

### Case 2 [LO22.6]

Marilyn's annual employee performance review is due next week. Her supervisor asks her to complete the Employee Review Input form. This is Marilyn's opportunity to provide her input about her job performance over the past year. She is asked to list her areas of weakness and her strengths. The employee is also asked to list continuing education that was completed over the past year. Marilyn realizes that she did not do any continuing education even though her employer requires at least 5 hours a year.

**1.** How should Marilyn respond to the continuing education section of the review?

_____

_____

_____

_____

**2.** Why do employers require medical personnel to participate in annual continuing education?

_____

_____

_____

_____

## Case 3 [LO22.3]

The practice manager has scheduled a training that will take place next week to update the employees on the use of MSDS forms. Being employed as an administrative medical assistant, Keith has never had to access these in the past and really does not understand their use.

**1.** How can Keith best prepare before attending this training?

_____

_____

_____

_____

**2.** What is the importance of understanding the use of MSDS forms in a medical practice?

_____

_____

_____

_____

# Demonstrate Your Knowledge

**Student Name:** _____

## Procedure 22–1: **Preparing an Agenda**

**GOAL:** To facilitate a meeting's organization and focus by providing a list of meeting topics, the name of the person reporting, and the order in which each topic will be addressed

**MATERIALS:** Paper and pen or computer, copy machine, minutes from last meeting

**METHOD:** To pass this procedure the minimum required score is _____ % or all elements must meet "satisfactory" ability on the final demonstration. The first box may be used as a practice or final demonstration, with the evaluator placing **S for Satisfactory** or **U for Unsatisfactory** if that is the grading criteria. The second box may be used as a final demonstration with a **grade point** written in the box.

| STEPS | POSSIBLE POINTS | S/U | POINTS EARNED |
|---|---|---|---|
| 1. Approximately 1 week before the meeting, e-mail or post a memo to staff offering them an opportunity to add items to the agenda. This is referred to as a *call for agenda items.* | 10 | | |
| 2. Place the following on top of the form used to create the agenda: <br>• Name of the practice <br>• Site name, if the practice has more than one location <br>• Title: "Staff Meeting Agenda" <br>• Date and time the meeting is scheduled to begin and end | 2<br><br>2<br>2<br><br>2 | | |
| 3. Many offices have standing topics that go on the agenda every month; add these to the agenda: <br>• Introduction of new staff members <br>• Approval of minutes if formal minutes are kept <br>• Staff news (promotions, birthdays, weddings, births, etc.) <br>• Quality assurance report <br>• Policy and procedure updates <br>• Committee reports <br>• Report from individuals who may have attended a conference | <br><br>1<br>1<br><br>1<br>1<br>1<br>1<br><br>1 | | |
| 4. Review the minutes from the previous meeting to determine any topics that required action with the person responsible. List these on the agenda under "Old Business." | 15 | | |
| 5. Add topics obtained from the *call for agenda items* and any new topics the manager wishes to discuss. List these under "New Business." | 10 | | |

*(Continued)*

| STEPS | POSSIBLE POINTS | S/U | POINTS EARNED |
|---|---|---|---|
| 6. Add "Other" on the agenda to allow for announcements or other brief information. | 5 | | |
| 7. Place the date and time of the next meeting at the end of the agenda. | 5 | | |
| 8. At least 1 week prior to the meeting, inform and verify people on the agenda who will present a topic at the meeting. | 15 | | |
| 9. Send agenda to staff members prior to the meeting. | 15 | | |
| 10. Make copies available at the staff meeting. | 10 | | |
| **Total Points (if applicable)** | 100 | | |

Comments: _____

_____

_____

Final Evaluator's Signature: _____

Date: _____

## CAAHEP Competencies Achieved

IV. C (9) Discuss applications of electronic technology in effective communication

V. P (7) Use Internet to access information related to the medical office

## ABHES Competencies Achieved

8. d. Apply concepts for office procedures

8. dd. Serve as a liaison between physician and others

8. hh. Receive, organize, prioritize, and transmit information expediently

8. ll. Apply electronic technology

Student Name: _____

## Procedure 22–2: Preparing a Travel Expense Report

Imagine that you attended the latest AAMA or AMT annual conference. Research the price of airfare from your locale to the city of the conference. Determine registration and other costs. Use these amounts to perform the procedure.

**GOAL:** To obtain reimbursement or account for pre-approved travel funds; to provide documentation of expenses for the medical office

**MATERIALS:** Travel expense form (Figure 22–6), pen receipts, conference Web site information, calculator (*Note:* A travel expense form is available at the end of this study guide.)

**METHOD:** To pass this procedure the minimum required score is _____% or all elements must meet "satisfactory" ability on the final demonstration. The first box may be used as a practice or final demonstration, with the evaluator placing **S for Satisfactory** or **U for Unsatisfactory** if that is the grading criteria. The second box may be used as a final demonstration with a **grade point** written in the box.

| STEPS | POSSIBLE POINTS | S/U | POINTS EARNED |
|---|---|---|---|
| 1. Ensure your travel has been approved. | 10 | | |
| 2. Save receipts from the event. | 10 | | |
| 3. Complete the personal identifying information on the form. | 10 | | |
| 4. Insert the purpose of the travel, the location, dates, and number of days. | 15 | | |
| 5. Place the amounts as labeled in the expense table. | 15 | | |
| 6. Total the amounts. | 10 | | |
| 7. Check the appropriate box to indicate if you missed work and the dates and amount of days. | 10 | | |
| 8. Sign and date the form. | 5 | | |
| 9. Attach receipts (generally, original receipts are submitted; keep copies for your own records). | 5 | | |
| 10. Submit completed form and receipts. | 10 | | |
| **Total Points (if applicable)** | 100 | | |

Comments: _____

_____

_____

Final Evaluator's Signature: _____

Date: _____

## CAAHEP Competencies Achieved

IV. C (9) Discuss applications of electronic technology in effective communication

V. P (7) Use Internet to access information related to the medical office

X. A (1) Apply ethical behaviors including honesty/integrity in the performance of medical assisting practice

## ABHES Competencies Achieved

8. d. Apply concepts for office procedures

8. hh. Receive, organize, prioritize, and transmit information expediently

8. ll. Apply electronic technology

Student Name: _____

## Procedure 22–3: Completing an Incident Report

**GOAL:** To provide documentation of an adverse occurrence or potential risk to facilitate investigation, correction, and aid in the avoidance of future occurrences

**MATERIALS:** Paper and pen, an incident report (Figure 22–9 may be used)
(*Note:* An incident report is available at the end of this study guide.)

**METHOD:** To pass this procedure the minimum required score is _____ % or all elements must meet "satisfactory" ability on the final demonstration. The first box may be used as a practice or final demonstration, with the evaluator placing **S for Satisfactory** or **U for Unsatisfactory** if that is the grading criteria. The second box may be used as a final demonstration with a **grade point** written in the box.

| STEPS | POSSIBLE POINTS | S/U | POINTS EARNED |
|---|---|---|---|
| After initial first aid and other appropriate assistive steps are taken: | | | |
| 1. Interview the person to whom the incident occurred, gathering the required facts as needed for the incident report, including contact information. | 25 | | |
| 2. Interview witnesses, gathering the required facts as needed for the incident report, including contact information. | 25 | | |
| 3. Ensure information is complete. | 10 | | |
| 4. Transfer the information to the incident report form. | 25 | | |
| 5. Review the form for accuracy and clarity. | 10 | | |
| 6. Submit the form to the appropriate supervisor. | 5 | | |
| **Total Points [if applicable]** | 100 | | |

Comments: _____

_____

_____

**Final Evaluator's Signature:** _____

**Date:** _____

## CAAHEP Competencies Achieved

X. A (1) Apply ethical behaviors including honesty/integrity in the performance of medical assisting practice

## ABHES Competencies Achieved

4. e. Perform risk management processes

8. d. Apply concepts for office procedures

8. hh. Receive, organize, prioritize, and transmit information expediently

# 23 Emergency Preparedness

## Test Your Knowledge

### Vocabulary Review

Match the key terms in the right column with the definitions in the left column by placing the letter of each correct answer in the space provided.

_____ **1.** the intentional release of a biologic agent with the intent to harm individuals

_____ **2.** a rolling device that holds emergency supplies and equipment

_____ **3.** the position a person is placed in after receiving first aid for choking or cardiopulmonary resuscitation

_____ **4.** to assess the urgency and types of conditions patients present as well as their immediate medical needs

_____ **5.** providing ventilation and blood circulation for a patient who shows none

_____ **6.** a condition that occurs when the blood supply to the brain is impaired; may cause temporary or permanent damage

_____ **7.** a network of qualified emergency services personnel who use community resources and equipment to provide emergency care to victims of injury or sudden illness

**a.** anaphylaxis [LO23.3]

**b.** automated external defibrillator (AED) [LO23.2]

**c.** bioterrorism [LO23.4]

**d.** cardiopulmonary resuscitation (CPR) [LO23.3]

**e.** crash cart [LO23.2]

**f.** emergency medical services (EMS) [LO23.1]

**g.** first aid [LO23.3]

**h.** recovery position [LO23.3]

**i.** stroke [LO23.3]

**j.** triage [LO23.3]

**k.** ventricular fibrillation (VF) [LO23.3]

_____ **8.** a severe allergic reaction, with symptoms that include respiratory distress, difficulty in swallowing, pallor, and a drastic drop in blood pressure that can lead to circulatory collapse

_____ **9.** immediate care given to someone who is injured or suddenly becomes ill, before complete medical care can be obtained

_____ **10.** an abnormal heart rhythm that is the most common cause of cardiac arrest

_____ **11.** a computerized defibrillator programmed to recognize lethal heart rhythms and deliver an electrical shock to restore a normal rhythm

## Multiple-Choice Certification Questions

There may be more than one answer; circle the letter of the choice that best completes each statement or answers each question.

**1.** [LO23.2] When you provide first aid to a patient who has an open cut on the hand, which of the following items do you need?
a. Sterile gauze and disposable gloves
b. Airway or mouthpiece
c. Ice pack and elastic bandages
d. Tweezers and scissors
e. Cold packs and antiseptic wipes

**2.** [LO23.3] The main symptom of choking is the
a. victim is having a seizure.
b. person is violently coughing.
c. victim is unable to speak.
d. victim's face is red.
e. victim's breathing is shallow and labored.

**3.** [LO23.4] During an emergency, what is the best way to remember how to operate a fire extinguisher?
a. Call the fire department and tell someone there that you need instructions immediately.
b. Find the safety manual and look up the instructions.
c. Ask a coworker who has been with the company for a long time how to operate it.
d. Remember the acronym "PASS," which stands for pull the pin, aim at the base of the fire, squeeze the trigger, and sweep side to side.
e. Locate the OSHA binder, determine what type of fire it is, then locate the instructions for use.

**4.** [LO23.3] If a patient has a fall from an examination table and cannot get up, you should
a. help the patient get up off the floor, then ask if they are hurt.
b. call EMS immediately.
c. instruct the patient not to move and get the physician in the exam room.
d. assist the patient off the floor and back to the exam table.
e. help the patient to a chair and document the incident in the patient's file.

5. **[LO23.3]** Why is it critical to control excessive external bleeding?
   a. The patient may experience an elevation of her blood pressure.
   b. Most offices do not have blood on hand for transfusion purposes.
   c. The patient may faint and fall down.
   d. It is hazardous to deal with excessive body fluids.
   e. The patient may go into shock due to the rapid blood loss.

6. **[LO23.3]** A patient who is hyperventilating may
   a. appear drowsy and lethargic.
   b. seem anxious and lightheaded.
   c. have slow, shallow breathing.
   d. appear normal and calm.
   e. have deep, slow breathing.

7. **[LO23.3]** Initial first aid for a nosebleed is to
   a. have the patient sit up and pinch the nostrils for at least 5 minutes.
   b. have the patient lie down so the blood will flow to the back of the throat.
   c. pack the nostrils with sterile gauze.
   d. apply ice to the back of the neck.
   e. place a cold compress on the forehead.

8. **[LO23.3]** Which of the following signs is *not* indicative of a foreign body airway obstruction in a responsive infant?
   a. Sudden onset of difficulty in breathing
   b. Inability to speak
   c. Inability to cry
   d. Blue lips
   e. Violent coughing

9. **[LO23.3]** The most significant problem for a patient experiencing anaphylactic shock is that the patient
   a. may have a weak pulse.
   b. will usually develop hives.
   c. becomes restless and has a headache.
   d. may have a life-threatening problem.
   e. may begin to experience swelling in the face.

10. **[LO23.3]** When a patient is vomiting, a serious complication might be
    a. nausea.
    b. chills.
    c. aspiration.
    d. fever.
    e. chest pain.

11. **[LO23.3]** The cardinal symptom of a heart attack is
    a. chest pain.
    b. pain in the abdomen.
    c. sweating.
    d. indigestion.
    e. jaw pain.

12. **[LO23.2]** Which of the following agencies provide CPR instruction?
    a. American Heart Association
    b. National Security Council
    c. American Red Cross
    d. Occupational Safety and Health Administration
    e. Answers (a) and (c).

13. **[LO23.3]** When a patient is in respiratory arrest, the patient will
   a. be choking.
   b. have shallow breathing.
   c. be hyperventilating.
   d. not be breathing.
   e. have difficulty breathing.

14. **[LO23.3]** When a patient collapses in the reception area and falls to the floor, you should first
   a. call EMS.
   b. check for responsiveness.
   c. start administering CPR.
   d. perform abdominal thrusts.
   e. put a pillow under the patient's head.

15. **[LO23.3]** When you administer CPR, the chest compressions should be delivered so the victim is receiving
   a. 60 compressions per minute.
   b. 80 compressions per minute.
   c. 90 compressions per minute.
   d. 100 compressions per minute.
   e. 120 compressions per minute.

16. **[LO23.4]** If there is a suspected bioterrorist attack in your facility, you should
   a. report to your local community command post.
   b. activate your fire alarm system.
   c. lock all the doors and go to your "shelter-in-place."
   d. inform your local health department of a suspected bioterrorism agent.
   e. turn off all electrical power to the facility.

17. **[LO23.4]** An example of an ideal location for the facility's "shelter-in-place" is
   a. an interior room with no windows.
   b. the lobby of the building.
   c. anywhere outside the building.
   d. the outside parking lot.
   e. none of the above.

18. **[LO23.2]** Which of the following is an electrical device that shocks the heart to restore normal beating?
   a. CVA
   b. MI
   c. AED
   d. PPE
   e. EMT

19. **[LO23.3]** Which of the following is the American Heart Association guideline for determining the age of a child or infant when administering first aid for choking?
   a. A child is between the ages of 7 and 11.
   b. An infant is a newborn up to 2 years of age.
   c. A child and infant are treated the same.
   d. An infant is younger than 1 year.
   e. A child is between the ages of 5 and 12.

20. **[LO23.2]** Which of the following would you *not* expect to find in the contents of a first aid kit?
   a. Analgesics, such as aspirin
   b. Benadryl
   c. Antiseptic spray
   d. Antibiotics, such as penicillin
   e. Glucose tablets or sugar source

**21.** [LO23.3] The most common abnormal rhythm that occurs during cardiac arrest is
   a. bradycardia.
   b. palpitation.
   c. tachycardia.
   d. atrial fibrillation.
   e. ventricular fibrillation.

**22.** [LO23.2] The primary reason for using PPE during an emergency is to
   a. be in compliance with state law.
   b. reduce the risk of exposing yourself to infection.
   c. follow the office protocol.
   d. be able to apply direct pressure to minimize blood loss.
   e. avoid post-exposure problems.

**23.** [LO23.3] Which of the following is the first sequential step in performing CPR?
   a. Check for breathing.
   b. Start compressions.
   c. Open the patient's airway.
   d. Start mouth-to-mouth breathing.
   e. Pinch the nose and administer two initial breaths.

**24.** [LO23.3] Which of the following is proper procedure when administering first aid for a choking infant?
   a. Position the infant on the back and administer five abdominal thrusts.
   b. Perform a blind finger sweep to see if you can feel the object in the infant's mouth.
   c. Administer back blows with the heel of your hand until the object is dislodged.
   d. Position the infant with the head higher than the chest and perform five chest thrusts.
   e. Alternate five back blows and five chest thrusts until the object is expelled.

**25.** [LO23.3] Which of the following would *not* be indicated for a patient who is vomiting?
   a. Administering intravenous fluids
   b. Putting on exam gloves
   c. Providing crackers and juice for the patient
   d. Documenting the characteristics of the vomit
   e. Determine if the patient is in pain or is nauseated

## True or False

Decide whether each statement is true or false. In the space at the left, write "T" for true or "F" for false. On the lines provided, rewrite the false statements to make them true.

_____ **1.** [LO23.3] The first sign of anaphylaxis usually comes from the patient's skin.

_____

_____ **2.** [LO23.3] A patient in the reception area may have chest pain that could indicate he is about to have a seizure.

_____

_____ **3.** [LO23.2] A pocket mask or mouth shield is necessary to use when performing the procedure to remove a foreign body airway obstruction in a responsive infant.

_____

_____ **4.** [LO23.3] If a choking victim is pregnant or obese, you will need to place your arms around the abdomen and perform thrusts until the object is expelled.

_____

_____ **5.** [LO23.3] After receiving first aid for choking or CPR, the person should be positioned in the recovery position.

_____

_____ **6.** [LO23.4] Bioterrorism is an intentional act of releasing a biologic agent that will cause harm to individuals.

_____

_____ **7.** [LO23.2] Smoking is not a fire hazard as long as it takes place in a designated smoking area.

_____

_____ **8.** [LO23.3] If a patient falls in the office but only has a small bump, be sure to notify the doctor, who will probably examine the patient.

_____

_____ **9.** [LO23.3] When a patient arrives at your medical facility with an open bleeding wound, you should determine the extent of the injury, send them to the local emergency room, and then notify your physician.

_____

_____ **10.** [LO23.3] It is inappropriate to perform a blind finger sweep on an adult who has a foreign body airway obstruction and is unconscious.

_____

## Sentence Completion

In the space provided, write the word or phrase that best completes each sentence.

**1.** [LO23.1] During an emergency, the administrative medical assistant will frequently be needed to contact the _____ _____ _____ or _____ the patient care given during an emergency.

**1.** _____

_____

**2.** [LO23.3] When administering first aid or emergency treatment, follow _____ _____ and assume that _____ blood and body fluids are _____ with bloodborne pathogens.

**2.** _____

_____

**3.** [LO23.4] When you perform triage during a disaster, you give each injured victim a tag that classifies the person as _____, needing immediate care; _____ needing care within several hours; _____, needing care when time is not critical; or _____.

**4.** [LO23.3] Choking occurs when food or a foreign object blocks a person's _____ or _____.

**5.** [LO23.4] In a medical facility, fire hazards can include _____ electrical wires, _____ outlets, and _____ grounded plugs.

**6.** [LO23.4] An evacuation route provides a safe way out of a building during an emergency, so you need to learn the location of fire _____, fire _____, and fire _____ in relation to the exam room.

**7.** [LO23.1] When you contact the EMS, do not hang up until the _____ gives you _____ to do so.

**8.** [LO23.2] When a patient falls from a chair or an examining table, you will document the _____, the _____, and the _____ in the patient's chart.

**9.** [LO23.3] When a person has severe vomiting, it can lead to _____ and dangerous changes in electrolyte levels.

**10.** [LO23.3] To properly perform abdominal thrusts on a responsive adult, position yourself behind the patient and place your fist against the _____ just above the navel and below the _____ _____.

**3.** _____

**4.** _____

**5.** _____

**6.** _____

**7.** _____

**8.** _____

**9.** _____

**10.** _____

# Apply Your Knowledge

## Short Answer

Write the answer to each question on the lines provided.

**1.** [LO23.3] List five benefits to providing prompt and appropriate first aid.

_____

_____

_____

**2.** [LO23.1] Provide six telephone numbers that you should have posted in your facility that might be required in an urgent or emergency situation.

_____

_____

_____

**3.** [LO23.2] List five items that need to be documented in the patient's chart following an emergency that resulted in the patient being transported to the hospital.

_____

_____

_____

**4.** [LO23.2] List three main guidelines you must adhere to when dealing with any emergency.

_____

_____

_____

**5.** [LO23.3] When an administrative medical assistant needs to take charge of an emergency, there are several items that help form a general impression of the patient. List five of these items.

_____

_____

_____

## Problem-Solving Activities

Follow the directions for each activity.

**1.** [LO23.3] Performing an Emergency Assessment
   a. Using the Progress Notes form on the facing page, chart the appropriate entry for the following scenario. Below the charting entry, explain how you handled the incident and what equipment, if any, was needed.
   b. Patient: Mary Burns, 46 years old, is seated in a chair in the reception area. As she got up from the chair, she tripped over her purse that was sitting on the floor, and she fell down, hitting her forehead on the coffee table. There were no other persons in the area at the time. You were the only one that witnessed the event. Ms. Burns has a bump on her forehead where she hit the coffee table. There is a small amount of blood on the floor. She states that she is light-headed and feels dizzy.

**Total Care Clinic**
Progress Notes

Name: _____ Chart #: _____

| DATE | |
|------|---|
| | |
| | |
| | |
| | |
| | |
| | |
| | |
| | |
| | |
| | |
| | |
| | |
| | |
| | |
| | |
| | |
| | |
| | |

2. **[LO23.3]** Controlling Bleeding
   a. Using the Progress Notes form below, chart the appropriate entry for the following scenario. Below the charting entry, explain how you handled the incident and what equipment, if any, was needed.
   b. There is construction work taking place in your medical building, and one of the workers rushes into your office with his hand wrapped in a handkerchief soaked with blood. He states that he just cut his hand with his circular saw. The reception area has several patients waiting to see the doctor.

**Total Care Clinic**
Progress Notes

Name: _____ Chart #: _____

| DATE | |
|------|---|
| | |
| | |
| | |
| | |
| | |
| | |
| | |
| | |
| | |
| | |
| | |
| | |
| | |
| | |
| | |
| | |
| | |
| | |
| | |

# Thinking Critically

Write your response to each case study question on the lines provided.

## Case 1 [LO23.3]

You and a co-worker are having lunch in a local restaurant. Across the dining room you hear a commotion at one of the tables. A man appears to be choking. A woman who is with him is slapping him on the back.

**1.** What, if anything, should you do?

_____

_____

_____

**2.** What are the typical signs or symptoms of choking?

_____

_____

_____

## Case 2 [LO23.3]

A patient has just seen the physician and is at the reception desk checking out. She states that her skin is itchy and she feels warm. Her face appears red and she is having difficulty breathing. You have a copy of her encounter form in your hand and see that she was treated for a sore throat, had a throat culture performed, and received an injection of penicillin.

**1.** What might be the cause of this patient's distress?

_____

_____

_____

**2.** How should you respond to assist the patient in this situation?

_____

_____

_____

## Case 3 [LO23.3]

Mrs. Miller has brought her 7-year-old son, Michael, to see the physician about his seasonal allergies. You do the preliminary charting and place them in an examination room to wait for the physician. In a few minutes the mother runs to the front desk and says her son has a nosebleed that won't stop. She said he is lying on the examination table and when he tries to sit up a lot of blood keeps flowing from his nose.

1. What should you do to assist Michael with the nosebleed?

_____

_____

_____

2. After you provide immediate care for the patient, what, if anything, needs to be documented?

_____

_____

_____

# Demonstrate Your Knowledge

**Student Name:** _____

## Procedure 23–1: Contacting Emergency Medical Services System

**GOAL:** To contact emergency medical services quickly and efficiently when an emergency occurs

**MATERIALS:** Telephone

**METHOD:** To pass this procedure the minimum required score is _____% or all elements must meet "satisfactory" ability on the final demonstration. The first box may be used as a practice or final demonstration, with the evaluator placing **S for Satisfactory** or **U for Unsatisfactory** if that is the grading criteria. The second box may be used as a final demonstration with a **grade point** written in the box.

| STEPS | POSSIBLE POINTS | S/U | POINTS EARNED |
|---|---|---|---|
| 1. Call 911 or the appropriate number. Emergency numbers should be posted by the telephone for quick access. | 10 | | |
| 2. Relax and speak clearly and calmly to the dispatcher. | 10 | | |
| 3. Be prepared to provide the following information: <br>a. Your name, telephone number, and location <br>b. Nature of the emergency <br>c. Number of people in need of help, condition of the injured or ill patient(s) <br>d. Summary of the first aid that has been given <br>e. Directions on how to reach the location of the emergency | 10<br>10<br><br>10<br><br>10<br><br>10 | | |
| 4. Ensure that the dispatcher has all needed information. | 10 | | |
| 5. Do not hang up until the dispatcher gives you permission to do so. | 10 | | |
| 6. Notify other personnel that the EMS has been contacted and when they are expected to arrive. | 10 | | |
| **Total Points (if applicable)** | 100 | | |

**Comments:** _____

_____

_____

**Final Evaluator's Signature:** _____

**Date:** _____

## CAAHEP Competencies Achieved

XI. A (1) Recognize the effects of stress on all persons involved in emergency situations

## ABHES Competencies Achieved

8. ee. Use proper telephone techniques

9. e. Recognize emergencies and treatments and minor office surgical procedures

## Procedure 23-2: Foreign Body Airway Obstruction in a Responsive Adult or Child

**GOAL:** To correctly relieve a foreign body from the airway of an adult or child

**OSHA GUIDELINES:** This procedure does not involve exposure to blood, body fluids, or tissues

**MATERIALS:** Choking adult or child patient.
Caution: *Never perform this procedure on someone who is not choking.*

**METHOD:** To pass this procedure the minimum required score is _____% or all elements must meet "satisfactory" ability on the final demonstration. The first box may be used as a practice or final demonstration, with the evaluator placing **S for Satisfactory** or **U for Unsatisfactory** if that is the grading criteria. The second box may be used as a final demonstration with a **grade point** written in the box.

| STEPS | POSSIBLE POINTS | S/U | POINTS EARNED |
|---|---|---|---|
| 1. Ask, "Are you choking?" If the answer is "Yes," indicated by a nod of the head or some other sign, ask, "Can you speak?" If the answer is "No," tell the patient that you can help. A choking person cannot speak, cough, or breathe, and exhibits the universal sign of choking. If the patient is coughing, observe him closely to see if he clears the object. If he is not coughing or stops coughing, use abdominal thrusts. | 10 | | |
| 2. Position yourself behind the patient. Place your fist against the abdomen just above the navel and below the xiphoid process. | 10 | | |
| 3. Grasp your fist with your other hand, and provide quick inward and upward thrusts into the patient's abdomen (Figure 23–6). The thrust should be sufficient to move enough air from the lungs so that the object can be displaced from the airway. Note: If a pregnant or obese person is choking, you will need to place your arms around the chest and perform thrusts over the center of the breastbone (Figure 23–7). | 10 | | |
| 4. Continue the thrusts until the object is expelled or the patient becomes unresponsive. | 15 | | |
| 5. If the patient becomes unresponsive, call EMS and position the patient on his back. | 15 | | |
| 6. Use the head tilt–chin lift to open the patient's airway. | 10 | | |

*(Continued)*

| STEPS | POSSIBLE POINTS | S/U | POINTS EARNED |
|---|---|---|---|
| 7. Look into the mouth. If you see the foreign body, remove it using your index finger. **Do not perform any blind finger sweeps on a child** (Figure 23–8). | 15 | | |
| 8. Open the airway and look, listen, and feel for breathing. If the patient is not breathing, attempt a rescue breath. Observe the chest. If it does not rise with the breath, reposition the airway and administer another rescue breath. If the chest does not rise after the second attempt, assume that the airway is still blocked and begin CPR (Procedure 23–5). | 15 | | |
| **Total Points (if applicable)** | 100 | | |

Comments: _____

_____

_____

Final Evaluator's Signature: _____

Date: _____

## CAAHEP Competencies Achieved

XI. P (9) Maintain provider/professional level CPR certification

XI. P (10) Perform first aid procedures

## ABHES Competencies Achieved

9. e. Recognize emergencies and treatments and minor office surgical procedures

9. o. Perform:

    (5) First aid and CPR

## Procedure 23-3: Foreign Body Airway Obstruction in a Responsive Infant

**GOAL:** To correctly relieve a foreign body from the airway of an infant

**OSHA GUIDELINES:** This procedure does not involve exposure to blood, body fluids, or tissues

**MATERIALS:** Choking infant.
Caution: *Never perform this procedure on an infant who is not choking.*

**METHOD:** To pass this procedure the minimum required score is _____ % or all elements must meet "satisfactory" ability on the final demonstration. The first box may be used as a practice or final demonstration, with the evaluator placing **S for Satisfactory** or **U for Unsatisfactory** if that is the grading criteria. The second box may be used as a final demonstration with a **grade point** written in the box.

| STEPS | POSSIBLE POINTS | S/U | POINTS EARNED |
|---|---|---|---|
| 1. Assess the infant for signs of severe or complete airway obstruction, which include<br>a. sudden onset of difficulty in breathing.<br>b. inability to speak, make sounds, or cry.<br>c. a high-pitched, noisy, wheezing sound, or no sounds while inhaling.<br>d. weak, ineffective coughs.<br>e. blue lips or skin. | 9 | | |
| 2. Hold the infant with his head down, supporting the body with your forearm. His legs should straddle your forearm, and you should support his jaw and head with your hand and fingers. This is best done in a sitting or kneeling position (Figure 23-9). | 9 | | |
| 3. Give up to five back blows with the heel of your free hand, as shown in Figure 23-9. Strike the infant's back forcefully between the shoulder blades. At any point if the object is expelled, discontinue the back blows. | 9 | | |
| 4. If the obstruction is not cleared, turn the infant over as a unit, supporting the head with your hands and the body between your forearms (Figure 23-10). | 9 | | |
| 5. Keep the head lower than the chest and perform five chest thrusts. Place two fingers over the breastbone (sternum), above the xiphoid. Give five quick chest thrusts about ½ to 1 inch deep. Stop the compressions if the object is expelled. | 9 | | |
| 6. Alternate five back blows and five chest thrusts until the object is expelled or until the infant becomes unconscious. If the infant becomes unconscious, call EMS or have someone do it for you. | 9 | | |

*(Continued)*

| STEPS | POSSIBLE POINTS | S/U | POINTS EARNED |
|---|---|---|---|
| 7. Open the infant's mouth by grasping both the tongue and the lower jaw between the thumb and fingers, and pull up the lower jawbone. *If you see the object, remove it using your smallest finger.* **Do not use blind finger sweeps on an infant. A blind finger sweep may push the object deeper into the airway.** | 9 | | |
| 8. Open the airway and attempt to provide rescue breaths. If the chest does not rise, reposition the airway (both head and chin) and try to provide another rescue breath. | 9 | | |
| 9. If the rescue breaths are unsuccessful, begin CPR. Hold the infant, supporting her body with your forearm and her head with your hand and fingers. Deliver 30 chest compressions about ½ to 1 inch deep. | 9 | | |
| 10. Open the infant's mouth and look for the foreign object. If you see an object, remove it with your smallest finger. | 10 | | |
| 11. Open the airway and attempt to provide rescue breaths. If the chest does not rise, continue CPR until the doctor or EMS arrives. | 9 | | |
| **Total Points (if applicable)** | 100 | | |

**Comments:** _____

_____

_____

**Final Evaluator's Signature:** _____

**Date:** _____

## CAAHEP Competencies Achieved

XI. P (9) Maintain provider/professional level CPR certification

XI. P (10) Perform first aid procedures

## ABHES Competencies Achieved

9. e. Recognize emergencies and treatments and minor office surgical procedures

9. o. Perform:

   (5) First aid and CPR

## Procedure 23-4: Caring for a Patient Who Is Vomiting

**GOAL:** To increase comfort and minimize complications, such as aspiration, for a patient who is vomiting

**MATERIALS:** Emesis basin, cool compress, cup of cool water, paper tissues or a towel, and (if ordered) intravenous fluids and electrolytes and an antinausea drug

**METHOD:** To pass this procedure the minimum required score is _____% or all elements must meet "satisfactory" ability on the final demonstration. The first box may be used as a practice or final demonstration, with the evaluator placing **S for Satisfactory** or **U for Unsatisfactory** if that is the grading criteria. The second box may be used as a final demonstration with a **grade point** written in the box.

| STEPS | POSSIBLE POINTS | S/U | POINTS EARNED |
|---|---|---|---|
| 1. Wash your hands and put on exam gloves and other PPE. | 12 | | |
| 2. Ask the patient when and how the vomiting started and how frequently it occurs. Find out whether she is nauseated or in pain. | 12 | | |
| 3. Give the patient an emesis basin to collect vomit. Observe and document its amount, color, odor, and consistency. Particularly note blood, bile, undigested food, or feces in the vomit. | 12 | | |
| 4. Place a cool compress on the patient's forehead to make her more comfortable. Offer water and paper tissues or a towel to clean her mouth. | 12 | | |
| 5. Monitor for signs of dehydration, such as confusion, irritability, and flushed, dry skin. Also monitor for signs of electrolyte imbalances, such as leg cramps or an irregular pulse. | 16 | | |
| 6. If requested, assist by laying out supplies and equipment for the physician to use in administering intravenous fluids and electrolytes. Administer an antinausea drug if prescribed. | 12 | | |
| 7. Prepare the patient for diagnostic tests if instructed. | 12 | | |
| 8. Remove the gloves and wash your hands. | 12 | | |
| **Total Points (if applicable)** | 100 | | |

**Comments:** _____

_____

_____

**Final Evaluator's Signature:** _____

**Date:** _____

## CAAHEP Competencies Achieved

III. P (3) Select appropriate barrier/personal protective equipment (PPE) for potentially infectious situations

IV. P (6) Prepare a patient for procedures and/or treatments

XI. P (10) Perform first aid procedures

## ABHES Competencies Achieved

9. e. Recognize emergencies and treatments and minor office surgical procedures

9. o. Perform:

    (5) First aid and CPR

9. q. Instruct patients with special needs

## Procedure 23–5: Performing Cardiopulmonary Resuscitation (CPR)

**GOAL:** To provide ventilation and blood circulation for a patient who shows none

**MATERIALS:** Mouth shield or, if not in the office, a piece of plastic with a hole for the mouth

**METHOD:** To pass this procedure the minimum required score is _____% or all elements must meet "satisfactory" ability on the final demonstration. The first box may be used as a practice or final demonstration, with the evaluator placing **S for Satisfactory** or **U for Unsatisfactory** if that is the grading criteria. The second box may be used as a final demonstration with a **grade point** written in the box.

| STEPS | POSSIBLE POINTS | S/U | POINTS EARNED |
|---|---|---|---|
| 1. Assess the area for safety, put on gloves if available. Check responsiveness. <br> • Tap shoulder <br> • Ask, "Are you OK?" | 10 | | |
| 2. Call 911 or the local emergency number, or have someone place the call for you, according to these guidelines. For sudden collapse: call EMS first, get AED, start CPR, use AED. For drowning or other arrest due to lack of oxygen: perform 2 minutes of CPR first, call EMS, resume CPR/AED. | 10 | | |
| 3. Place the heel of one hand on the patient's sternum between the nipples. Place your other hand over the first, interlacing your fingers (Figure 23–11). | 10 | | |
| 4. Give 30 chest compressions at least 2 inches deep. You should compress the chest hard and fast (at least 100 compressions per minute) (Figure 23–12). Give compressions of sufficient depth and rate and allow chest recoil with minimal interruptions in compressions. Rapid chest compression increases the likelihood of blood reaching the brain and other vital tissues. | 15 | | |
| 5. Open the patient's airway. <br> • Tilt the patient's head back, using the head tilt-chin lift maneuver (Figure 23–13). <br> • For a trauma victim, use jaw thrust to open airway; only use head tilt-chin lift if jaw thrust is not effective. <br> Simply opening the airway may cause the patient to start breathing again. | 15 | | |

*(Continued)*

| STEPS | POSSIBLE POINTS | S/U | POINTS EARNED |
|---|---|---|---|
| 6. Check for breathing.<br> • If the patient is not breathing or has inadequate breathing, position the patient on his back and give two rescue breaths, each one second long. Each breath should cause the chest to rise. When giving rescue breaths, use one of three methods:<br> a. Mouth-to-mouth or mouth-to-nose rescue breathing (Figures 23–14 and 23–15). Using a face shield, place your mouth around the patient's mouth and pinch the nose, or close the patient's mouth and place your mouth around the patient's nose.<br> b. Mouth to mask device (Figure 23–16)<br> c. Bag-mask ventilation (Figure 23–17). Ensure the adequate rise and fall of the patient's chest. If his chest does not rise, reposition the airway and try again. If on the second attempt the chest does not rise, your patient may have an airway obstruction. See Procedure 23–2. Rapid chest compression increases the likelihood of blood reaching the brain and other vital tissues. | 15 | | |
| 7. Continue cycles of 30:2 until the patient begins to move, an AED is available, qualified help arrives, or you are too exhausted to continue. | 15 | | |
| 8. If the patient starts moving, check for breathing. If the patient is breathing adequately, put him in the recovery position and monitor him until the doctor or EMS arrives. | 10 | | |
| **Total Points (if applicable)** | 100 | | |

Comments: _____

_____

_____

**Final Evaluator's Signature:** _____

**Date:** _____

## CAAHEP Competencies Achieved

XI. P (9) Maintain provider/professional level CPR certification

XI. P (10) Perform first aid procedures

## ABHES Competencies Achieved

9. e. Recognize emergencies and treatments and minor office surgical procedures

9. o. Perform:

   (5) First aid and CPR

Student Name: _____

## Procedure 23–6: Assisting with Triage in a Disaster

**GOAL:** To prioritize disaster victims

**MATERIALS:** Disaster tag and pen

**METHOD:** To pass this procedure the minimum required score is _____% or all elements must meet "satisfactory" ability on the final demonstration. The first box may be used as a practice or final demonstration, with the evaluator placing **S for Satisfactory** or **U for Unsatisfactory** if that is the grading criteria. The second box may be used as a final demonstration with a **grade point** written in the box.

| STEPS | POSSIBLE POINTS | S/U | POINTS EARNED |
|---|---|---|---|
| 1. Wash your hands and put on exam gloves and other PPE if available. | 10 | | |
| 2. Tag victims by type of injury and need for care, classifying them as emergent, urgent, nonurgent, or dead. Sorting of the victims, completed by clinical personnel, allows for rapid treatment based on need. | 20 | | |
| 3. Label the emergent patients no. 1, and send them to appropriate treatment stations immediately. Emergent patients, such as those who are in shock or who are hemorrhaging, need immediate care. | 20 | | |
| 4. Label the urgent patients no. 2, and send them to basic first-aid stations. Urgent patients need care within the next several hours. Such patients may have lacerations that can be dressed quickly to stop the bleeding but can wait for suturing. | 20 | | |
| 5. Label nonurgent patients no. 3, and send them to volunteers who will be empathic and provide refreshments. Nonurgent patients are those for whom timing of treatment is not critical, such as patients who have no physical injuries but who are emotionally upset. | 15 | | |
| 6. Label patients who are dead no. 4. Ensure that the bodies are moved to an area where they will be safe until they can be identified and proper action can be taken. | 15 | | |
| **Total Points (if applicable)** | 100 | | |

**Comments:** _____

_____

_____

**Final Evaluator's Signature:** _____

**Date:** _____

### CAAHEP Competency Achieved

XI. P (6) Participate in a mock environmental exposure event with documentation of steps taken

### ABHES Competencies Achieved

2. c. Assist the physician with the regimen of diagnostic and treatment modalities as they relate to each body system

9. e. Recognize emergencies and treatments and minor office surgical procedures

# 24 The Externship and Employment Search

## Test Your Knowledge

### Vocabulary Review

Match the key terms in the right column with the definitions in the left column by placing the letter of each correct answer in the space provided.

_____ **1.** making contacts with relatives, friends, and acquaintances that may have information about finding a job in your field

_____ **2.** a résumé that is focused on a specific job

_____ **3.** a recommendation for employment

_____ **4.** experiential learning by students having an opportunity to hone skills in the work setting while earning school credit

_____ **5.** a type of critique aimed at giving an individual feedback to improve performance

_____ **6.** a mentor or teacher

_____ **7.** the representative of the school who ensures scheduling and monitoring of students for a practicum

_____ **8.** a contract between the school and externship site

_____ **9.** groups considered at risk for coercion and exploitation such as children, elderly, and persons with special needs

**a.** targeted résumé [LO24.4]

**b.** constructive criticism [LO24.2]

**c.** externship coordinator [LO24.1]

**d.** preceptor [LO24.1]

**e.** reference [LO24.3]

**f.** networking [LO24.3]

**g.** affiliation agreement [LO24.1]

**h.** externship [LO24.1]

**i.** vulnerable populations [LO24.5]

# Multiple-Choice Certification Questions

There may be more than one answer; circle the letter of the choice that best completes each statement or answers each question.

**1.** [LO24.1] Two of the recognized accrediting agencies for allied health programs are
  a. AHIMA and CAAHEP.
  b. the AMA and ABHES.
  c. CAAHEP and the CDC.
  d. OSHA and ABHES.
  e. ABHES and CAAHEP.

**2.** [LO24.3] Most classified ads for an administrative medical assistant position will include
  a. the expected salary for the position.
  b. a copy of the job description.
  c. the experience preferred for the position.
  d. the type and name of insurance provided by the employer.
  e. the number of paid holidays offered to the employee.

**3.** [LO24.3] One of the easiest and most effective ways to network is to
  a. become a member of a church group.
  b. call former classmates who are also unemployed.
  c. search the Internet on Craigslist.
  d. join a professional organization and attend its meetings.
  e. talk with your neighbors.

**4.** [LO24.4] Which of the following is information that should be included on your résumé to help a prospective employer know who you are and what you can offer?
  a. Your favorite hobbies and pastimes
  b. The number of children you have and their ages
  c. Your physical characteristics such as height and weight
  d. Awards and honors you have received related to your career
  e. Your personal travel experiences

**5.** [LO24.1] When an educational institution partners with a medical facility to provide an externship experience for a student, they will sign a contract known as a/an
  a. liability agreement.
  b. externship contract.
  c. affiliation agreement.
  d. indemnity clause.
  e. contractual agreement.

**6.** [LO24.1] A practicum is another term for
  a. coordinator.
  b. externship.
  c. instructor.
  d. supervisor.
  e. preceptor.

**7.** [LO24.2] When an externship coordinator is placing students at externship sites, one of the most important criteria to consider is whether
  a. the office is open 5 days a week.
  b. the clinic can provide a minimum of 40 hours per week.
  c. the facility staff will sign the student's time card.
  d. the site is best suited for the student.
  e. the site will give the student a passing grade and evaluation.

**8.** [LO24.2] If an extern student knows that he will be absent on a particular day during the externship course, the student should
   a. ask to be pulled off the site and be assigned to a new site.
   b. not show up on that day but talk to the preceptor the next day.
   c. notify the preceptor in advance of the planned absence.
   d. call the externship coordinator when he returns to the site the next day.
   e. notify another student in the class and have that person contact the school.

**9.** [LO24.2] Of the following procedures, which one cannot be compromised at all while at the externship site?
   a. Wearing the school badge
   b. Completing a minimum of 40 hours a week
   c. Asking only the externship coordinator if there are questions about the facility's policies
   d. Maintaining perfect attendance with no absences or being late
   e. Observing HIPAA compliance

**10.** [LO24.2] Which of the following actions would be considered an act of fraud?
   a. Hanging up on an angry patient
   b. Falsifying a time card
   c. Claiming that you don't know the answer to a patient's question
   d. Forgetting to call your preceptor when you are going to be absent
   e. Performing a procedure without the preceptor observing you

**11.** [LO24.2] Which of the following guidelines would benefit the externship student?
   a. Bringing breakfast to the extern office so as not to be late
   b. Sitting back and waiting to be asked to participate in a procedure
   c. Utilizing time management skills
   d. Working outside your scope of practice
   e. Being aggressive, not assertive, with the office staff to get your hours completed

**12.** [LO24.2] It is appropriate to discuss the patients from your externship
   a. with your preceptor at the medical facility.
   b. at home because your family probably does not personally know the patients.
   c. with other students back at school.
   d. at a local restaurant with your friends.
   e. with the career services personnel at your school.

**13.** [LO24.2] As an extern, if you are uncomfortable about the way a procedure is performed at the site, you should
   a. not ask the preceptor because this will appear as if you are argumentative.
   b. talk with another student from the school to confirm the performance of the procedure.
   c. discuss the procedure with the externship coordinator.
   d. look up the information on the Internet.
   e. tell the preceptor that you can only perform it the way you were taught at school.

**14.** [LO24.4] The purpose of a cover letter is to
   a. state your salary expectations.
   b. recap your work experience.
   c. list your references.
   d. introduce your résumé.
   e. list your available times for an interview.

**15.** [LO24.3] Appropriate references include all the following *except*
   a. your preceptor.
   b. a family member.
   c. an instructor.
   d. the extern site physician.
   e. a former employer.

**16.** [LO24.5] The appropriate time to discuss the employment salary is
   a. when you are offered the job.
   b. after the interview.
   c. before you schedule the interview.
   d. after you accept the job.
   e. when you call inquiring about the job.

**17.** [LO24.5] Which of the following is an inappropriate question for an interviewer to ask?
   a. What shifts are you available to work?
   b. How well do you work under pressure?
   c. What are your long-term goals?
   d. Are you able to work overtime occasionally?
   e. Do you have plans to start a family?

**18.** [LO24.3, 24.5] Your references should be
   a. listed on the résumé after your education information.
   b. included on a separate sheet of paper.
   c. contacted during the interview.
   d. discussed during the interview, stating what they would say about you.
   e. sent in a cover letter and résumé to familiarize the employer with your work history.

**19.** [LO24.4] In your cover letter, you should
   a. restate what is on your résumé.
   b. list your references.
   c. discuss your academic history including high school.
   d. refer to the enclosed résumé.
   e. tell the reader that you will stop by to meet him or her and schedule an interview.

**20.** [LO24.4] Which of the following is the best example of a professional objective for an administrative medical assistant?
   a. To secure a position where I can gain increasing responsibility
   b. To fulfill my immediate need for a job
   c. To work with patients in need
   d. To understand the field of medicine and diseases
   e. To work with physicians

**21.** [LO24.4] Characteristics of a good résumé include
   a. at least six references listed at the beginning of the first page.
   b. a list of memberships and affiliations connected to the field of application.
   c. your education background listing your high school first and your highest level of education at the bottom of the list.
   d. a full narrative overview of each position you have held, including those unconnected to the field in which you are applying.
   e. your signature at the end of the résumé verifying the truthfulness of the information.

**22.** [LO24.1] When an externship coordinator is determining the adequacy of a site for externship, one major consideration is the
   a. type of insurance the facility accepts.
   b. safety of the medical environment.
   c. brand of EHR software the facility uses.
   d. type of public transportation available to the site.
   e. site's willingness to hire the student upon completion.

# True or False

Decide whether each statement is true or false. In the space at the left, write "T" for true or "F" for false. On the lines provided, rewrite the false statements to make them true.

_____ **1.** **[LO24.1]** Extern students are not paid but usually receive educational credit for completion of the course.

_____

_____ **2.** **[LO24.1]** The externship must be completed at the end of the program.

_____

_____ **3.** **[LO24.1]** The externship site is responsible for retaining complete care of the patient.

_____

_____ **4.** **[LO24.2]** The extern student is required to maintain professional behavior most of the time.

_____

_____ **5.** **[LO24.3]** Employment services are an excellent way to gain experience and select a position.

_____

_____ **6.** **[LO24.4]** As you learn new administrative skills, you should update your résumé to reflect these skills.

_____

_____ **7.** **[LO24.3]** Joining a professional organization and attending conferences are the most difficult ways to network.

_____

_____ **8.** **[LO24.2]** Poor behaviors should be addressed prior to the externship, and students should not believe that improvement will be made while on-site.

_____

_____ **9.** **[LO24.2]** If an extern student is uncertain about her progress, she should wait until the end of the extern course and then discuss her progress with the externship coordinator.

_____

_____ **10.** **[LO24.2, 24.5]** Personal cell phones should be turned off at all times except during lunch and breaks.

_____

## Sentence Completion

In the space provided, write the word or phrase that best completes each sentence.

1. **[LO24.4]** Cover letters are as important as your _____ in your job search.

2. **[LO24.3]** It is professional to always _____ before you list someone as a reference.

3. **[LO24.4]** The appropriate colored paper for a résumé is _____, _____, or _____.

4. **[LO24.1]** The _____, the _____, and the _____ all have responsibilities associated with the externship.

5. **[LO24.2]** Externs with the best hands-on skills have been unsuccessful and given poor evaluations due to _____ in the "_____ _____" or professional behaviors.

6. **[LO24.5]** Focus on how you can benefit the organization, and do not ask about _____, or _____ until you are offered the position.

1. _____
   _____

2. _____
   _____

3. _____
   _____

4. _____
   _____

5. _____
   _____

6. _____
   _____

# Apply Your Knowledge

## Short Answer

Write the answer to each question on the lines provided.

1. **[LO24.2]** Explain the significance of grading professional behaviors demonstrated during the externship.

   _____

   _____

   _____

   _____

2. **[LO24.3]** List five resources to use in a job search.

   _____

   _____

   _____

   _____

**3.** [LO24.1] List five responsibilities of the student during the externship experience.

_____

_____

_____

_____

**4.** [LO24.4] Explain why a cover letter is essential to include with a mailed résumé.

_____

_____

_____

_____

**5.** [LO24.5] List five reasons why a person would not be hired.

_____

_____

_____

_____

## Problem-Solving Activities

Follow the directions for each activity.

1. **[LO24.2]** Completing an Externship Time Card
   a. On the following externship time card form, fill in the appropriate hours completed for a 1-week time period, total the number of hours, and review for submission to the preceptor for signature.
   b. Monday, September 6—arrived at clinic at 7:50 A.M., put away personal items, checked in with preceptor at 8:00 A.M. Took lunch break from 12:30 P.M. to 1:30 P.M. Left clinic at 4:50 P.M.
   c. Tuesday, September 7—arrived at clinic at 7:45 A.M., checked in with preceptor at 7:45 A.M. to learn how to remove clinic telephones from answering service. Lunch break from 11:30 A.M. to 12:30 P.M., left at 5:15 P.M. after last patient checked out.
   d. Wednesday, September 8—arrived at clinic at 8:15 A.M., left at 11:45 A.M., went home for the day due to illness.
   e. Thursday, September 9—arrived at clinic at 7:55 A.M., lunch break 12:00 P.M. to 12:45 P.M., left clinic at 5:00 P.M.
   f. Friday, September 10—arrived at school at 7:00 A.M. to meet with extern coordinator, arrived at clinic at 8:15 A.M., lunch break 1:00 P.M. to 1:30 P.M., left clinic at 5:30 P.M.

| DAY/DATE | HOURS | DAILY | IN/OUT |
|---|---|---|---|
| Mon |  | Total | In |
|  |  |  | Out |
|  |  |  | In |
|  |  |  | Out |
| Tue |  | Total | In |
|  |  |  | Out |
|  |  |  | In |
|  |  |  | Out |
| Wed |  | Total | In |
|  |  |  | Out |
|  |  |  | In |
|  |  |  | Out |
| Thurs |  | Total | In |
|  |  |  | Out |
|  |  |  | In |
|  |  |  | Out |
| Fri |  | Total | In |
|  |  |  | Out |
|  |  |  | In |
|  |  |  | Out |
|  |  | Weekly Total Hours Completed | |

_____
Preceptor Signature

**2.** **[LO24.4]** Employment Worksheet
   a. When you start to draft a résumé, it is suggested that you start by completing a worksheet. It will allow you to organize the information that you want to use on your résumé.
   b. Complete the Employment Worksheet below providing your specific information for each section. The worksheet will help you remember things that need to be included on your résumé.

---

### EMPLOYMENT WORKSHEET

Job Title _____

Dates _____

Employer _____

City, State _____

Major Duties _____

_____

_____

_____

_____

_____

_____

_____

_____

Special Projects _____

_____

_____

_____

Accomplishments _____

_____

_____

_____

_____

_____

_____

_____

_____

---

# Thinking Critically

Write your response to each case study question on the lines provided.

## Case 1 [LO24.5]

You are the administrative medical assistant and are covering the reception desk. There are several candidates scheduled to come in today for interviews for the one position open for a medical records filing assistant. All the candidates were asked to arrive 15 minutes prior to their interview time so they could complete the job application. One of the candidates arrives 10 minutes late and, as she is completing the application, states that she has another interview in 30 minutes and asks if she will be able to get "in and out" of the interview within the next 20 minutes.

1. When your office manager asks you about your initial opinion of the candidates, what should you tell her about this candidate?

_____

_____

_____

_____

2. What should this candidate have done differently to plan her schedule?

_____

_____

_____

_____

## Case 2 [LO24.2, 24.5]

Brianna is a recent graduate trying to secure permanent employment as an administrative medical assistant. Since graduation she has completed 10 interviews. She is quite shy and does not make good eye contact with people she doesn't know. Her voice is very soft and shaky when she tries to answer questions during interviews. She has good skills, dresses appropriately, and has good references.

1. Why do you think Brianna has not been able to secure a job?

_____

_____

_____

_____

**2.** What can Brianna do to improve her interview skills?

_____

_____

_____

_____

## Case 3 [LO24.2, 24.5]

Rhonda completed her externship at an internal medicine clinic where, according to her preceptor, she did a mediocre job. She is trying to get a job in the field and only has the externship preceptor to list as an employment reference. When a prospective employer calls the preceptor for information about Rhonda's work, the preceptor states that Rhonda completed her work, but does not describe her overall quality of work. Rhonda believes this is prohibiting her from getting a job.

**1.** What can Rhonda do during an interview to address the preceptor's possible response?

_____

_____

_____

_____

**2.** Why is it critical to approach the externship as if it were a paid position?

_____

_____

_____

_____

# Demonstrate Your Knowledge

**Student Name:** _____

## Procedure 24–1: Writing Thank-You Notes

**GOAL:** To develop an appropriate, professional thank-you note after an interview or externship

**MATERIALS:** Paper, pen, dictionary, thesaurus, computer, #10 business envelope

**METHOD:** To pass this procedure the minimum required score is _____ % or all elements must meet "satisfactory" ability on the final demonstration. The first box may be used as a practice or final demonstration, with the evaluator placing **S for Satisfactory** or **U for Unsatisfactory** if that is the grading criteria. The second box may be used as a final demonstration with a **grade point** written in the box.

| STEPS | POSSIBLE POINTS | S/U | POINTS EARNED |
|---|---|---|---|
| 1. Be prompt to complete the letter within 2 days of the interview or completion of the externship so the interviewer or employer will remember you. Begin by typing the date at the top of the letter. | 5 | | |
| 2. Type the name of the person who interviewed you (or who was your mentor in the externship if that is who you are thanking). Include credentials and title, such as "Dr." or "Director of Client Services." Include the complete address of the office or organization. | 5 | | |
| 3. Start the letter with "Dear Dr., Mr., Mrs., Miss, *or* Ms. _____,". | 5 | | |
| 4. In the first paragraph, thank the interviewer for his time and for granting the interview. Discuss some specific impressions, for example, "I found the interview and tour of the facilities an enjoyable experience. I would welcome the opportunity to work in such a state-of-the-art medical setting." If you are writing to thank your mentor for her time during your externship and for allowing you to perform your externship at her office, practice, or clinic, discuss the knowledge and experience you gained during the externship. | 25 | | |
| 5. In the second paragraph, mention the aspects of the job or externship that you found most interesting or challenging. For a job interview thank-you note, state how your skills and qualifications will make you an asset to the staff. When preparing an externship thank-you letter, mention interest in any future positions. | 25 | | |

*(Continued)*

| STEPS | POSSIBLE POINTS | S/U | POINTS EARNED |
|---|---|---|---|
| 6. In the last paragraph, thank the interviewer for considering you for the position. Ask to be contacted at his earliest convenience regarding his employment decision. | 25 | | |
| 7. Close the letter with "Sincerely," and type your name. Leave enough space above your typewritten name to sign your name. | 5 | | |
| 8. Type your return address in the upper left corner of the #10 business envelope. Then type the interviewer's name and address in the envelope's center, apply the proper postage, and mail the letter. You can also e-mail your thank-you letter. Proper letter format and professional tone and appearance still apply. Send the thank-you letter as an attachment. | 5 | | |
| **Total Points (if applicable)** | 100 | | |

**Comments:** _____

_____

_____

**Final Evaluator's Signature:** _____

**Date:** _____

## CAAHEP Competencies Achieved

IV. C (8) Recognize elements of fundamental writing skills

IV. P (10) Compose professional/business letters

## ABHES Competency Achieved

11. a. Perform the essential requirements for employment such as résumé writing, effective interviewing, dressing professionally, and following up appropriately

## Procedure 24–2: **Completing a Job Application**

**GOAL:** To complete an accurate and legible job application

**MATERIALS:** Job application (paper or electronic), personal and reference information including dates and contact information or completed sample application. See the Sample Application for Employment (Figure 24–8 in your student text) at the end of this study guide.

**METHOD:** To pass this procedure the minimum required score is _____% or all elements must meet "satisfactory" ability on the final demonstration. The first box may be used as a practice or final demonstration, with the evaluator placing **S for Satisfactory** or **U for Unsatisfactory** if that is the grading criteria. The second box may be used as a final demonstration with a **grade point** written in the box.

| STEPS | POSSIBLE POINTS | S/U | POINTS EARNED |
|---|---|---|---|
| 1. Review the application form completely before beginning. Directions may be on the last page. | 10 | | |
| 2. Complete the personal information carefully. Following all directions.<br>• For paper applications, look at the fine print. For example, some forms require the last name to be written first or may request that all information be printed. A black ink pen should be used unless the directions state otherwise. Pens cannot be erased so go slowly and be precise.<br>• For electronic forms, read each direction before you begin to input the information. Be careful not to hit the Tab or Enter key until you have checked your entry into each space of the form. | 10 (paper or electronic) | | |
| 3. Complete the rest of the application, referring to your completed sample application or list of personal and reference information. | 10 | | |
| 4. Complete all the requested information. Do not leave any blanks. Finish the application once you have all the requested information. This may require you to cancel the process electronically or take the application home. | 10 | | |
| 5. List your most recent employment first, and be certain to include all education such as vocations training certification or other courses you may have taken. | 10 | | |
| 6. List any skills you have that are relevant to the position. Be specific. | 10 | | |
| 7. When completing salary requirements, either include a range or insert "negotiable" or "flexible." These can be discussed in more detail once you are offered the job. | 10 | | |

*(Continued)*

| STEPS | POSSIBLE POINTS | S/U | POINTS EARNED |
|---|---|---|---|
| 8. Include complete information about your references. References do not always have to be professional. If you have volunteered, you can use members of the organizations that you have helped. You may want to ask teachers or your supervisor at your externship site. In all cases, ask for permission prior to using the person for a reference. | 10 | | |
| 9. Review your application for completeness, accuracy, spelling, grammar, and legibility. | 10 | | |
| 10. Sign and date your application and submit to the appropriate person or electronically. | 10 | | |
| **Total Points (if applicable)** | 100 | | |

**Comments:** _____

_____

_____

**Final Evaluator's Signature:** _____

**Date:** _____

## CAAHEP Competencies Achieved

IV. C (8) Recognize elements of fundamental writing skills

## ABHES Competency Achieved

11. a. Perform the essential requirements for employment such as résumé writing, effective interviewing, dressing professionally, and following up appropriately

## Procedure 24–3: Writing a Résumé

**GOAL:** To develop a résumé that defines your career objective and highlights your skills

**MATERIALS:** Pen, dictionary, thesaurus, computer

**METHOD:** To pass this procedure the minimum required score is _____% or all elements must meet "satisfactory" ability on the final demonstration. The first box may be used as a practice or final demonstration, with the evaluator placing **S for Satisfactory** or **U for Unsatisfactory** if that is the grading criteria. The second box may be used as a final demonstration with a **grade point** written in the box.

| STEPS | POSSIBLE POINTS | S/U | POINTS EARNED |
|---|---|---|---|
| 1. Type your full name, address (temporary and permanent, if you have both), telephone number with area code, and e-mail address (if you have one). | 10 | | |
| 2. List your general career objective. You may also choose to summarize your skills. | 20 | | |
| 3. List the highest level of education or the most recently obtained degree first. Include the school name, degree earned, and date of graduation. Be sure to list any special projects, courses, or participation in overseas study programs. | 20 | | |
| 4. Summarize your work experience. List your most recent or most relevant employment first. Describe your responsibilities, and list job titles, company names, and dates of employment. Summer employment, volunteer work, and student externships may also be included. Use short sentences with strong action words such as "directed," "designed," "developed," and "organized." For example, condense a responsibility into "Processed insurance and billing" or "Drafted correspondence as requested." | 20 | | |
| 5. List any memberships and affiliations with professional organizations. List them alphabetically or by order of importance. | 20 | | |
| 6. Do not list references on your résumé. It is easier to update your reference list if you maintain it in a separate file. | 0 | | |
| 7. Do not list the salary you wish to receive in a medical assisting position. Salary requirements should not be discussed until a job offer is received. | 0 | | |

*(Continued)*

| STEPS | POSSIBLE POINTS | S/U | POINTS EARNED |
|---|---|---|---|
| 8. Print your résumé on an 8½ by 11 inch sheet of high-quality white, off-white, or other light-colored bond paper. Carefully check your résumé for spelling, punctuation, and grammatical errors. Have someone else double-check your résumé whenever possible. | 10 | | |
| **Total Points (if applicable)** | 100 | | |

**Comments:** _____

_____

_____

**Final Evaluator's Signature:** _____

**Date:** _____

## CAAHEP Competencies Achieved

IV. C (8) Recognize elements of fundamental writing skills

IV. P (10) Compose professional/business letters

## ABHES Competency Achieved

11. a. Perform the essential requirements for employment such as résumé writing, effective interviewing, dressing professionally, and following up appropriately

# Procedure/Documentation Forms

Use these forms while performing procedures that require documentation.

# Procedure 2–1: Professional Behaviors Assessment Rubric

PROFESSIONAL BEHAVIORS ASSESSMENT

Student's Name: _____

Be honest as you complete this self-assessment. It is for your benefit.

Rate yourself on each behavior. Create an improvement plan for behaviors that are questionable or unacceptable.

Decide on specific time intervals to review your progress, for example every week or every month.

You may ask a classmate to assess you and compare that student's ratings with your own.

| BEHAVIOR | 1<br>*Unacceptable* | 2<br>*Questionable* | 3<br>*Acceptable* | 4<br>*Super* | 5<br>*Rating* | 6<br>*Comments* |
|---|---|---|---|---|---|---|
| **COMPREHENSION**<br>Ability to learn, retain, and process information in a reasonable time | Responds slowly and with poor understanding or does not retain information. | Is inconsistent in learning or retaining information.<br><br>Sometimes does well and other times not. | Learns information in reasonable time.<br><br>Retention is adequate. | Understands all concepts and details; learns new things easily.<br><br>Retention is excellent. | | |
| **PERSISTENCE**<br>Ability to continue in spite of difficulty; determined; tenacious | Fails to finish work on time, gives up easily, or puts forth little effort. | Sometimes does not finish work as assigned or has a tendency to give up easily. | Follows through on assignments. | Follows through on assignments despite challenges; never gives up. | | |
| **SELF-CONFIDENCE**<br>Believes in oneself; assured | Overconfident; unaware of own limitations or inability to act Independently. | Indecisive, cannot proceed without reassurance. | Generally acts independently with minimal reassurance. | Approaches assignments with full knowledge and no hesitation; checks when appropriate. | | |
| **JUDGMENT**<br>Ability to evaluate, come to appropriate conclusion, and act; critical thinking | Frequently does not evaluate, reach appropriate conclusion, or act; never or seldom thinks critically. | Does not consistently evaluate or come to appropriate conclusion; limited critical thinking. | Evaluates, reaches appropriate conclusion, and acts; uses critical thinking. | Consistently analyzes situations; performs well in complex situations. | | |
| **KNOWLEDGE**<br>Understanding through study and experience; associating theory with practice | Poor understanding or difficulty associating theory with practice. | Inadequate understanding or inability to consistently associate theory with practice. | Possesses adequate understanding; associates theory with practice. | Demonstrates superior understanding and ability to associate theory with practice. | | |

Comment Section:

*(Continued)*

# Procedure 2–1: Professional Behaviors Assessment Rubric *(continued)*

| BEHAVIOR | 1<br>*Unacceptable* | 2<br>*Questionable* | 3<br>*Acceptable* | 4<br>*Super* | 5<br>*Rating* | 6<br>*Comments* |
|---|---|---|---|---|---|---|
| **ORGANIZATION**<br>Independent tasks are planned and completed properly and orderly in a given time | Poor or no planning with extra steps.<br><br>Improper performance.<br><br>Delay.<br><br>Work area in disorder. | Occasional poor planning or performance.<br><br>Delay.<br><br>Work area in disorder. | Sequences steps as directed.<br><br>Ability to coordinate more than one task.<br><br>Work area in order. | Anticipates future work.<br><br>Performs multiple tasks simultaneously and systematically.<br><br>Work area impeccable. | | |
| **COMMUNICATION**<br>Ability to give and receive clear, accurate Information | Difficulty due to inability to encode, decode; language or other barriers. | Does not consistently communicate adequately or clearly. | Standard communication. | Consistently uses good encoding and decoding with extreme tact and professionalism. | | |
| **INTEGRITY**<br>Sound and honest decision making within acceptable code of values* | Likely to make poor decisions or inability to function within acceptable code of values. | Actions suggest personal considerations may outweigh code of values. | Trustworthy.<br><br>Makes appropriate decisions. | Role model for code of values. | | |
| **GROWTH**<br>Continual striving to improve and learn new material | Puts forth little effort or interest in improving or personal responsibility. | Tries to improve when asked to do so; content with passing grades but can do better. | Consistently puts forth effort to learn and Improve.<br><br>Accepts criticism. | Always striving for improvement; seeks feedback; has career plan. | | |
| **COOPERATION**<br>Appropriately and willingly works with others in the best interest of the work | Uncooperative when asked to perform a task; irritates others; is inclined to be quarrelsome. | Does not consistently cooperate with others. | Cooperates with others in agreeable manner. | Always appropriately helpful; others enjoy working with him/her; uses tact in getting job done. | | |
| **ACCEPTANCE OF CRITICISM**<br>Willing to consider suggestions and observations | Frequently rejects or is defensive of appropriate criticism.<br><br>Demonstrates hostility. | Sometimes defensive of appropriate criticism from faculty or peers. | Accepts most criticism. | Accepts and appreciates appropriate criticism.<br><br>Offers suggestions for correction. | | |

* Code of values refers to student handbook, catalog syllabus, other guidelines.
Comment Section:

# Procedure 2–1: Professional Behaviors Assessment Rubric *(concluded)*

| **BEHAVIOR** | **1** <br> *Unacceptable* | **2** <br> *Questionable* | **3** <br> *Acceptable* | **4** <br> *Super* | **5** <br> *Rating* | **6** <br> *Comments* |
|---|---|---|---|---|---|---|
| **RELATIONS WITH OTHERS** <br> Ability to appropriately get along with others | Shows lack of respect or patience or avoids others or disruptive. | Has occasional difficulty in routine program relationships. | Gets along with others; handles routine interactions appropriately. | Has superior ability to deal with others; is respected by peers and faculty; respects all. | | |
| **QUALITY OF WORK** <br> Striving for excellence in performing work | Work contains an unacceptable % of errors or shows evidence of minimal effort. | Does not seem to have quite enough concern about the quality of his/her work. | Quality of work is adequate. | Work is consistently close to perfection. | | |
| **PUNCTUALITY AND ATTENDANCE** <br> Coming to work/class on appointed days and times | Chronically late or absences excessive to expectations* or takes "extended" breaks. | Occasionally late or absent or takes "extended" break. | Never late or absent with the exception of a rare emergency; takes appropriate breaks. | Never late or absent; takes appropriate breaks. | | |
| **PROFESSIONAL APPEARANCE** <br> Adherence to dress code; practices good hygiene | Very untidy. <br><br> Doesn't follow dress code. <br><br> Has hygiene issues or inappropriate body art.** | Sometimes untidy and careless about appearance or hygiene. <br><br> Problem with body art. | Generally neat and clean. <br><br> Adheres to dress code. <br><br> Body art appropriately covered. | Always impeccable personal appearance. <br><br> Properly attired all of the time. <br><br> No body art. | | |

*Expectations are defined in syllabi and policies and procedures.
**As described in program policies.

Comments:

Reviewed _____ Date: _____

Reviewed _____ Date: _____

Reviewed _____ Date: _____

## TOTAL CARE CLINIC, PC

**Notice of Privacy Practices**

I understand that *Total Care Clinic* creates and maintains medical records describing my health history, symptoms, examinations, test results, diagnoses, treatments, and plans for my future care and/or treatment. I further understand that this information may be used for any of the following:

1. Plan and document my care and treatment
2. Communicate with health professionals involved in my care and treatment
3. Verify insurance coverage for planned procedures and/or treatments for the applicable diagnoses
4. Application of any medical or surgical procedures and diagnoses (codes) to my medical insurance claim forms as application for payment of services rendered
5. Assessment of quality of care and utilization review of the health care professionals providing my care

Additionally, it has been explained to me that:

1. A complete description of the use and disclosure of this information is included in a *Notice of Information of Privacy Practices* which has been provided to me
2. I have had a right to review this information prior to signing this consent
3. _____ has the right to change this notice and their practices
4. Any revision of this notice will be mailed to me at the address I provided to them prior to its implementation
5. I may object to the use of my health information for specific purposes
6. I may request restrictions as to the manner my information may be used or disclosed in order to carry out treatment, payment, or health information
7. I understand that it is not required that my requested restrictions be honored
8. I may revoke this consent in writing, except for those disclosures which may have taken place prior to the receipt of my revocation

At the time of the document signing, I request the following restrictions to disclosure or use of my health information: _____

_____

_____        _____
Printed Name of Patient or Legal Guardian        Signature of Parent or Legal Guardian

_____        _____
Printed Name of Witness/Title        Signature of Witness/Title

Date: _____

## TOTAL CARE CLINIC, PC

**Privacy Violation Complaint Form**

As per our Privacy Policies and Procedures, we are providing this form for individuals who feel they have a complaint regarding how their protected health information was handled by our office. You have the right to make a complaint and we may take no retaliatory actions against you because of it. We will respond to this complaint within 30 days of its receipt.

Patient Name: _____

Address: _____

DOB: _____ Date of Complaint: _____

Phone: H _____ Cell _____ Work _____

Best time to reach you: _____

Reason for the complaint (Please be as specific as possible, attaching additional documentation as necessary): _____

_____

_____

_____

_____

_____        _____
              Signature                                   Date

-----------------------------------------------------------------------------------

Office Use Only

Received by: _____        Date_____

Follow-up Started on (date): _____

TOTAL CARE CLINIC, PC

**Authorization to Release Health Information**

I, _____ residing at

_____ and DOB

of _____ give permission to (name of practice) _____

_____ to release to _____

_____ of Total Care Clinic the following information:

_____

_____

_____

Reason for the request:

_____

_____

_____

Signature of Patient or Legal Guardian _____

Printed Name of Patient or Legal Guardian _____

If Guardian, relationship to Patient _____

This authorization will expire on: _____

**YOU MAY REFUSE TO SIGN THIS AUTHORIZATION.** You may revoke this authorization at any time by notifying Total Care Clinic in writing. Revocation will have no effect on actions taken prior to receipt of any revocation. Any disclosure of information carries the potential for unauthorized redisclosure and the information may not be protected by federal confidentiality rules.

# Procedure 7–1: Patient Registration Form

## TOTAL CARE CLINIC, PC

### Patient Registration Form

Date: _____

Last name: _____ First name: _____ MI: _____

Address: _____ Birth date: ____/____/____

City/St/Zip: _____ SSN: _____

Marital status: (please circle) Single   Married   Divorced   Widowed   **Pt. language:** _____

Home phone: _____ Cell phone: _____ E-mail: _____

Referred by: _____ Patient's employer: _____

Employer's address:  _____ City/St/Zip: _____

Primary insurance: _____ Phone: _____

Group name: _____ Group #: _____ ID #: _____

Subscriber's name: _____ Subscriber's birth date: ____/____/____

Secondary insurance: _____ Phone: _____

Group name: _____ Group #: _____ ID #: _____

Subscriber's name: _____ Subscriber's birth date: ____/____/____

Relative emergency contact: _____ Relationship: _____

Address: _____ Phone: _____

I have reviewed the above information and, to the best of my knowledge, it is correct.

Printed name of patient or legal representative: _____

Signature of patient or legal representative: _____

## TOTAL CARE CLINIC, PC

342 East Park Blvd
Funton, XY 12345-6789
Tel: 521-234-0001
Fax: 521-234-0002
www.totalcareclinic.org

***Instruction to Office Staff: Scan in as "Release" with date***

**PATIENT NAME:** _____

**Date of Birth:** _____

**Today's Date:** _____

## AUTHORIZATION TO RELEASE INFORMATION

I hereby authorize the Total Care Clinic (TCC) to release any medical information necessary to process insurance claims relating to the medical care rendered by the physicians and staff of TCC.

Signature:_____     Date: _____

## ASSIGNMENT OF BENEFITS

I authorize payment of medical benefits to the Total Care Clinic for any medical care rendered to myself or to my dependents.

Signature:_____     Date: _____

## FINANCIAL RESPONSIBILITY

I understand that payment of the portion of the bill that is my responsibility is due on the date service is rendered (any copay, unsatisfied deductible, no-show, less than 24-hour cancellation and co-insurance; if a cash pay patient, the full amount of the bill). I also understand that any service not covered by my insurance is my responsibility subject to the terms of any contract between the insurance plan and the Total Care Clinic.

Signature:_____     Date: _____

# Procedure 8–1: Typical Supplies in a Medical Office

| ADMINISTRATIVE SUPPLIES | CLINICAL SUPPLIES | GENERAL SUPPLIES |
|---|---|---|
| Appointment books, daybooks (still used in noncomputerized offices) | Alcohol swabs | Liquid hypoallergenic soap |
| Back-to-school/back-to-work slips | Applicators | Paper cups |
| Clipboards | Bandaging materials: adhesive tape, gauze pads, gauze sponges, elastic bandages, adhesive bandages, roller bandages (gauze and elastic) | Paper towels |
| Computer supplies | Cloth or paper gowns and drapes | Tampons and sanitary pads |
| Copy and facsimile (fax) machine paper | Cotton, cotton swabs | Tissues: facial, toilet |
| File folders, coding tabs | Culture tubes | |
| HIPAA forms (Notice of Privacy Practices, authorization forms, disclosure logs, request to inspect and copy medical record forms, request for amendment forms, acknowledgment of request for amendment forms) | 50% dextrose solution | |
| History and physical examination sheet cards | Disposable sheaths for thermometers | |
| Insurance forms: disability, HMO and other third-party payers, life insurance examinations, Veterans Administration, workers' compensation | Disposable tips for otoscopes | |
| Insurance manuals | Gloves: sterile, examination | |
| Local welfare department forms | Hemoccult test kits | |
| Patient education materials | Iodine or Betadine pads | |
| Pens, pencils, erasers | Lancets | |
| Prescription pads | Lubricating jelly | |
| Rubber bands, paper clips | Microscopic slides and fixative | |
| Registration forms | Needles, syringes | |
| Social Security forms | Nitroglycerin tablets | |
| Stamps | Safety pins | |
| Stationery: appointment cards, bookkeeping supplies (ledgers, statement, billing forms), letterhead, second sheets, envelopes, business cards, prescription pads, notebooks, notepads, telephone memo pads | Silver nitrate sticks | |
| | Sutures removal kits | |
| | Sutures | |
| | Table covers (examination) | |
| | Tongue depressors | |
| | Topical skin freeze | |
| | Urinalysis test sticks | |
| | Urine containers | |
| | Injectable medications as appropriate to the type of practice | |
| | Other medicines, chemicals, solutions, ointments, lotions, and disinfectants, as needed | |

# Procedure 8–2: Requisition Order

## REQUISITION

Funton Business Supplies
1021 North 1st Street
Funton, XY 12345-6789
Tel: 521-454-5211
Fax: 521-454-5212

SHIP TO: Total Care Clinic, PC
342 E. Park Blvd
Funton, XY 12345-6789
Accountant #: 0060812 MD
Date ordered: 08/05/XX

| Item # | Description | Unit Quantity | Price per unit | Total |
|--------|-------------|---------------|----------------|--------|
| 65245 | Toner | 2 | $65.00 | $130.00 |
| 78769 | Paper | 3 boxes | $36.00 | $108.00 |
| Subtotal | | | | $238.00 |
| Tax | | | | $10.10 |
| Shipping | | | | waived |
| Total | | | | $248.10 |

# Procedure 8–2: Packing Slip

## PACKING SLIP

Funton Business Supplies
1021 North 1st Street
Funton, XY 12345-6789
Tel: 521-454-5211
Fax: 521-454-5212

Date ordered: 08/05/XX
Date shipped: 08/06/XX
Order #: 0056211

SHIP TO: Total Care Clinic, PC
342 E. Park Blvd
Funton, XY 12345-6789
Accountant #: 0060812 MD

| Item # | Description | Unit Quantity | Price per unit | Total |
|--------|-------------|---------------|----------------|-------|
| 65245 | Toner | 2 | $65.00 | Backorder to ship 08/15/XX |
| 78769 | Paper | 3 boxes | $36.00 | $108.00 |
| Subtotal | | | | $108.00 |
| Tax | | | | $3.60 |
| Shipping | | | | waived |
| Total | | | | $111.60 |

# Procedure 8–2: Invoice

## INVOICE

Funton Business Supplies
1021 North 1st Street
Funton, XY 12345-6789
Tel: 521-454-5211
Fax: 521-454-5212

Date ordered: 08/05/XX
Date shipped: 08/06/XX
Order #: 0056211
Remit in full within 30 days
to avoid late charge

SHIP TO: Total Care Clinic, PC
342 E. Park Blvd
Funton, XY 12345-6789
Accountant #: 0060812 MD

| Item # | Description | Unit Quantity | Price per unit | Total |
|--------|-------------|---------------|----------------|---------|
| 78769 | Paper | 3 boxes | $36.00 | $108.00 |
| Subtotal | | | | $108.00 |
| Tax | | | | $3.60 |
| Shipping | | | | waived |
| Total | | | | $111.60 |

# Procedure 8—4: Daily Checklist for Opening the Office

| DAILY CHECKLIST: OPENING FACILITY (INITIAL WHEN COMPLETED) DATE: FROM _____ TO _____ | | | | | | | | | | |
|---|---|---|---|---|---|---|---|---|---|---|
| | M | T | W | TH | F | M | T | W | TH | F |
| 1. Security system disarmed | | | | | | | | | | |
| 2. Messages/answering services retrieved | | | | | | | | | | |
| 3. Messages routed and ready for callback | | | | | | | | | | |
| 4. Fax machine checked | | | | | | | | | | |
| 5. Appointment book and insurance rosters checked | | | | | | | | | | |
| 6. Charts pulled and paperwork attached | | | | | | | | | | |
| 7. Equipment working properly | | | | | | | | | | |
| 8. Rooms supplied and ready | | | | | | | | | | |
| 9. Refrigerator temperature checked | | | | | | | | | | |
| 10. Emergency supplies including O2 checked | | | | | | | | | | |
| 11. Reception area in order and patient education material available | | | | | | | | | | |
| 12. Lab specimens from day before were picked up | | | | | | | | | | |

# Procedure 8–4: Daily Checklist for Closing the Office

| DAILY CHECKLIST: CLOSING FACILITY<br>(INITIAL WHEN COMPLETED)<br>DATE: FROM _____ TO _____ | M | T | W | TH | F | M | T | W | TH | F |
|---|---|---|---|---|---|---|---|---|---|---|
| 1. Computers are logged out and off | | | | | | | | | | |
| 2. Contaminated supplies/equipment are properly disposed | | | | | | | | | | |
| 3. Areas are restocked | | | | | | | | | | |
| 4. Patient's charts are pulled or reviewed for next day and any test results, etc., are available | | | | | | | | | | |
| 5. Laboratory specimens are in pick-up receptacle | | | | | | | | | | |
| 6. All equipment (i.e., coffee pot, EKG machine) is turned off | | | | | | | | | | |
| 7. Reception area is organized | | | | | | | | | | |
| 8. Calls are forwarded to voicemail/answering machine | | | | | | | | | | |
| 9. Medical records are secured | | | | | | | | | | |
| 10. All doors and windows are locked | | | | | | | | | | |
| 11. Security system is armed | | | | | | | | | | |

# Procedure 12–1: Appointment Book Matrix

## APPOINTMENT RECORD

| 12 November Tuesday | | DOCTOR | 13 November Wednesday | |
|---|---|---|---|---|
| | | **AM** | | |
| | | 8:00 | | |
| | | 8:15 | | |
| | | 8:30 | | |
| | | 8:45 | | |
| | | 9:00 | | |
| | | 9:15 | | |
| | | 9:30 | | |
| | | 9:45 | | |
| | | 10:00 | | |
| | | 10:15 | | |
| | | 10:30 | | |
| | | 10:45 | | |
| | | 11:00 | | |
| | | 11:15 | | |
| | | 11:30 | | |
| | | 11:45 | | |
| | | 12:00 | | |
| | | 12:15 | | |
| | | 12:30 | | |
| | | 12:45 | | |
| | | **PM** | | |
| | | 1:00 | | |
| | | 1:15 | | |
| | | 1:30 | | |
| | | 1:45 | | |
| | | 2:00 | | |
| | | 2:15 | | |
| | | 2:30 | | |
| | | 2:45 | | |
| | | 3:00 | | |
| | | 3:15 | | |
| | | 3:30 | | |
| | | 3:45 | | |
| | | 4:00 | | |
| | | 4:15 | | |
| | | 4:30 | | |
| | | 4:45 | | |
| | | 5:00 | | |
| | | 5:15 | | |
| | | 5:30 | | |
| | | 5:45 | | |

REMARKS & NOTES _____

# Procedure 12–4: Appointment Card

TOTAL CARE CLINIC, PC
342 E. Park Blvd
Funton, XY 12345-6789

Patient Name: _____

Date: _____
           Month    Day    Year

Time: _____  A.M.  P.M.

Appointment with: _____

# Procedure 13–1: Letterhead

## TOTAL CARE CLINIC, PC

342 East Park Blvd
Futon, XY 12345-6789
Tel: 521-234-0001    Fax: 521-234-0002
www.totalcareclinic.org

# Procedure 15–1: Patient Registration Form

**TOTAL CARE CLINIC, PC**

342 East Park Blvd
Funton, XY   12345-6789
521-234-0001   Fax: 521-234-0002

## Patient Registration
### Patient Information

Name: _____ Today's Date: _____

Address: _____

City: _____ State: _____ Zip Code: _____

Telephone (Home): _____ (Work): _____ (Cell): _____

Birthdate: _____ Age: _____ Sex:  M   F   No. of Children _____ Marital Status:  M   S   W   D

Social Security Number: _____ Employer: _____ Occupation: _____

Primary Physician: _____

Referred by: _____

Person to Contact in Emergency: _____

Emergency Telephone: _____

Special Needs: _____

## Responsible Party

Party Responsible for Payment:        Self          Spouse          Parent          Other

Name (If Other Than Self): _____

Address: _____

City: _____ State: _____ Zip Code: _____

## Primary Insurance

Primary Medical Insurance: _____

Insured party:        Self        Spouse     Parent     Other

ID#/Social Security No.: _____ Group/Plan No.: _____

Name (If Other Than Self): _____

Address: _____

City: _____ State: _____ Zip Code: _____

## Secondary Insurance

Secondary Medical Insurance: _____

Insured party:        Self        Spouse     Parent     Other

ID#/Social Security No.: _____ Group/Plan No.: _____

Name (If Other Than Self): _____

Address: _____

City: _____ State: _____ Zip Code: _____

# Procedure 15–1: Medical History Form

## Total Care Clinic, PC
### Medical History

Name _____ Age _____ Sex _____ S M W D
Address _____ Phone _____ Date _____

Occupation _____ Ref. by _____
Chief Complaint _____

Present Illness _____
_____
_____
_____
_____
_____

History —Military _____
       —Social _____
       —Family _____
       —Marital _____
       —Menstrual _____ Menarche _____ Para. _____ LMP _____
       —Illness  Measles  Pert.  Var.  Pneu.  Pleur.  Typh.  Mal.  Rh. Fev.  Sc. Fev.  Diphth.  Other
       —Surgery _____
       —Allergies _____
       —Current Medications _____

### Physical Examination

Temp. _____ Pulse _____ Resp. _____ BP _____ Ht. _____ Wt. _____
General Appearance _____ Skin _____ Mucous Membrane _____
Eyes: _____ Vision _____ Pupil _____ Fundus _____
Ears: _____
Nose: _____
Throat: _____ Pharynx _____ Tonsils _____
Chest: _____ Breasts _____
Heart: _____
Lungs: _____
Abdomen: _____
Genitalia: _____
Rectum: _____
Pelvic: _____
Extremities: _____ Pulses _____
Lymph Nodes: ____ Neck ____ Axilla ____ Inguinal ____ Abdominal ____
Neurological: _____
Diagnosis: _____
_____
_____

Treatment: _____
_____
_____

Laboratory Findings: _____
Date _____ Blood _____
_____
_____
_____

Date _____ Urine _____
_____
_____
_____
_____
_____

# Procedure 15–1: Progress Note

| DATE | PROGRESS NOTES |
|------|----------------|
|      |                |

Form OMB-1243

# Procedure 16–1: Patient Record with Medications Listed

Name: _Jennifer Haddix_    DOB _12/05/84_    Date _08/28/12_

ALLERGIES: _Bee Stings, Penicillin_    Note

### Review of Systems

| Systems | NL | Note | Systems | NL | Note |
|---|---|---|---|---|---|
| Constitutional | | | Musculoskeletal | | |
| Eyes | | | Skin/breasts | | |
| ENT/mouth | | | Neurologic | | |
| Cardiovascular | | | Psychiatric | | |
| Respiratory | | | Endocrine | | |
| GI | | | Hem/lymph | | |
| GU | | | Allergy/immun | | |

| Current Medicines | Date | Current Diagnosis |
|---|---|---|
| ClaritinD prN  MVI T qd  Ortho Novum 7/7/7 T qd | | |

H: _5'7"_    W: _140_    T: _97.8_    P: _88_    R: _20_

B/P Sitting _122/78_ or Standing _____ Supine _____

Last Tetanus _06/12/09_

L.M.P. _08/20/12_

O2 Sat: _98%_  Pain Scale: _6/10_

| Social Habits | Yes | No |
|---|---|---|
| Tobacco | | ✓ |
| Alcohol | ✓ | ooo |
| Rec. Drugs | | ✓ |

CC: Ⓛ Shoulder pain X 3 days due to fall.
"Sharp pain that hurts when I move"

HPI:

# Procedure 16–2: DEA Form 224

**Form-224**

## APPLICATION FOR REGISTRATION
### Under the Controlled Substances Act

APPROVED OMB NO 1117-0014
FORM DEA-224 (10-06)
Previous editions are obsolete

| | |
|---|---|
| **INSTRUCTIONS** | **Save time—apply on-line at *www.deadiversion.usdoj.gov*** |

1. To apply by mail complete this application. Keep a copy for your records.
2. Print clearly, using black or blue ink, or use a typewriter.
3. Mail this form to the address provided in Section 7 or use enclosed envelope.
4. Include the correct payment amount. FEE IS NON-REFUNDABLE.
5. If you have any questions call 800-882-9539 prior to submitting your application.

IMPORTANT: DO NOT SEND THIS APPLICATION AND APPLY ON-LINE.

**DEA OFFICIAL USE:**

Do you have other DEA registration numbers?
☐ NO        ☐ YES

**MAIL-TO ADDRESS** — Please print mailing address changes to the right of the address in this box.

**FEE FOR THREE (3) YEARS IS $551**
**FEE IS NON-REFUNDABLE**

---

**SECTION 1     APPLICANT IDENTIFICATION**     ☐ Individual Registration     ☐ Business Registration

Name 1     (Last Name of individual -OR- Business or Facility Name)

Name 2     (First Name and Middle Name of individual -OR- Continuation of business name)

Street Address Line 1 (if applying for fee exemption, this must be address of the fee exempt institution)

Address Line 2

City                    State     Zip Code

Business Phone Number          Point of Contact

Business Fax Number            Email Address

**DEBT COLLECTION INFORMATION**
Mandatory pursuant to Debt Collection Improvements Act

Social Security Number (*if registration is for individual*)

Provide **SSN** or **TIN.**
See additional information note #3 on page 4.

Tax Identification Number (*if registration is for business*)

**FOR Practitioner or MLP ONLY:**

Professional Degree: *select from list only*

Professional School:

Year of Graduation:

National Provider Identification:

Date of Birth (*MM-DD-YYYY*):

---

**SECTION 2**
**BUSINESS ACTIVITY**

Check one business activity box only

☐ Central Fill Pharmacy
☐ Retail Pharmacy
☐ Nursing Home
☐ Automated Dispensing System

☐ Practitioner (DDS, DMD, DO, DPM, DVM, MD or PHD)
☐ Practitioner Military (DDS, DMD, DO, DPM, DVM, MD or PHD)
☐ Mid-level Practitioner (MLP) (DOM, HMD, MP, ND, NP, OD, PA, or RPH)
☐ Euthanasia Technician

☐ Ambulance Service
☐ Animal Shelter
☐ Hospital/Clinic
☐ Teaching Institution

FOR Automated Dispensing System (ADS) ONLY:

DEA Registration # of Retail Pharmacy for this ADS

An ADS is automatically fee-exempt.
Skip Section 6 and Section 7 on page 2.
You must attach a notarized affidavit.

---

**SECTION 3**
**DRUG SCHEDULES**

Check all that apply

☐ Schedule II Narcotic
☐ Schedule II Non-Narcotic

☐ Schedule III Narcotic
☐ Schedule III Non-Narcotic

☐ Schedule IV
☐ Schedule V

*(Continued)*

# Procedure 16–2: DEA Form 224 *(concluded)*

**SECTION 4**

**STATE LICENSE(S)**

Be sure to include both state license numbers if applicable

You MUST be currently authorized to prescribe, distribute, dispense, conduct research, or otherwise handle the controlled substances in the schedules for which you are applying under the laws of the **state** or jurisdiction in which you are operating or propose to operate.

State License Number (required)

Expiration Date (required)    /    /    MM - DD - YYYY

What state was this license issued in? _____

State Controlled Substance License Number (if required)

Expiration Date    /    /    MM - DD - YYYY

What state was this license issued in? _____

---

**SECTION 5**

**LIABILITY**

**IMPORTANT**

All questions in this section must be answered.

1. Has the applicant ever been **convicted of a crime** in connection with controlled substance(s) under state or federal law, or is any such action pending?     YES ☐   NO ☐

   Date(s) of incident MM-DD-YYYY: ☐☐ – ☐☐ – ☐☐☐☐

2. Has the applicant ever surrendered (for cause) or had a **federal** controlled substance registration revoked, suspended, restricted, or denied, or is any such action pending?     YES ☐   NO ☐

   Date(s) of incident MM-DD-YYYY: ☐☐ – ☐☐ – ☐☐☐☐

3. Has the applicant ever surrendered (for cause) or had a **state** professional license or controlled substance registration revoked, suspended, denied, restricted, or placed on probation, or is any such action pending?     YES ☐   NO ☐

   Date(s) of incident MM-DD-YYYY: ☐☐ – ☐☐ – ☐☐☐☐

4. If the applicant is a **corporation** (other than a corporation whose stock is owned and traded by the public), association, partnership, or pharmacy, has any officer, partner, stockholder, or proprietor been **convicted of a crime** in connection with controlled substance(s) under state or federal law, or ever surrendered, for cause, or had a **federal** controlled substance registration revoked, suspended, restricted, denied, or ever had a **state** professional license or controlled substance registration revoked, suspended, denied, restricted or placed on probation, or is any such action pending?     YES ☐   NO ☐

   Date(s) of incident MM-DD-YYYY: ☐☐ – ☐☐ – ☐☐☐☐   *Note: If question 4 does not apply to you, be sure to mark 'NO'. It will slow down processing of your application if you leave it blank.*

---

**EXPLANATION OF "YES" ANSWERS**

Applicants who have answered "YES" to any of the four questions above **must provide a statement to explain each "YES" answer.**

Use this space or attach a separate sheet and return with application

Liability question # _____      Location(s) of incident: _____

Nature of incident:

Disposition of incident:

---

**SECTION 6**   **EXEMPTION FROM APPLICATION FEE**

☐ Check this box if the applicant is a federal, state, or local government official or institution. Does not apply to contractor-operated institutions.

Business or Facility Name of Fee Exempt Institution. **Be sure to enter the address of this exempt institution in Section 1.**

**FEE EXEMPT CERTIFIER**

Provide the name and phone number of the certifying official

The undersigned hereby certifies that the applicant named hereon is a federal, state or local government official or institution, and is exempt from payment of the application fee.

_____ Signature of certifying official (other than applicant)      Date _____

_____ Print or type name and title of certifying official      Telephone No. (required for verification) _____

---

**SECTION 7**

**METHOD OF PAYMENT**

Check one form of payment only

Sign if paying by credit card

☐ Check   Make check payable to: **Drug Enforcement Administration** See page 4 of instructions for important information.

☐ American Express   ☐ Discover   ☐ Master Card   ☐ Visa

Credit Card Number      Expiration Date

_____ Signature of Card Holder

_____ Printed Name of Card Holder

*Mail this form with payment to:*

U.S. Department of Justice
Drug Enforcement Administration
P.O. Box 28083
Washington, DC 20038-8083

**FEE IS NON-REFUNDABLE**

---

**SECTION 8**

**APPLICANTS SIGNATURE**

Sign in ink

I certify that the foregoing information furnished on this application is true and correct.

_____ **Signature of applicant (sign in ink)**      Date _____

_____ Print or type name and title of applicant

**WARNING:** Section 843(a)(4)(A) of Title 21, United States Code states that any person who knowingly or intentionally furnishes false or fraudulent information in this application is subject to imprisonment for not more than four years, a fine of not more than $30,000,00 or both.

# Procedure 16–2: DEA Form 222

**DEA Form-222**
**(Oct. 1992)**

**U.S. OFFICIAL ORDER FORMS - SCHEDULES I & II**
Drug Enforcement Administration
**SUPPLIER'S Copy 1**

**See Reverse of PURCHASER'S Copy for Instructions**

No order form may be issued for Schedule I and II substances unless a completed application form has been received. (21 CFR 1305.04).

**OMB APPROVAL No. 1117-0010**

To: (Name of Supplier)

Street Address

Address

City                                              State

Date (MM-DD-YYYY)

Suppliers DEA Registration No.

To Be Filled in By **PURCHASER**

| Line No. | No. of Packages | Size of Package | Name of Item |
|---|---|---|---|
| 1 | | | |
| 2 | | | |
| 3 | | | |
| 4 | | | |
| 5 | | | |
| 6 | | | |
| 7 | | | |
| 8 | | | |
| 9 | | | |
| 10 | | | |

To Be Filled in By **SUPPLIER**

| National Drug Code | Packages Shipped | Date Shipped |
|---|---|---|
| | | |
| | | |
| | | |
| | | |
| | | |
| | | |
| | | |
| | | |
| | | |
| | | |

◄ **LAST LINE COMPLETED**    *(MUST BE 10 OR LESS)*

Signature of **PURCHASER** or Attorney or Agent

Date Issued

DEA Registration No.

Schedules

Name and Address of Registrant

Registered As a

No. of This Order Form

# Procedure 16–2: DEA Form 41

| OMB Approval No. 1117-0007 | U.S. Department of Justice/Drug Enforcement Administration **REGISTRANTS INVENTORY OF DRUGS SURRENDERED** | PACKAGE NO. |
|---|---|---|

The following schedule is an inventory of controlled substances which is hereby surrendered to you for proper disposition.

**FROM:** *(Include Name, Street, City, State and ZIP Code in space provided below.)*

Signature of applicant or authorized agent

Registrant's DEA Number

Registrant's Telephone Number

**NOTE:** CERTIFIED MAIL (Return Receipt Requested) IS REQUIRED FOR SHIPMENTS OF DRUGS VIA U.S. POSTAL SERVICE. See instructions on reverse (page 2) of form.

| NAME OF DRUG OR PREPARATION — Registrants will fill in Columns 1, 2, 3, and 4 ONLY. | Number of Containers | CONTENTS (Number of grams, tablets, ounces or other units per container) | Controlled Substance Content, (Each Unit) | FOR DEA USE ONLY DISPOSITION | QUANTITY GMS. | MGS. |
|---|---|---|---|---|---|---|
| *1* | *2* | *3* | *4* | *5* | *6* | *7* |
| 1 | | | | | | |
| 2 | | | | | | |
| 3 | | | | | | |
| 4 | | | | | | |
| 5 | | | | | | |
| 6 | | | | | | |
| 23 | | | | | | |
| 24 | | | | | | |

The controlled substances surrendered in accordance with Title 21 of the Code of Federal Regulations, Section 1307.21, have been received in _____ packages purporting to contain the drugs listed on this inventory and have been: **(1) Forwarded tape-sealed without opening; (2) Destroyed as indicated and the remainder forwarded tape-sealed after verifying contents; (3) Forwarded tape-sealed after verifying contents.

DATE _____

**Strike out lines not applicable.*

DESTROYED BY: _____

WITNESSED BY: _____

## INSTRUCTIONS

1. List the name of the drug in column 1, the number of containers in column 2, the size of each container in column 3, and in column 4 the controlled substance content of each unit described in column 3; e.g., morphine sulfate tabs., 3 pkgs., 100 tabs., 1/4 gr. (16 mg.) or morphine sulfate tabs., 1 pkg., 83 tabs., 1/2 gr. (32 mg.), etc.
2. All packages included on a single line should be identical in name, content and controlled substance strength.
3. Prepare this form in quadruplicate. Mail two (2) copies of this form to the Special Agent in Charge, under separate cover. Enclose one additional copy in the shipment with the drugs. Retain one copy for your records. One copy will be returned to you as a receipt. No further receipt will be furnished to you unless specifically requested. Any further inquiries concerning these drugs should be addressed to the DEA District Office which serves your area.
4. There is no provision for payment for drugs surrendered. This is merely a service rendered to registrants enabling them to clear their stocks and records of unwanted items.
5. Drugs should be shipped tape-sealed via prepaid express or certified mail (**return receipt requested**) to Special Agent in Charge, Drug Enforcement Administration, of the DEA District Office which serves your area.

### PRIVACY ACT INFORMATION

AUTHORITY: Section 307 of the Controlled Substances Act of 1970 (PL 91-513).
PURPOSE: To document the surrender of controlled substances which have been forwarded by registrants to DEA for disposal.
ROUTINE USES: This form is required by Federal Regulations for the surrender of unwanted Controlled Substances. Disclosures of information from this system are made to the following categories of users for the purposes stated.
    A. Other Federal law enforcement and regulatory agencies for law enforcement and regulatory purposes.
    B. State and local law enforcement and regulatory agencies for law enforcement and regulatory purposes.
EFFECT: Failure to document the surrender of unwanted Controlled Substances may result in prosecution for violation of the Controlled Substances Act.

Under the Paperwork Reduction Act, a person is not required to respond to a collection of information unless it displays a currently valid OMB control number. Public reporting burden for this collection of information is estimated to average 30 minutes per response, including the time for reviewing instructions, searching existing data sources, gathering and maintaining the data needed, and completing and reviewing the collection of information. Send comments regarding this burden estimate or any other aspect of this collection of information, including suggestions for reducing this burden, to the Drug Enforcement Administration, FOI and Records Management Section, Washington, D.C. 20537; and to the Office of Management and Budget, Paperwork Reduction Project no. 1117-0007, Washington, D.C. 20503.

# Procedure 16–4: Progress Note

**Total Care Clinic, PC**
Progress Notes

Name: _____ Chart #: _____

| DATE | |
|------|---|
| | |
| | |
| | |
| | |
| | |
| | |
| | |
| | |
| | |
| | |
| | |
| | |
| | |
| | |
| | |
| | |
| | |
| | |
| | |
| | |

Name _____     DOB _____     Date _____

ALLERGIES: _____     Note

### Review of Systems

| Systems | NL | Note | Systems | NL | Note |
|---|---|---|---|---|---|
| Constitutional | | | Musculoskeletal | | |
| Eyes | | | Skin/breasts | | |
| ENT/mouth | | | Neurologic | | |
| Cardiovascular | | | Psychiatric | | |
| Respiratory | | | Endocrine | | |
| GI | | | Hem/lymph | | |
| GU | | | Allergy/immun | | |

| Current Medicines | Date | Current Diagnosis |
|---|---|---|
| | | |

H: _____     W: _____     T: _____     P: _____     R: _____

B/P Sitting _____     or Standing _____     Supine _____

Last Tetanus _____          Social Habits   Yes   No

L.M.P. _____               Tobacco   ___   ___

                                 Alcohol   ___   ___

O2 Sat: _____   Pain Scale: _____   Rec. Drugs   ___   ___

CC:

HPI:

# Procedure 16–5: Referral Form

---

## REQUEST FOR SERVICES

Facility: _____

Provider: _____

Address: _____

_____

Phone: _____ Fax: _____

### PATIENT INFORMATION

Patient name _____ TCC# _____

Date of Birth _____ Home Phone _____ Alt Phone _____

### REASON FOR REQUEST

Reason for request / Specific question(s) to be answered:

1. _____

2. _____

History / Symptoms / Specific question(s) to be answered: _____

_____

_____

_____

☐ Check here if additional clinical information is included with this request.

### SERVICES REQUESTED

☐ Abnormal Weight Gain
☐ Adolescent Medicine/Teen Health Center
☐ Aerodigestive
☐ Allergy Clinic
☐ Audology (Hearing)
☐ Behavioral Medcine & Clinical Psychology
☐ Brachial Plexus Clinic
☐ Breast Feeding Clinic
☐ Cardiology
☐ Cardiothoracic Surgery
☐ Cerebral Palsy Center
☐ Chronic Pain Management
☐ Colorectal Surgery
☐ Comprehensive Weight Management Center
☐ Craniofacial Center
☐ Dentistry
☐ Dermatology

☐ Developmental & Behavioral Pediatrics
☐ Diabetes
☐ Diagnostic Clinic
☐ Endocrinology
☐ ENT (Otolaryngology)
☐ Feeding Team
☐ Fetal Surgery
☐ Gastroenterology-GI
☐ Gynecology
☐ Healthworks
☐ Hemangioma & Vascular Malformation Team
☐ Hematology-Oncology
☐ Human Genetics
☐ Hypertension / Cholesterol Clinic
☐ Infectious Diseases-ID
☐ International Adoption Center-IAC
☐ Nephrology

☐ Neurology
☐ Neurosurgery
☐ Nutrition
☐ Ophthalmology / Eye Clinic
☐ Orthopaedics
☐ Physical Medicine & Rehabilitation
☐ Plastic Surgery
☐ Psychiatry
☐ Pulmonary Medicine
☐ Rheumatology
☐ Safe & Healthy Children Center
☐ Sleep Center
☐ Sports Medicine
☐ Surgery (General & Thoracic Surgery)
☐ Urology
☐ Other_____

### REQUESTING PRACTITIONER / GROUP

**TOTAL CARE CLINIC, PC**
342 East Park Blvd.
Futon, XY 12345-6789
www.totalcareclinic.org

Physician Name _____

Tel: 521-234-0001
Fax: 521-234-0002

# Procedure 16–5: Laboratory Requisition Form

## Account Information

| TCC Account Number | | | |
|---|---|---|---|
| **Patient Account Number** | | | |
| **Address - Street** | | | |
| **City** | | **State** | **ZIP Code** |

**Ship to: Total Care Laboratories**
**1400 West Park Blvd.**
**Funton, XY 12345-6789**

TCC Internal Use

Place Barcode Label Here

## Patient Information

| Patient Name (Print Clearly)-Last | First | Middle Initial | Gender | Birth Date (mm/dd/yyyy) | Age |
|---|---|---|---|---|---|
| | | | ☐ Male<br>☐ Female | | |
| **Patient Number** | **Sample or Hospital Number** | | **Collection Date (mm/dd/yyyy)** | | **Collection Time**<br>☐ AM<br>☐ PM |
| **Referring Physician (Print Clearly)-Last** | **First** | **Middle Initial** | **Phone or Fax (Area Code and Number)** | | |

## Call Back information - Complete ONLY if CALL BACK is required

| Phone or Fax for Call Back - Select One<br>☐ Phone  ☐ Fax - number given must be from a fax machine that complies with applicable HIPAA regulations | Phone or Fax (Area Code and Number) |
|---|---|
| | |

## Test(s) Requested

| Test Number | Test Name |
|---|---|
| | |
| | |
| | |
| | |
| | |
| | |
| | |
| | |
| Source/<br>Specimen Type | If Urine<br>TV- |

# Procedure 17–3: Insurance Claim Register

| Patient Name | Insurance Company | Claim Filing | | Insurance Response Pd, Denied, Rejct, Suspd, Info Req | Date Resubmitted | Payment | | Patient Balance | Date Patient Billed |
|---|---|---|---|---|---|---|---|---|---|
| | | Date | Amount | Date | | Date | Amount | | |
| | | | | | | | | | |
| | | | | | | | | | |
| | | | | | | | | | |
| | | | | | | | | | |
| | | | | | | | | | |
| | | | | | | | | | |
| | | | | | | | | | |
| | | | | | | | | | |
| | | | | | | | | | |
| | | | | | | | | | |
| | | | | | | | | | |
| | | | | | | | | | |
| | | | | | | | | | |
| | | | | | | | | | |
| | | | | | | | | | |
| | | | | | | | | | |
| | | | | | | | | | |
| | | | | | | | | | |
| | | | | | | | | | |
| | | | | | | | | | |
| | | | | | | | | | |
| | | | | | | | | | |
| | | | | | | | | | |
| | | | | | | | | | |
| | | | | | | | | | |
| | | | | | | | | | |
| | | | | | | | | | |
| | | | | | | | | | |
| | | | | | | | | | |
| | | | | | | | | | |
| | | | | | | | | | |
| | | | | | | | | | |
| | | | | | | | | | |
| | | | | | | | | | |
| | | | | | | | | | |
| | | | | | | | | | |
| | | | | | | | | | |
| | | | | | | | | | |

## 1500

## HEALTH INSURANCE CLAIM FORM

APPROVED BY NATIONAL UNIFORM CLAIM COMMITTEE 08/05

| | PICA | | | | | | | | PICA | |

**CARRIER**

1. MEDICARE  MEDICAID  TRICARE CHAMPUS  CHAMPVA  GROUP HEALTH PLAN  FECA BLK LUNG  OTHER
(Medicare #)  (Medicaid #)  (Sponsor's SSN)  (Member ID#)  (SSN or ID)  (SSN)  (ID)

1a. INSURED'S I.D. NUMBER  (For Program in Item 1)

2. PATIENT'S NAME (Last Name, First Name, Middle Initial)

3. PATIENT'S BIRTH DATE  MM  DD  YY  SEX  M  F

4. INSURED'S NAME (Last Name, First Name, Middle Initial)

5. PATIENT'S ADDRESS (No., Street)

6. PATIENT RELATIONSHIP TO INSURED  Self  Spouse  Child  Other

7. INSURED'S ADDRESS (No., Street)

CITY  STATE

8. PATIENT STATUS  Single  Married  Other

CITY  STATE

ZIP CODE  TELEPHONE (Include Area Code)  (     )

Employed  Full-Time Student  Part-Time Student

ZIP CODE  TELEPHONE (Include Area Code)  (     )

9. OTHER INSURED'S NAME (Last Name, First Name, Middle Initial)

10. IS PATIENT'S CONDITION RELATED TO:

11. INSURED'S POLICY GROUP OR FECA NUMBER

a. OTHER INSURED'S POLICY OR GROUP NUMBER

a. EMPLOYMENT? (Current or Previous)  YES  NO

a. INSURED'S DATE OF BIRTH  MM  DD  YY  SEX  M  F

b. OTHER INSURED'S DATE OF BIRTH  MM  DD  YY  SEX  M  F

b. AUTO ACCIDENT?  PLACE (State)  YES  NO

b. EMPLOYER'S NAME OR SCHOOL NAME

c. EMPLOYER'S NAME OR SCHOOL NAME

c. OTHER ACCIDENT?  YES  NO

c. INSURANCE PLAN NAME OR PROGRAM NAME

d. INSURANCE PLAN NAME OR PROGRAM NAME

10d. RESERVED FOR LOCAL USE

d. IS THERE ANOTHER HEALTH BENEFIT PLAN?  YES  NO  *If yes*, return to and complete item 9 a-d.

**READ BACK OF FORM BEFORE COMPLETING & SIGNING THIS FORM.**

12. PATIENT'S OR AUTHORIZED PERSON'S SIGNATURE  I authorize the release of any medical or other information necessary to process this claim. I also request payment of government benefits either to myself or to the party who accepts assignment below.

SIGNED _____  DATE _____

13. INSURED'S OR AUTHORIZED PERSON'S SIGNATURE  I authorize payment of medical benefits to the undersigned physician or supplier for services described below.

SIGNED _____

**PATIENT AND INSURED INFORMATION**

14. DATE OF CURRENT:  MM  DD  YY  ILLNESS (First symptom) OR INJURY (Accident) OR PREGNANCY(LMP)

15. IF PATIENT HAS HAD SAME OR SIMILAR ILLNESS.  GIVE FIRST DATE  MM  DD  YY

16. DATES PATIENT UNABLE TO WORK IN CURRENT OCCUPATION  MM  DD  YY  FROM  TO  MM  DD  YY

17. NAME OF REFERRING PROVIDER OR OTHER SOURCE

17a.

17b. NPI

18. HOSPITALIZATION DATES RELATED TO CURRENT SERVICES  MM  DD  YY  FROM  TO  MM  DD  YY

19. RESERVED FOR LOCAL USE

20. OUTSIDE LAB?  YES  NO  $ CHARGES

21. DIAGNOSIS OR NATURE OF ILLNESS OR INJURY (Relate Items 1, 2, 3 or 4 to Item 24E by Line)

1. L___ . ___
2. L___ . ___
3. L___ . ___
4. L___ . ___

22. MEDICAID RESUBMISSION  CODE  ORIGINAL REF. NO.

23. PRIOR AUTHORIZATION NUMBER

| 24. A. DATE(S) OF SERVICE | | | | | | B. PLACE OF SERVICE | C. EMG | D. PROCEDURES, SERVICES, OR SUPPLIES (Explain Unusual Circumstances) | | E. DIAGNOSIS POINTER | F. $ CHARGES | G. DAYS OR UNITS | H. EPSDT Family Plan | I. ID. QUAL. | J. RENDERING PROVIDER ID. # |
|---|---|---|---|---|---|---|---|---|---|---|---|---|---|---|---|
| From | | | To | | | | | CPT/HCPCS | MODIFIER | | | | | | |
| MM | DD | YY | MM | DD | YY | | | | | | | | | | |
| 1 | | | | | | | | | | | | | | NPI | |
| 2 | | | | | | | | | | | | | | NPI | |
| 3 | | | | | | | | | | | | | | NPI | |
| 4 | | | | | | | | | | | | | | NPI | |
| 5 | | | | | | | | | | | | | | NPI | |
| 6 | | | | | | | | | | | | | | NPI | |

25. FEDERAL TAX I.D. NUMBER  SSN  EIN

26. PATIENT'S ACCOUNT NO.

27. ACCEPT ASSIGNMENT? (For govt. claims, see back)  YES  NO

28. TOTAL CHARGE  $

29. AMOUNT PAID  $

30. BALANCE DUE  $

31. SIGNATURE OF PHYSICIAN OR SUPPLIER INCLUDING DEGREES OR CREDENTIALS (I certify that the statements on the reverse apply to this bill and are made a part thereof.)

SIGNED _____  DATE _____

32. SERVICE FACILITY LOCATION INFORMATION

a. NPI  b.

33. BILLING PROVIDER INFO & PH #  (     )

a. NPI  b.

**PHYSICIAN OR SUPPLIER INFORMATION**

NUCC Instruction Manual available at: www.nucc.org

APPROVED OMB-0938-0999 FORM CMS-1500 (08/05)

# Procedure 17–5: Superbill

**Total Care Clinic, PC**
342 East Park Blvd
Funton, XY 12345-6789

☐ PRIVATE ☐ BLUECROSS ☐ IND. ☐ MEDICARE ☐ MEDICAID ☐ HMO ☐ PPO

| PATIENT'S LAST NAME | FIRST | ACCOUNT # | BIRTHDATE / / | SEX ☐ MALE ☐ FEMALE | TODAY'S DATE / / |
|---|---|---|---|---|---|
| INSURANCE COMPANY | | SUBSCRIBER | PLAN # | SUB. # | GROUP |

| ASSIGNMENT: I hereby assign my insurance benefits to be paid directly to the undersigned physician. I am financially responsible for non-covered services. SIGNED: (Patient, or Parent, if Minor)    DATE:  /  / | RELEASE: I hereby authorize the physician to release to my insurance carrers any information required to process this claim. SIGNED: (Patient, or Parent, if Minor)    DATE:  /  / |
|---|---|

| ✔ | DESCRIPTION | M/Care | CPT/Mod | DxRe | FEE | ✔ | DESCRIPTION | M/Care | CPT/Mod | DxRe | FEE | ✔ | DESCRIPTION | M/Care | CPT/Mod | DxRe | FEE |
|---|---|---|---|---|---|---|---|---|---|---|---|---|---|---|---|---|---|
| | OFFICE CARE | | | | | | PROCEDURES | | | | | | INJECTIONS/IMMUNIZATIONS | | | | |
| | NEW PATIENT | | | | | | Tread Mill (In Office) | | 93015 | | | | Tetanus/Diphtheria | | 90718 | | |
| | Brief | | 99201 | | | | 24 Hour Holter | | 93224 | | | | MMR | | 90707 | | |
| | Limited | | 99202 | | | | If Medicare (Set up Fee) | | 93225 | | | | Pneumococcal | | 90732 | | |
| | Intermediate | | 99203 | | | | Physician Interpret | | 93227 | | | | Influenza | | 90656 | | |
| | Extended | | 99204 | | | | EKG w/Interpretation | | 93000 | | | | TB Skin Test (PPD) | | 86580 | | |
| | Comprehensive | | 99205 | | | | EKG (tracing only) | | 93005 | | | | Antigen Injection-Single | | 95115 | | |
| | | | | | | | Sigmoidoscopy | | 45300 | | | | Multiple | | 95117 | | |
| | ESTABLISHED PATIENT | | | | | | Sigmoidoscopy, Flexible | | 45330 | | | | B12 Injection | J3420 | 90782 | | |
| | Minimal | | 99211 | | | | Sigmoidos. , Flex. w/Bx. | | 45331 | | | | Injection, IM | | 90782 | | |
| | Brief | | 99212 | | | | Spirometry, FEV/FVC | | 94010 | | | | Compazine | J0780 | 90782 | | |
| | Limited | | 99213 | | | | Spirometry, Post-Dilator | | 94060 | | | | Demerol | J2175 | 90782 | | |
| | Intermediate | | 99214 | | | | | | | | | | Vistaril | J3410 | 90782 | | |
| | Extended | | 99215 | | | | | | | | | | Susphrine | J0170 | 90782 | | |
| | Comprehensive | | 99215 | | | | LABORATORY | | | | | | Decadron | J0890 | 90782 | | |
| | | | | | | | Blood Draw Fee | | 36415 | | | | Estradiol | J1000 | 90782 | | |
| | CONSULTATION-OFFICE | | | | | | Urinalysis, Chemical | | 81000 | | | | Testosterone | J1080 | 90782 | | |
| | Focused | | 99241 | | | | Throat Culture | | 87081 | | | | Lidocaine | J2000 | 90782 | | |
| | Expanded | | 99242 | | | | Occult Blood | | 82270 | | | | Solumedrol | J2920 | 90782 | | |
| | Detailed | | 99243 | | | | Pap Handling Charge | | 99000 | | | | Solucortef | J1720 | 90782 | | |
| | Comprehensive 1 | | 99244 | | | | Pap Life Guard | | 88150-90 | | | | Hydeltra | J1690 | 90782 | | |
| | Comprehensive 2 | | 99245 | | | | Gram Stain | | 87205 | | | | | | | | |
| | MCR Pts - use E/M codes | | | | | | Hanging Drop | | 87210 | | | | INJECTIONS - JOINT/BURSA | | | | |
| | Case Management | | 98900 | | | | Urine Drug Screen | | 80100 | | | | Small Joints | | 20600 | | |
| | | | | | | | | | | | | | Intermediate | | 20605 | | |
| | Post-op Exam | | 99024 | | | | SUPPLIES | | | | | | Large Joints | | 20610 | | |
| | | | | | | | | | | | | | Trigger Point | | 20552 | | |
| | | | | | | | | | | | | | MISCELLANEOUS | | | | |

| DIAGNOSIS: | ICD-9 | | | | | | |
|---|---|---|---|---|---|---|---|
| Abdominal Pain | 789.0 | Gout | 274.0 | C.V.A. - Acute | 436. | Electrolyte Dis. | 276.9 | Herpes Simplex | 054.9 |
| Abscess (Site) | 682.9 | Asthma | 493.90 | Cere. Vas. Accid. (Old) | 438 | Fatigue | 780.7 | Herpes Zoster | 053.9 |
| Adverse Drug Rx | 995.2 | Asthmatic Bronchitis | 493.90 | Cerumen | 380.4 | Fibrocys. Br. Dis | 610.1 | Hydrocele | 603.9 |
| Alcohol Detox | 291.8 | Atrial Fib. | 427.31 | Chestwall Pain | 786.59 | Fracture (Site) | 829.0 | Hyperlipidemia | 272.4 |
| Alcoholism | 303.90 | Atrial Tachi. | 427.0 | Cholecystitis | 575.0 | Open/Close | | Hypertension | 401.9 |
| Allergic Rhinitis | 477 | Bowel Obstruct. | 560.9 | Cholelithiasis | 574.00 | Fungal Infect. (Site) | 110.8 | Hyperthyroidism | 242.9 |
| Allergy | 995.3 | Breast Mass | 611.72 | COPD | 492.8 | Gastric Ulcer | 531.90 | Hypothyroidism | 244.9 |
| Alzheimer's Dis. | 290.1 | Bronchitis | 490 | Cirrhosis | 571.5 | Gastritis | 535.0 | Labyrinthitis | 386.30 |
| Anemia | 285.9 | Bursitis | 727.3 | Cong. Heart Fail. | 428.9 | Gastroenteritis | 558.9 | Lipoma (Site) | 214.9 |
| Anemia - Pernicious | 281.0 | Cancer, Breast (Site) | 174.9 | Conjunctivitis | 372.30 | G.I. Bleeding | 578.9 | Lymphoma | 202.8 |
| Angina | 413.9 | Metastatic (Site) | 199.1 | Contusion (Site) | 924.9 | Glomerulonephritis | 583.9 | Mit. Valve Prolapse | 424.0 |
| Anxiety Synd. | 300.00 | Colon | 153.9 | Costochondritis | 733.99 | Headache | 784.0 | Myocard. Infarction (Area) | 410.9 |
| Appendicitis | 541 | Cancer, Rectal | 154.1 | Depression | 311. | Headache, Tension | 307.81 | M.I., Old | 412 |
| Arterioscl. H.D. | 414.0 | Lung (Site) | 162.9 | Dermatitis | 692.9 | Migraine (Type) | 346.9 | Myositis | 729.1 |
| Arthritis, Osteo. | 715.90 | Skin (Site) | 173.9 | Diabetes Mellitus | 250.00 | Hemorrhoids | 455.6 | Nausea/Vomiting | 787.0 |
| Rheumatoid | 714.0 | Card. Arrhythmia (Type) | 427.9 | Diabetic Ketosis | 250.1 | Hernia, Hiatal | 553.3 | Neuralgia | 729.2 |
| Lupus | 710.0 | Cardiomyopathy | 425.4 | Diverticulitis | 562.11 | Inguinal | 550.9 | Nevus (Site) | 216.9 |
| | | Cellulitis (Site) | 682.9 | Diverticulosis | 562.10 | Hepatitis | 573.3 | Obesity | 278.0 |

DIAGNOSIS: (IF NOT CHECKED ABOVE)

| SERVICES PERFORMED AT: ☐ Office ☐ E.R. ☐ CLAIM CONTAINS NO ORDERED REFERRING SERVICE ☐ Rodriguez Patel ☐ Fredericks Kacharski ☐ Wiley | REFERRING PHYSICIAN & I.D. NUMBER |
|---|---|

| RETURN APPOINTMENT INFORMATION: 5 - 10 - 15 - 20 - 30 - 40 - 60  [  DAYS] [  WKS.] [  MOS.] [  PRN] | NEXT APPOINTMENT M - T - W - TH - F - S  DATE / / TIME: | AM PM | ACCEPT ASSIGNMENT? ☐ YES ☐ NO | DOCTOR'S SIGNATURE |
|---|---|---|---|---|

| INSTRUCTIONS TO PATIENT FOR FILING INSURANCE CLAIMS: | | |
|---|---|---|
| 1. Complete upper portion of this form, sign and date. 2. Attach this form to your own insurance company's form for direct reimbursement. **MEDICARE PATIENTS - DO NOT SEND THIS TO MEDICARE. WE WILL SUBMIT THE CLAIM FOR YOU.** | ☐ CASH ☐ CHECK # _____ ☐ VISA ☐ MC ☐ CO-PAY | TOTAL TODAY'S FEE ___ OLD BALANCE ___ TOTAL DUE ___ AMOUNT REC'D. TODAY ___ |

INSUR-A-BILL ® BIBBERO SYSTEMS, INC. • PETALUMA, CA • UP. SUPER. © 6/94 (BIBB/STOCK)

# Procedure 17–6: Age Analysis

## ACCOUNTS RECEIVABLE–AGE ANALYSIS

Date: _____

| Patient | Balance | Date of Charges | Most Recent Payment | 30 days | 60 days | 90 days | 120 days | Remarks |
|---------|---------|-----------------|---------------------|---------|---------|---------|----------|---------|
|         |         |                 |                     |         |         |         |          |         |
|         |         |                 |                     |         |         |         |          |         |
|         |         |                 |                     |         |         |         |          |         |
|         |         |                 |                     |         |         |         |          |         |
|         |         |                 |                     |         |         |         |          |         |
|         |         |                 |                     |         |         |         |          |         |
|         |         |                 |                     |         |         |         |          |         |

# Procedure 19–1: Superbill

**Total Care Clinic, PC**
342 East Park Blvd
Funton, XY 12345-6789

☐ PRIVATE  ☐ BLUECROSS  ☐ IND.  ☐ MEDICARE  ☐ MEDICAID  ☐ HMO  ☐ PPO

| PATIENT'S LAST NAME | FIRST | ACCOUNT # | BIRTHDATE / / | SEX ☐ MALE ☐ FEMALE | TODAY'S DATE / / |
|---|---|---|---|---|---|
| INSURANCE COMPANY | SUBSCRIBER | | PLAN # | SUB. # | GROUP |

ASSIGNMENT: I hereby assign my insurance benefits to be paid directly to the undersigned physician. I am financially responsible for non-covered services.
SIGNED: (Patient, or Parent, if Minor)     DATE: / /

RELEASE: I hereby authorize the physician to release to my insurance carrers any information required to process this claim.
SIGNED: (Patient, or Parent, if Minor)     DATE: / /

| ✔ | DESCRIPTION | M/Care | CPT/Mod | DxRe | FEE | ✔ | DESCRIPTION | M/Care | CPT/Mod | DxRe | FEE | ✔ | DESCRIPTION | M/Care | CPT/Mod | DxRe | FEE |
|---|---|---|---|---|---|---|---|---|---|---|---|---|---|---|---|---|---|
| | OFFICE CARE | | | | | | PROCEDURES | | | | | | INJECTIONS/IMMUNIZATIONS | | | | |
| | NEW PATIENT | | | | | | Tread Mill (In Office) | | 93015 | | | | Tetanus/Diphtheria | | 90718 | | |
| | Brief | | 99201 | | | | 24 Hour Holter | | 93224 | | | | MMR | | 90707 | | |
| | Limited | | 99202 | | | | If Medicare (Set up Fec) | | 93225 | | | | Pneumococcal | | 90732 | | |
| | Intermediate | | 99203 | | | | Physician Interpret | | 93227 | | | | Influenza | | 90656 | | |
| | Extended | | 99204 | | | | EKG w/Interpretation | | 93000 | | | | TB Skin Test (PPD) | | 86580 | | |
| | Comprehensive | | 99205 | | | | EKG (tracing only) | | 93005 | | | | Antigen Injection-Single | | 95115 | | |
| | | | | | | | Sigmoidoscopy | | 45300 | | | | Multiple | | 95117 | | |
| | ESTABLISHED PATIENT | | | | | | Sigmoidoscopy, Flexible | | 45330 | | | | B12 Injection | J3420 | 90782 | | |
| | Minimal | | 99211 | | | | Sigmoidos. , Flex. w/Bx. | | 45331 | | | | Injection, IM | | 90782 | | |
| | Brief | | 99212 | | | | Spirometry, FEV/FVC | | 94010 | | | | Compazine | J0780 | 90782 | | |
| | Limited | | 99213 | | | | Spirometry, Post-Dilator | | 94060 | | | | Demerol | J2175 | 90782 | | |
| | Intermediate | | 99214 | | | | | | | | | | Vistaril | J3410 | 90782 | | |
| | Extended | | 99215 | | | | | | | | | | Susphrine | J0170 | 90782 | | |
| | Comprehensive | | 99215 | | | | LABORATORY | | | | | | Decadron | J0890 | 90782 | | |
| | | | | | | | Blood Draw Fee | | 36415 | | | | Estradiol | J1000 | 90782 | | |
| | CONSULTATION-OFFICE | | | | | | Urinalysis, Chemical | | 81000 | | | | Testosterone | J1080 | 90782 | | |
| | Focused | | 99241 | | | | Throat Culture | | 87081 | | | | Lidocaine | J2000 | 90782 | | |
| | Expanded | | 99242 | | | | Occult Blood | | 82270 | | | | Solumedrol | J2920 | 90782 | | |
| | Detailed | | 99243 | | | | Pap Handling Charge | | 99000 | | | | Solucortef | J1720 | 90782 | | |
| | Comprehensive 1 | | 99244 | | | | Pap Life Guard | | 88150-90 | | | | Hydeltra | J1690 | 90782 | | |
| | Comprehensive 2 | | 99245 | | | | Gram Stain | | 87205 | | | | | | | | |
| | MCR Pts - use E/M codes | | | | | | Hanging Drop | | 87210 | | | | INJECTIONS - JOINT/BURSA | | | | |
| | Case Management | | 98900 | | | | Urine Drug Screen | | 80100 | | | | Small Joints | | 20600 | | |
| | | | | | | | | | | | | | Intermediate | | 20605 | | |
| | Post-op Exam | | 99024 | | | | | | | | | | Large Joints | | 20610 | | |
| | | | | | | | SUPPLIES | | | | | | Trigger Point | | 20552 | | |
| | | | | | | | | | | | | | MISCELLANEOUS | | | | |

**DIAGNOSIS:**

| | | ICD-9 | | | | | | | | | | | |
|---|---|---|---|---|---|---|---|---|---|---|---|---|---|
| | Abdominal Pain | 789.0 | | Gout | 274.0 | | C.V.A. - Acute | 436. | | Electrolyte Dis. | 276.9 | | Herpes Simplex | 054.9 |
| | Abscess (Site) | 682.9 | | Asthma | 493.90 | | Cere. Vas. Accid. (Old) | 438 | | Fatigue | 780.7 | | Herpes Zoster | 053.9 |
| | Adverse Drug Rx | 995.2 | | Asthmatic Bronchitis | 493.90 | | Cerumen | 380.4 | | Fibrocys. Br. Dis | 610.1 | | Hydrocele | 603.9 |
| | Alcohol Detox | 291.8 | | Atrial Fib. | 427.31 | | Chestwall Pain | 786.59 | | Fracture (Site) | 829.0 | | Hyperlipidemia | 272.4 |
| | Alcoholism | 303.90 | | Atrial Tachi. | 427.0 | | Cholecystitis | 575.0 | | Open/Close | | | Hypertension | 401.9 |
| | Allergic Rhinitis | 477 | | Bowel Obstruct. | 560.9 | | Cholelithiasis | 574.00 | | Fungal Infect. (Site) | 110.8 | | Hyperthyroidism | 242.9 |
| | Allergy | 995.3 | | Breast Mass | 611.72 | | COPD | 492.8 | | Gastric Ulcer | 531.90 | | Hypothyroidism | 244.9 |
| | Alzheimer's Dis. | 290.1 | | Bronchitis | 490 | | Cirrhosis | 571.5 | | Gastritis | 535.0 | | Labyrinthitis | 386.30 |
| | Anemia | 285.9 | | Bursitis | 727.3 | | Cong. Heart Fail. | 428.9 | | Gastroenteritis | 558.9 | | Lipoma (Site) | 214.9 |
| | Anemia - Pernicious | 281.0 | | Cancer, Breast (Site) | 174.9 | | Conjunctivitis | 372.30 | | G.I. Bleeding | 578.9 | | Lymphoma | 202.8 |
| | Angina | 413.9 | | Metastatic (Site) | 199.1 | | Contusion (Site) | 924.9 | | Glomerulonephritis | 583.9 | | Mit. Valve Prolapse | 424.0 |
| | Anxiety Synd. | 300.00 | | Colon | 153.9 | | Costochondritis | 733.99 | | Headache | 784.0 | | Myocard. Infarction (Area) | 410.9 |
| | Appendicitis | 541 | | Cancer, Rectal | 154.1 | | Depression | 311. | | Headache, Tension | 307.81 | | M.I., Old | 412 |
| | Arterioscl. H.D. | 414.0 | | Lung (Site) | 162.9 | | Dermatitis | 692.9 | | Migraine (Type) | 346.9 | | Myositis | 729.1 |
| | Arthritis, Osteo. | 715.90 | | Skin (Site) | 173.9 | | Diabetes Mellitus | 250.00 | | Hemorrhoids | 455.6 | | Nausea/Vomiting | 787.0 |
| | Rheumatoid | 714.0 | | Card. Arrhythmia (Type) | 427.9 | | Diabetic Ketosis | 250.1 | | Hernia, Hiatal | 553.3 | | Neuralgia | 729.2 |
| | Lupus | 710.0 | | Cardiomyopathy | 425.4 | | Diverticulitis | 562.11 | | Inguinal | 550.9 | | Nevus (Site) | 216.9 |
| | | | | Cellulitis (Site) | 682.9 | | Diverticulosis | 562.10 | | Hepatitis | 573.3 | | Obesity | 278.0 |

DIAGNOSIS: (IF NOT CHECKED ABOVE)

SERVICES PERFORMED AT: ☐ Office ☐ E.R.  ☐ CLAIM CONTAINS NO ORDERED REFERRING SERVICE

☐ Rodriguez Patel  ☐ Fredericks Kacharski  ☐ Wiley

REFERRING PHYSICIAN & I.D. NUMBER

| RETURN APPOINTMENT INFORMATION: 5 - 10 - 15 - 20 - 30 - 40 - 60  [ DAYS] [ WKS.] [ MOS.] [ PRN] | NEXT APPOINTMENT  M - T - W - TH - F - S  DATE / / TIME: | ACCEPT ASSIGNMENT? AM ☐ YES PM ☐ NO | DOCTOR'S SIGNATURE |
|---|---|---|---|

**INSTRUCTIONS TO PATIENT FOR FILING INSURANCE CLAIMS:**

1. Complete upper portion of this form, sign and date.
2. Attach this form to your own insurance company's form for direct reimbursement.

**MEDICARE PATIENTS - DO NOT SEND THIS TO MEDICARE. WE WILL SUBMIT THE CLAIM FOR YOU.**

☐ CASH
☐ CHECK  #
☐ VISA
☐ MC
☐ CO-PAY

| TOTAL TODAY'S FEE | |
|---|---|
| OLD BALANCE | |
| TOTAL DUE | |
| AMOUNT REC'D. TODAY | |

INSUR-A-BILL ® BIBBERO SYSTEMS, INC. • PETALUMA, CA • UP. SUPER. © 6/94 (BIBB/STOCK)

# Procedure 21–1: Daily Log

**Dr.** _____   **Date** _____

| Hour | Patient | Service Provided | Charge | Payment | Adj | Balance |
|------|---------|------------------|--------|---------|-----|---------|
|      | 1       |                  |        |         |     |         |
|      | 2       |                  |        |         |     |         |
|      | 3       |                  |        |         |     |         |
|      | 4       |                  |        |         |     |         |
|      | 5       |                  |        |         |     |         |
|      | 6       |                  |        |         |     |         |
|      | 7       |                  |        |         |     |         |
|      | 8       |                  |        |         |     |         |
|      | 9       |                  |        |         |     |         |
|      | 10      |                  |        |         |     |         |
|      | 11      |                  |        |         |     |         |
|      | 12      |                  |        |         |     |         |
|      | 13      |                  |        |         |     |         |
|      | 14      |                  |        |         |     |         |
|      | 15      |                  |        |         |     |         |
|      | 16      |                  |        |         |     |         |
|      |         |                  |        | *Totals* |     |         |

# Procedure 21–1: Patient Ledger Card

**TOTAL CARE CLINIC, PC**
342 East Park Blvd
Funton, XY 12345-6789

Patient's Name _____

Home Phone _____ **Work Phone** _____

Social Security No. _____

Employer _____

Insurance _____

Policy # _____

**Person Responsible for Charges (if Different from Patient)** _____

| Date | Reference | Description | Charge | Credits | | Current Balance |
|------|-----------|-------------|--------|---------|-----|-----------------|
|      |           |             |        | Payments | Adj. |                 |
|      |           | Balance Forward ——→ |  |  |  |                 |
|      |           |             |        |         |     |                 |
|      |           |             |        |         |     |                 |
|      |           |             |        |         |     |                 |
|      |           |             |        |         |     |                 |
|      |           |             |        |         |     |                 |
|      |           |             |        |         |     |                 |
|      |           |             |        |         |     |                 |
|      |           |             |        |         |     |                 |
|      |           |             |        |         |     |                 |
|      |           |             |        |         |     |                 |
|      |           |             |        |         |     |                 |
|      |           |             |        |         |     |                 |
|      |           |             |        |         |     |                 |
|      |           |             |        |         |     |                 |
|      |           |             |        |         |     |                 |
|      |           |             |        |         |     |                 |
|      |           |             |        |         |     |                 |
|      |           |             |        |         |     |                 |

Please Pay Last Amount in This Column

OV—Office Visit       C—Consultation       EX—Examination
X—X-ray               NC—No Charge         INS—Insurance
ROA—Received on Account   MA—Missed Appointment

# Procedure 21–2: Daily Log

| Hour | Patient | Service Provided | Charge | Payment | Adj | Balance |
|------|---------|------------------|--------|---------|-----|---------|
| Dr. _____   Date _____ | | | | | | |
| | 1 | | | | | |
| | 2 | | | | | |
| | 3 | | | | | |
| | 4 | | | | | |
| | 5 | | | | | |
| | 6 | | | | | |
| | 7 | | | | | |
| | 8 | | | | | |
| | 9 | | | | | |
| | 10 | | | | | |
| | 11 | | | | | |
| | 12 | | | | | |
| | 13 | | | | | |
| | 14 | | | | | |
| | 15 | | | | | |
| | 16 | | | | | |
| | | | | Totals | | |

# Procedure 21–2: Patient Ledger Card

TOTAL CARE CLINIC, PC
342 East Park Blvd
Funton, XY 12345-6789

**Patient's Name** _____

**Home Phone** _____ **Work Phone** _____

**Social Security No.** _____

**Employer** _____

**Insurance** _____

**Policy #** _____

**Person Responsible for Charges (if Different from Patient)** _____

| Date | Reference | Description | Charge | Credits | | Current Balance |
|------|-----------|-------------|--------|---------|-----|-----------------|
|      |           |             |        | Payments | Adj. |                 |
|      |           | Balance Forward ⟶ |   |         |     |                 |
|      |           |             |        |         |     |                 |
|      |           |             |        |         |     |                 |
|      |           |             |        |         |     |                 |
|      |           |             |        |         |     |                 |
|      |           |             |        |         |     |                 |
|      |           |             |        |         |     |                 |
|      |           |             |        |         |     |                 |
|      |           |             |        |         |     |                 |
|      |           |             |        |         |     |                 |
|      |           |             |        |         |     |                 |
|      |           |             |        |         |     |                 |
|      |           |             |        |         |     |                 |
|      |           |             |        |         |     |                 |
|      |           |             |        |         |     |                 |
|      |           |             |        |         |     |                 |
|      |           |             |        |         |     |                 |
|      |           |             |        |         |     |                 |
|      |           |             |        |         |     |                 |
|      |           |             |        |         |     |                 |

Please Pay Last Amount in This Column ▲

OV—Office Visit          C—Consultation          EX—Examination
X—X-ray                  NC—No Charge            INS—Insurance
ROA—Received on Account  MA—Missed Appointment

# Procedure 21–3: Daily Log

| | | | | | | |
|---|---|---|---|---|---|---|
| Dr. _____ | | | Date _____ | | | |

| Hour | Patient | Service Provided | Charge | Payment | Adj | Balance |
|---|---|---|---|---|---|---|
| | 1 | | | | | |
| | 2 | | | | | |
| | 3 | | | | | |
| | 4 | | | | | |
| | 5 | | | | | |
| | 6 | | | | | |
| | 7 | | | | | |
| | 8 | | | | | |
| | 9 | | | | | |
| | 10 | | | | | |
| | 11 | | | | | |
| | 12 | | | | | |
| | 13 | | | | | |
| | 14 | | | | | |
| | 15 | | | | | |
| | 16 | | | | | |
| | | | | Totals | | |

# Procedure 21–3: Patient Ledger Card

**TOTAL CARE CLINIC, PC**
342 East Park Blvd
Funton, XY 12345-6789

**Patient's Name** _____

**Home Phone** _____ **Work Phone** _____

**Social Security No.** _____

**Employer** _____

**Insurance** _____

**Policy #** _____

**Person Responsible for Charges (if Different from Patient)** _____

| Date | Reference | Description | Charge | Credits | | Current Balance |
|------|-----------|-------------|--------|---------|-----|-----------------|
| | | | | Payments | Adj. | |
| | | Balance Forward ⟶ | | | | |
| | | | | | | |
| | | | | | | |
| | | | | | | |
| | | | | | | |
| | | | | | | |
| | | | | | | |
| | | | | | | |
| | | | | | | |
| | | | | | | |
| | | | | | | |
| | | | | | | |
| | | | | | | |
| | | | | | | |
| | | | | | | |
| | | | | | | |
| | | | | | | |
| | | | | | | |
| | | | | | | |

Please Pay Last Amount in This Column ▲

OV—Office Visit          C—Consultation          EX—Examination
X—X-ray                  NC—No Charge             INS—Insurance
ROA—Received on Account  MA—Missed Appointment

# Procedure 21–4: Patient Ledger Card

**TOTAL CARE CLINIC, PC**
342 East Park Blvd
Funton, XY 12345-6789

**Patient's Name** _____

**Home Phone** _____  **Work Phone** _____

**Social Security No.** _____

**Employer** _____

**Insurance** _____

**Policy #** _____

**Person Responsible for Charges (if Different from Patient)** _____

| Date | Reference | Description | Charge | Credits | | Current Balance |
|------|-----------|-------------|--------|---------|------|-----------------|
| | | | | Payments | Adj. | |
| | | Balance Forward ⟶ | | | | |
| | | | | | | |
| | | | | | | |
| | | | | | | |
| | | | | | | |
| | | | | | | |
| | | | | | | |
| | | | | | | |
| | | | | | | |
| | | | | | | |
| | | | | | | |
| | | | | | | |
| | | | | | | |
| | | | | | | |
| | | | | | | |
| | | | | | | |
| | | | | | | |
| | | | | | | |

Please Pay Last Amount in This Column ▲

OV—Office Visit          C—Consultation          EX—Examination
X—X-ray                  NC—No Charge            INS—Insurance
ROA—Received on Account  MA—Missed Appointment

**DEPOSIT TICKET**

**TOTAL CARE CLINIC, PC**

342 East Park Blvd
Funton, XY 12345-6789

DATE _____**20**____
*DEPOSITS MAY NOT BE AVAILABLE FOR IMMEDIATE WITHDRAWAL*

_____

| CASH | CURRENCY | | |
|------|----------|--|--|
| | COIN | | |
| LIST CHECKS SINGLY | | | |
| | | | |
| | | | |
| | | | |
| | TOTAL | | |
| → | LESS CASH RECEIVED | | |
| | NET DEPOSIT | | |

89-852
―――
622

BE SURE EACH ITEM IS
PROPERLY ENDORSED

## FIRST NATIONAL BANK

### CLINTON BRANCH

⑆062208525⑆ 526 6612 ⑈ 0789

CHECKS AND OTHER ITEMS ARE RECEIVED FOR DEPOSIT SUBJECT TO THE PROVISIONS OF THE UNIFORM COMMERCIAL CODE OR ANY APPLICABLE COLLECTION AGREEMENT

| CHECKS LIST SINGLY | DOLLARS | CENTS |
|--------------------|---------|-------|
| 1 | | |
| 2 | | |
| 3 | | |
| 4 | | |
| 5 | | |
| 6 | | |
| 7 | | |
| 8 | | |
| 9 | | |
| 10 | | |
| 11 | | |
| 12 | | |
| 13 | | |
| 14 | | |
| 15 | | |
| TOTAL | | |

ENTER TOTAL ON THE FRONT SIDE OF THIS TICKET

# Procedure 21–6: Bank Reconciliation Form

## BANK RECONCILIATION

CLIENT NAME: _____  MONTH OF: _____

BANK: _____  ACCOUNT NO. : _____

| GENERAL LEDGER | | BALANCE PER BANK STATEMENT | |
|---|---|---|---|
| ACCOUNT BALANCE............................. | | AS OF: | |
| ADD DEBITS: | | ADD DEPOSITS IN TRANSIT: | |
| | | | |
| | | | |
| | | | |
| | | | |
| | | | |
| TOTAL DR............. | | | |
| TOTAL................................ | | TOTAL IN TRANSIT | |
| | | TOTAL................................. | |
| LESS CREDITS: | | | |
| Checks | | | |
| Auto Withdrawals | | | |
| Bank Fees | | | |
| | | LESS CHECKS OUTSTANDING: | |
| | | (SEE LIST BELOW) | |
| TOTAL CR............. | | TOTAL................. | |
| BANK BAL PER GENERAL LEDGER.. | | BANK BALANCE PER REC.................. | |

**CHECKS:**

| NUMBER | AMOUNT | NUMBER | NUMBER | NUMBER | AMOUNT |
|---|---|---|---|---|---|
| | | | | | |
| | | | | | |
| | | | | | |
| | | | | | |
| | | | | | |
| | | | | | |
| | | | | | |
| | | | | | |
| | | | | | |
| | | | | | |
| | | | | | |
| | | | | | TOTAL |
| TOTAL | | TOTAL | | GRAND TOTAL | |

# Procedure 21–7: Record of Office Disbursements

**Record of Office Disbursements**
_____ 2012

| DATE | PAYEE | CK. NO. | TOTAL AMOUNT | RENT | UTILITIES | POSTAGE | LAB./ X-RAY | MEDICAL SUPPLIES | OFFICE SUPPLIES | WAGES | INSURANCE | TAXES | TRAVEL | MISC. |
|------|-------|---------|--------------|------|-----------|---------|-------------|------------------|-----------------|-------|-----------|-------|--------|-------|
| | | | | | | | | | | | | | | |

**TYPES OF EXPENSES**

# Procedure 21–8: Employee Earnings Record

| | | | | | | | | | | | | |
|---|---|---|---|---|---|---|---|---|---|---|---|---|

Name _____  Soc. Sec. No. _____  Dependents _____ Year _____

Address _____  Birth Date _____  Deductions _____

_____  Job Title _____  Pay Rate _____

_____  Employed on _____

Spouse _____  Terminated on _____  Record of Changes

Phone _____  Reason _____

| Date | Rate |
|---|---|
| | |
| | |

| Check Number | Period Number | Earnings | | | Deductions | | | | | Net Pay | Cumulative FICA |
|---|---|---|---|---|---|---|---|---|---|---|---|
| | | Regular | OT | Total | FICA | Fed. Tax | State | SUI | SDI | | |
| | | | | | | | | | | | |
| | | | | | | | | | | | |
| | | | | | | | | | | | |
| | | | | | | | | | | | |
| | | | | | | | | | | | |
| | | | | | | | | | | | |
| | | | | | | | | | | | |
| | | | | | | | | | | | |
| 1st Quarter Total | | | | | | | | | | | |
| | | | | | | | | | | | |
| | | | | | | | | | | | |
| | | | | | | | | | | | |
| | | | | | | | | | | | |
| | | | | | | | | | | | |
| | | | | | | | | | | | |
| | | | | | | | | | | | |
| | | | | | | | | | | | |
| 2d Quarter Total | | | | | | | | | | | |
| | | | | | | | | | | | |
| | | | | | | | | | | | |
| | | | | | | | | | | | |
| | | | | | | | | | | | |
| | | | | | | | | | | | |
| | | | | | | | | | | | |
| | | | | | | | | | | | |
| | | | | | | | | | | | |
| 3d Quarter Total | | | | | | | | | | | |
| | | | | | | | | | | | |
| | | | | | | | | | | | |
| | | | | | | | | | | | |
| | | | | | | | | | | | |
| | | | | | | | | | | | |
| | | | | | | | | | | | |
| 4th Quarter Total | | | | | | | | | | | |

# Procedure 21–8: Payroll Register

Pay Period 6/1–6/14

| Emp. No. | Name | Earnings to date | Hrly. Rate | Reg. Hrs. | OT Hrs. | OT Earnings | TOTAL GROSS | Earnings Subject to Unemp. | Earnings Subject to FICA | Social Security (FICA) | Medicare | Federal W/H | State W/H | Health Ins. | Net Pay | Check No. |
|---|---|---|---|---|---|---|---|---|---|---|---|---|---|---|---|---|
| | | | | | | | | | | | | | | | | |
| | | | | | | | | | | | | | | | | |
| | | | | | | | | | | | | | | | | |
| | | | | | | | | | | | | | | | | |
| | | | | | | | | | | | | | | | | |
| | | | | | | | | | | | | | | | | |
| | | | | | | | | | | | | | | | | |

**TOTAL CARE CLINIC, PC**

342 East Park Blvd
Funton, XY 12345-6789
Tel: 521-234-0001
Fax: 521-234-0002

## TRAVEL EXPENSE REPORT
### (Travel with estimated expenses must be approved prior to the event)

Applicant's name: _____ Date: _____

Applicant's address: _____

Applicant's cell phone and home phone: _____

Name of activity and type (example: professional meeting, conference; attach Web or brochure information): _____

Purpose of travel: _____

Location of activity: _____

Dates: _____ Number of days: _____

| | |
|---|---|
| **Registration fee** | $ |
| **Transportation: *indicate major mode of travel** _____ | $ |
| Airport shuttle or parking | $ |
| Taxi | $ |
| **Lodging (daily rate_____ × _____number of days)** | $ |
| **Meals ($30 per day × _____ number of days)** | $ |
| **Other (explain)** | $ |
| **Total** | $ |

Did you miss work days:  ☐ NO  ☐ YES (If "YES" include dates and number of days)

Dates: _____ Number of days: _____

Signature: _____

*If using your own vehicle, mileage is reimbursed at the current rate. Check with your supervisor prior to travel.

*This form must be submitted with receipts in 10 working days upon return. Noncompliance may result in denial of reimbursement or if funds were previously awarded, payroll deduction may occur to recover the amount.*

---

### For Management Use Only

☐  Not approved   ☐  Approved   Amount:_____

Name (print):_____ Date:_____

Signature:_____

# Procedure 22–3: Incident Report

## TOTAL CARE CLINIC, PC

342 E. Park Blvd
Funton, XY 12345-6789
Tel: 521-234-0001
Fax: 521-234-0002

### Incident Report
**(Only for Internal Use)**

Date/time of incident: _____  Location: _____

**Name of injured or at risk party:**_____

**Circle one:**      **Patient**      **Staff Member**      **Other (complete blank)** _____

**Address of above party:**_____

**Phone numbers of above party: home**_____ cell _____

**Describe the incident (use back of sheet if additional space needed):** _____

_____

_____

_____

**Describe action(s) taken and by whom:** _____

_____

_____

_____

**Name(s)/contact information of witnesses:** _____

_____

_____

**Name(s)/time of parties notified:** _____

_____

**Name of person completing report:** _____  Date/time: _____

**Report submitted to:** _____  Date/time: _____

**(Submit form to immediate supervisor of area where the incident occurred)**

# Procedure 24–2: Sample Application for Employment

## APPLICATION FOR EMPLOYMENT

**PERSONAL INFORMATION**          DATE OF APPLICATION: _____

**Name:** ...................................................................................................................
                Last                First              Middle

**Address:** ...............................................................................................................
          Street          (Apt)        City, State        Zip

**Alternate Address:** ...............................................................................................
         Street                  City, State        Zip

**Contact Information:**   **( )**        **( )** ....................................
                Home Telephone      Mobile        E-mail

*How did you learn about our facility?*

**POSITION SOUGHT:** _____   **Available Start Date:** _____

**Desired Pay Range:** _____   **Are you currently employed?** _____
             By Hour or Salary

**EDUCATION**

|  | Name and Location | Graduate?—Degree? | Major/Subjects of Study |
|---|---|---|---|
| **High School** | | | |
| **College or University** | | | |
| **Specialized Training, Trade School, etc.** | | | |
| **Other Education** | | | |

**Please list your areas of highest proficiency, special skills, or other items that may contribute to your abilities in performing the above-mentioned position.**

.....................................................................................................................................

.....................................................................................................................................

.....................................................................................................................................

*(Continued)*

# Procedure 24–2: Sample Application for Employment *(concluded)*

## PREVIOUS EXPERIENCE

Please list, beginning from most-recent [add pages if needed].

| Dates Employed | Company Name | Location | Role/Title |
|---|---|---|---|
| | | | |

**Job notes, tasks performed, and reason for leaving:**

| Dates Employed | Company Name | Location | Role/Title |
|---|---|---|---|
| | | | |

**Job notes, tasks performed, and reason for leaving:**

## REFERENCES

Provide names and contact information.

**Name:**                                         **Job Title or Relationship:**

**Address:**
        Street        (Apt)        City, State        Zip

**Contact Information:**  (  )      (  )
        Phone        Fax        E-mail

**Name:**                                         **Job Title or Relationship:**

**Address:**
        Street        (Apt)        City, State        Zip

**Contact Information:**  (  )      (  )
        Phone        Fax        E-mail

**Name:**                                         **Job Title or Relationship:**

**Address:**
        Street        (Apt)        City, State        Zip

**Contact Information:**  (  )      (  )
        Phone        Fax        E-mail

**Applicant's Signature:**_____ **Date:**_____

*[For Office Use Only]* Date: _____ Initials: _____ Follow-Up: _____

# Practice Application Forms

Use these forms to complete the practice application activities from the textbook or the study guide. Make additional copies for extra practice.

# Appointment Sheet

## APPOINTMENT RECORD

| *12* November<br>Tuesday | | AM | *13* November<br>Wednesday | |
|---|---|---|---|---|
| | | **AM** | | |
| | | 8:00 | | |
| | | 8:15 | | |
| | | 8:30 | | |
| | | 8:45 | | |
| | | 9:00 | | |
| | | 9:15 | | |
| | | 9:30 | | |
| | | 9:45 | | |
| | | 10:00 | | |
| | | 10:15 | | |
| | | 10:30 | | |
| | | 10:45 | | |
| | | 11:00 | | |
| | | 11:15 | | |
| | | 11:30 | | |
| | | 11:45 | | |
| | | 12:00 | | |
| | | 12:15 | | |
| | | 12:30 | | |
| | | 12:45 | | |
| | | **PM** | | |
| | | 1:00 | | |
| | | 1:15 | | |
| | | 1:30 | | |
| | | 1:45 | | |
| | | 2:00 | | |
| | | 2:15 | | |
| | | 2:30 | | |
| | | 2:45 | | |
| | | 3:00 | | |
| | | 3:15 | | |
| | | 3:30 | | |
| | | 3:45 | | |
| | | 4:00 | | |
| | | 4:15 | | |
| | | 4:30 | | |
| | | 4:45 | | |
| | | 5:00 | | |
| | | 5:15 | | |
| | | 5:30 | | |
| | | 5:45 | | |

REMARKS & NOTES _____

# Medical History/Examination Form

**Total Care Clinic, PC**
## Medical History

Name _____ Age _____ Sex _____ S  M  W  D

Address _____ Phone _____ Date _____

Occupation _____ Ref. by _____

Chief Complaint _____

Present Illness _____

_____

_____

_____

_____

_____

History —Military _____

—Social _____

—Family _____

—Marital _____

—Menstrual _____ Menarche _____ Para. _____ LMP _____

—Illness  Measles  Pert.  Var.  Pneu.  Pleur.  Typh.  Mal.  Rh. Fev.  Sc. Fev.  Diphth.  Other

—Surgery _____

—Allergies _____

—Current Medications _____

## Physical Examination

Temp. _____ Pulse _____ Resp. _____ BP _____ Ht. _____ Wt. _____

General Appearance _____ Skin _____ Mucous Membrane _____

Eyes: _____ Vision _____ Pupil _____ Fundus _____

Ears: _____

Nose: _____

Throat: _____ Pharynx _____ Tonsils _____

Chest: _____ Breasts _____

Heart: _____

Lungs: _____

Abdomen: _____

Genitalia: _____

Rectum: _____

Pelvic: _____

Extremities: _____ Pulses _____

Lymph Nodes: _____ Neck _____ Axilla _____ Inguinal _____ Abdominal _____

Neurological: _____

Diagnosis: _____

_____

_____

Treatment: _____

_____

_____

Laboratory Findings: _____

Date _____ Blood _____

_____

_____

Date _____ Urine _____

_____

_____

_____

_____

_____

# Referral Form

## REQUEST FOR SERVICES

Facility:_____

Provider:_____

Address:_____

_____

Phone:_____ Fax:_____

### PATIENT INFORMATION

Patient name _____ TCC# _____

Date of Birth _____ Home Phone _____ Alt Phone _____

### REASON FOR REQUEST

Reason for request / Specific question(s) to be answered:

1._____

2._____

History / Symptoms / Specific question(s) to be answered: _____

_____

_____

_____

☐ Check here if additional clinical information is included with this request.

### SERVICES REQUESTED

☐ Abnormal Weight Gain
☐ Adolescent Medicine/Teen Health Center
☐ Aerodigestive
☐ Allergy Clinic
☐ Audology (Hearing)
☐ Behavioral Medcine & Clinical Psychology
☐ Brachial Plexus Clinic
☐ Breast Feeding Clinic
☐ Cardiology
☐ Cardiothoracic Surgery
☐ Cerebral Palsy Center
☐ Chronic Pain Management
☐ Colorectal Surgery
☐ Comprehensive Weight Management Center
☐ Craniofacial Center
☐ Dentistry
☐ Dermatology

☐ Developmental & Behavioral Pediatrics
☐ Diabetes
☐ Diagnostic Clinic
☐ Endocrinology
☐ ENT (Otolaryngology)
☐ Feeding Team
☐ Fetal Surgery
☐ Gastroenterology-GI
☐ Gynecology
☐ Healthworks
☐ Hemangioma & Vascular Malformation Team
☐ Hematology-Oncology
☐ Human Genetics
☐ Hypertension / Cholesterol Clinic
☐ Infectious Diseases-ID
☐ International Adoption Center-IAC
☐ Nephrology

☐ Neurology
☐ Neurosurgery
☐ Nutrition
☐ Ophthalmology / Eye Clinic
☐ Orthopaedics
☐ Physical Medicine & Rehabilitation
☐ Plastic Surgery
☐ Psychiatry
☐ Pulmonary Medicine
☐ Rheumatology
☐ Safe & Healthy Children Center
☐ Sleep Center
☐ Sports Medicine
☐ Surgery (General & Thoracic Surgery)
☐ Urology
☐ Other_____

### REQUESTING PRACTITIONER / GROUP

**TOTAL CARE CLINIC, PC**
342 East Park Blvd.
Futon, XY 12345-6789
www.totalcareclinic.org

Physician Name _____

Tel: 521-234-0001
Fax: 521-234-0002

# Laboratory Requisition Form

## Account Information

| TCC Account Number |
|---|
| |

| Patient Account Number |
|---|
| |

| Address - Street |
|---|
| |

| City | State | ZIP Code |
|---|---|---|
| | | |

**Ship to: Total Care Laboratories**
**1400 West Park Blvd.**
**Funton, XY 12345-6789**

TCC Internal Use

Place Barcode Label Here

## Patient Information

| Patient Name (Print Clearly)-Last | First | Middle Initial | Gender | Birth Date (mm/dd/yyyy) | Age |
|---|---|---|---|---|---|
| | | | ☐ Male ☐ Female | | |

| Patient Number | Sample or Hospital Number | Collection Date (mm/dd/yyyy) | Collection Time |
|---|---|---|---|
| | | | ☐ AM ☐ PM |

| Referring Physician (Print Clearly)-Last | First | Middle Initial | Phone or Fax (Area Code and Number) |
|---|---|---|---|
| | | | |

## Call Back information - Complete ONLY if CALL BACK is required

| Phone or Fax for Call Back - Select One | Phone or Fax (Area Code and Number) |
|---|---|
| ☐ Phone  ☐ Fax - number given must be from a fax machine that complies with applicable HIPAA regulations | |

## Test(s) Requested

| Test Number | Test Name |
|---|---|
| | |
| | |
| | |
| | |
| | |
| | |
| | |

| Source/ Specimen Type | | If Urine TV- |
|---|---|---|
| | | |

# Laboratory Results

**Morris A. Turner, MD**

## TCP LAB

**Total Care Laboratories**
1400 West Park Blvd.
Funton, XY 12345-6789

*C.L.I.A. #21-1862*

| | | | |
|---|---|---|---|
| WELLS, KARLA<br>Patient Name | 09/12/12<br>Date Drawn | 09/12/12<br>Date Received | 09/13/12<br>Date of Report |
| F   43<br>Sex   Age | Linda F. Wiley, PA-C<br>342 East Park Blvd.<br>Funton, XY 12345-6789 | 23341<br>ID Number | 67294<br>Account Number |
| 166241809<br>Patient ID/Soc. Sec. Number | | | 897211<br>Specimen Number |

| TEST NAME | RESULT ABNORMAL | RESULT NORMAL | UNITS | REFERENCE RANGE |
|---|---|---|---|---|
| **CHEM-SCREEN PANEL** | | | | |
| GLUCOSE | | 76.0 | MG/DL | 65.0–115 |
| SODIUM | | 139.0 | MMOL/L | 134–143 |
| POTASSIUM | | 4.00 | MMOL/L | 3.60–5.10 |
| CHLORIDE | | 107.0 | MMOL/L | 96.0–107 |
| BUN | | 17.0 | MG/DL | 6.00–19.0 |
| BUN/CREATININE RATIO | | 14.2 | | |
| URIC ACID | | 4.30 | MG/DL | 2.20–6.20 |
| PHOSPHATE | | 2.40 | MG/DL | 2.40–4.50 |
| CALCIUM | | 9.50 | MG/DL | 8.60–10.0 |
| MAGNESIUM | | 1.75 | MEG/L | 1.40–2.00 |
| CHOLESTEROL | 237.0 | | MG/DL | 130–200 |
| CHOL. PERCENTILE | 90.0 | | PERCENTILE | 1.00–75.0 |
| HDL CHOLESTEROL | 41.0 | | MG/DL | 48.0–89.0 |
| CHOL./HDL RATIO | | 5.80 | | |
| LDL CHOL., CALCULATED | 175.0 | | MG/DL | 65.5–130 |
| TRIGLYCERIDES | | 104.0 | MG/DL | 00.0–200 |
| TOTAL PROTEIN | | 6.60 | GM/DL | 6.40–8.00 |
| ALBUMIN | | 4.10 | GM/DL | 3.70–4.80 |
| GLOBULIN | | 2.50 | GM/DL | 2.20–3.60 |
| ALB/GLOB RATIO | | 1.64 | | 1.10–2.10 |
| TOTAL BILIRUBIN | | 0.80 | MG/DL | 0.20–1.30 |
| DIRECT BILIRUBIN | | 0.15 | MG/DL | 0.00–0.20 |
| ALK. PHOSPHATASE | | 44.0 | UNITS/L | 25.0–125 |
| G-GLUTAMYL TRANSPEP. | | 8.00 | UNITS/L | 1.00–63.0 |
| AST (SGOT) | | 21.0 | IU/L | 1.00–40.0 |
| ALT (SGPT) | | 14.0 | IU/L | 1.00–50.0 |
| LD | | 134.0 | IU/L | 90.0–250 |
| IRON | | 130.0 | MCG/DL | 35.0–180 |

# Disbursements Journal

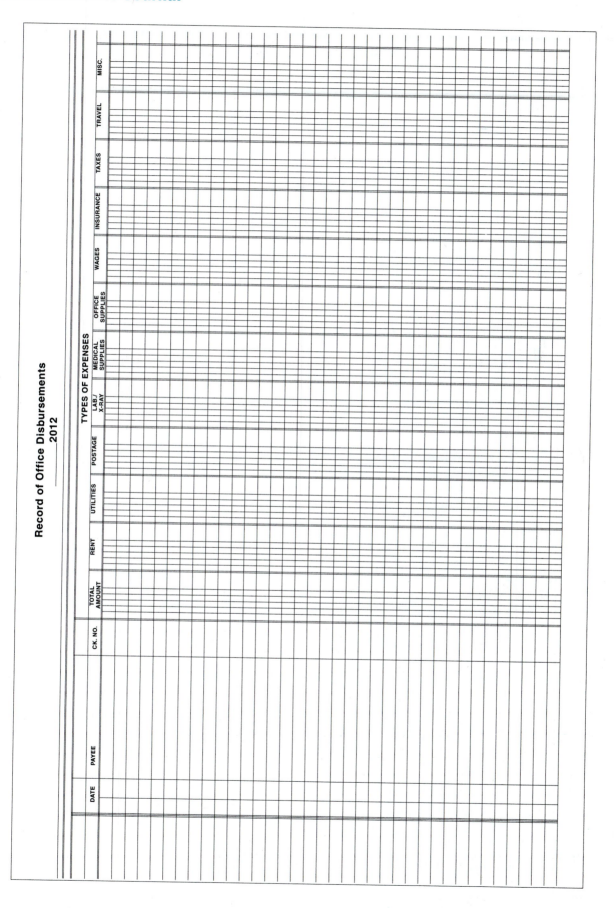

**Record of Office Disbursements**
_____ 2012

| DATE | PAYEE | CK. NO. | TOTAL AMOUNT | RENT | UTILITIES | POSTAGE | LAB./ X-RAY | MEDICAL SUPPLIES | OFFICE SUPPLIES | WAGES | INSURANCE | TAXES | TRAVEL | MISC. |
|------|-------|---------|--------------|------|-----------|---------|-------------|------------------|-----------------|-------|-----------|-------|--------|-------|
|      |       |         |              |      |           |         |             |                  |                 |       |           |       |        |       |

TYPES OF EXPENSES

# The Problem-Solving Process

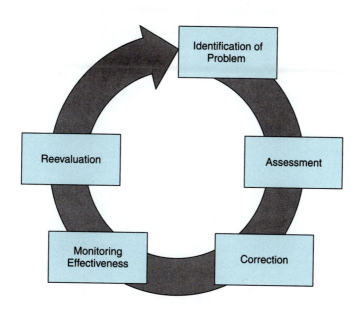

# Employee Handbook Topics

| | | |
|---|---|---|
| Welcome message | EEOC statement | Performance reviews and improvement plans |
| Organization's mission | Employment applications | Personal communications |
| ADA statements | Equipment and facility use | Personnel records |
| Attendance policies | Grievance process | Probationary period |
| Benefits | Holidays | Risk management and incident reports |
| Bereavement | Job Descriptions | Safety and security |
| Confidentiality and HIPAA | Jury duty | Schedules, accountability and requests for time off |
| Continuing education and tuition reimbursement | Leaves of Absence | Sexual harassment guidelines |
| Disability benefits | On the job injuries | Smoking policy |
| Disaster preparedness and emergency response | Orientation | Substance abuse |
| Dress code | OSHA | Subpoenas |
| Drug testing | Overtime | |
| Electronic communication and device use | Payroll periods | Wage increases and adjustments |

# Guidelines for a Successful Externship

1. Review your manual prior to the start of your externship; know the expectations and skills you must complete.

2. Avoid scheduling personal appointments, vacations, or any time off during the externship.

3. Ensure you have reliable transportation and child-care arrangements including sick-child care (Figure 24–3).

4. If you are unsure or uncomfortable with a skill, attempt to improve it prior to proceeding to the site.

5. Arrive on time and ready to work (not with a doughnut and coffee in hand). Notify both your clinical site preceptor and the school externship coordinator if you are late or absent.

6. Make sure your cell phone is OFF at all times with the exception of lunch and breaks.

7. Ensure your appearance is clean and neat and meets the standards of the school and facility. Wear your designated name badge at all times.

8. Demonstrate your willingness to learn. DO NOT sit back and wait to be asked to participate.

9. Use your time wisely. If there are slow periods, perhaps there is medical literature or an interesting case study available or filing you can do.

10. Adhere to confidentiality and HIPAA requirements AT ALL TIMES. Do not discuss patients at home or in public places.

11. Stay within the scope of practice.

12. Call the externship coordinator in a timely manner if there are any questions, concerns, or problems.

13. Be appropriately assertive but not aggressive about completing the required skills; e.g., if appointment scheduling is done in another department, check with your preceptor about going to that department to perform the competency.

14. Keep up with the required documentation. Murphy's Law guarantees that the person you need to sign off on hours or procedures will be on an extensive leave if you wait.

15. Attitude is almost everything; demonstrate a responsible positive attitude at all times.

16. Avoid "office politics." DO NOT gossip or take sides in disagreements among staff, and do not ask about or discuss salaries with staff.

17. **Remember, you represent your school and yourself. The health-care community is a small world. Do not, in any way, act in an unprofessional manner. It may come back to haunt you when you least expect it (perhaps when you are applying for that ideal job). It may also influence the site's willingness to accept future externs from your school.**